ANGLO-EUROPEAN COLLEGE OF CHIROPRACTIC

Fundamentals of
Complementary and
Alternative Medicine

Fundamentals of Complementary and Alternative Medicine

Edited by

Marc S. Micozzi, MD, PhD

Executive Director
The College of Physicians of Philadelphia
Adjunct Professor of Physical Medicine
Department of Rehabilitation Medicine
University of Pennsylvania
Philadelphia, Pennsylvania

With Foreword by
C. Everett Koop, MD, ScD

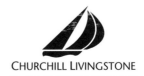

CHURCHILL LIVINGSTONE

New York, Edinburgh, London, Madrid, Melbourne, San Francisco, Tokyo

Library of Congress Cataloging-in-Publication Data

Fundamentals of complementary and alternative medicine / edited by
  Marc S. Micozzi ; with foreword by C. Everett Koop.
      p.   cm.— (Complementary and alternative medicine)
    Includes bibliographical references and index.
    ISBN 0-443-05355-3
    1. Alternative Medicine.   I. Micozzi, Marc S., DATE.
  II. Series.
    [DNLM: 1. Alternative Medicine.   WB 890 F981 1996]
  R733.F86   1996
  615.5—dc20
  DNLM/DLC
  for Library of Congress   95-39128
                                                              CIP

Distributed in the United Kingdom by Churchill Livingstone, Robert Stevenson House, 1–3 Baxter's Place, Leith Walk, Edinburgh EH1 3AF, and by associated companies, branches, and representatives throughout the world.

Accurate indications, adverse reactions, and dosage schedules for drugs are provided in this book, but it is possible that they may change. The reader is urged to review the package information data of the manufacturers of the medications mentioned.

The Publishers have made every effort to trace the copyright holders for borrowed material. If they have inadvertently overlooked any, they will be pleased to make the necessary arrangements at the first opportunity.

Acquisitions Editor: *Inta Ozols*
Production Editor: *Kamely Dahir Hayes*
Production Supervisor: *Sharon Tuder*
Cover Design: *Jeannette Jacobs*

Printed in the United States of America

First published in 1996   7   6   5   4   3   2

To my teachers at the University of Pennsylvania School of Medicine and in the Greater Philadelphia medical community who taught me both the art and science of medicine, and who maintain the traditions on which American medicine was founded and upon which the future of American medicine will be built.

Contributors

Gerard C. Bodeker, EdD

Chairman, Global Initiative for Traditional Systems of Health, Department of Dermatology, Churchill Hospital, Headington, Oxford, England

Claire Monod Cassidy, PhD

Research Director, Traditional Acupuncture Institute, Columbia, Maryland

Effie Poi Yew Chow, PhD, RN, CA

President and Chief Nurse Acupuncturist and Qigong Master, General Clinic, Qigong Institute, East West Academy of Healing Arts, San Francisco, California

Kevin V. Ergil, MA, MS, LAc, PhDcand

Dean and Director, Pacific Institute of Oriental Medicine, New York, New York

Jennifer Jacobs, MD, MPH

Clinical Assistant Professor, Department of Epidemiology, University of Washington School of Public Health and Community Medicine, Seattle, Washington; Private Practice, Family Medicine, The Evergreen Clinic, Edmonds, Washington

Ted J. Kaptchuk, OMD

Associate Director, Center for Alternative Medicine Research, Beth Israel Hospital, Boston, Massachusetts

Charles T. McGee, MD

Private Practice, Coeur d'Alene, Idaho

Lisa Meserole, MS, RD, ND

Chair, Department of Botanical Medicine, Bastyr University; Naturopathic Physician, Seattle Healing Arts Clinic, Seattle, Washington

Marc S. Micozzi, MD, PhD

Executive Director, The College of Physicians of Philadelphia, Philadelphia, Pennsylvania; formerly Founding Director National Museum of Health and Medicine, Washington, DC

Richard Moskowitz, MD

Instructor, Homeopathic Philosophy, National Center for Homeopathy, Alexandria, Virginia; Private Practice, Family Medicine, Watertown, Massachusetts

Joseph E. Pizzorno, Jr, ND

President, Natural Health Clinic, Bastyr University, Seattle, Washington

Daniel Redwood, DC

Chiropractic Physician, Atlantic Chiropractic, Virginia Beach, Virginia

Kenneth Sancier, PhD

Co-President and Director of Research, Qigong Institute, East West Academy of Healing Arts, San Francisco, California

Hari M. Sharma, MD

Professor Emeritus, Department of Pathology, Director, Division of Cancer Prevention and Natural Products Research, Department of Pathology, The Ohio State University College of Medicine, Columbus, Ohio

Victoria E. Slater, RN, MSN, PhDcand

Doctoral Candidate, University of Tennessee College of Nursing; Certified Healing Touch Instructor, Certified Integrative Hypnotherapist, Third Degree Reiki Master Practitioner, Private Practice, Energetic Healing, Knoxville, Tennessee

Caroline J. Stevensen, BA Hons

Macmillan Specialist and Lecturer in Complementary Therapies, Academic Unit, Royal London Homeopathic Hospital NHS Trust, London, England

Michael Terman, PhD

Associate Professor, Department of Psychiatry, Columbia University Collage of Physicians and Surgeons; Director, Clinical Chronobiology Program, New York State Psychiatric Institute; President, Center for Environmental Therapeutics, New York, New York

Robert T. Trotter II, PhD

Department of Anthropology, Northern Arizona University, Flagstaff, Arizona

Glenn N. Wagner, DO

Deputy Director, Armed Forces Institute of Pathology, Washington, DC

Alan D. Watkins, MD

MRC Fellow, University Medicine, Southampton General Hospital, Southampton, United Kingdom

Kenneth G. Zysk, PhD

Assistant Professor, Department of Asian Studies, New York University Faculty of Arts and Sciences, New York, New York

The Art and Science of Medicine

For over forty years I have tried to identify the mix of personal attributes and technical skills that make one an outstanding doctor. I am sure that most physicians in the United States have pondered the same question. Now, through the work of the C. Everett Koop Institute at Dartmouth I have an opportunity to influence the way medical students are trained. The Institute, working in partnership with the Dartmouth Medical School and the Dartmouth-Hitchcock Medical Center, is actively engaged in training physicians for the next century.

Since doctors must remain abreast of a growing volume of new information, our medical schools help both their graduates and society by producing physicians who are computer literate and comfortable with telemedicine. As a scientific pursuit, medicine should take advantage of the technologic innovations that allow us to better serve the lifetime learning needs of physicians as well as the health education needs of patients. Nonetheless since medicine is also an art, doctors still need to listen to their patients. This aspect of medical practice has not changed.

As I travel across the country many of the people I meet are eager to share their ideas for improving the nation's health care system. The most common complaint I hear focusses on poor communication in the doctor–patient relationship. Too many patients feel that their physician does not really listen to them. When the patient attempts to explain his or her problem, the doctor interrupts. Subsequently, when the doctor tries to explain what conditions the patient has and attempts to outline a treatment regimen, the patient is confused because the physician does not communicate to the level of the patient's understanding.

From my perspective, medical students need to master the art of listening to and communicating with their patients just as much as they need to learn the fundamentals of human biology. We have found at the Koop Institute that a student's communication skills are greatly improved by having to explain the first principles of health promotion and disease prevention to second graders. Medical students who choose to participate in programs sponsored by the Koop Institute work in and with local communities from their very first year. Some choose to advise junior high and high school students on the risks associated with alcohol, tobacco, and sexually transmitted diseases; others help rural physicians take better advantage of the computer revolution.

Just as a physician should be sensitive to the feelings of a patient and the needs of the community, he or she must be conversant with major trends and developments in society. I would like to tell you about one current trend that is of interest to me. Three years ago, a study conducted at Harvard Medical School and reported in the *New England Journal of Medicine* focussed on attitudes toward complementary and alternative medicine in the United States. The study indicated that one third of adult Americans regularly use some kind of complementary or alternative treatment even though it was not covered by insurance and they had to pay for it themselves. This is an opportune time for us to take a second look at such alternative treatment approaches as acupuncture, botanical medicine, homeopathy, and others; not to offer these treatment modalities blindly but to expose them to the scientific method. Physicians have to depend on facts—on empirical data—when they determine treatment strategy for a particular patient. Today we do not have a lot of data on the potential of alternative approaches to help or harm human health. It is time to discover the value of these treatment regimens. We can conduct the necessary studies and assemble the data that doctors and health policymakers need; a type of biomedical research that would be a prudent long-term investment.

In my lifetime we have achieved great successes in the fight against infectious diseases. We have more work to do in our effort to improve the quality of life and make people more comfortable as they endure chronic health problems such as cancer, heart disease, and arthritis. Drugs and surgery can be useful tools in the effort to treat these diseases, but when possible I would like to see us increase the range of approaches that can be used. My experience as a doctor has taught me that often a mix of different approaches is necessary to achieve success. We need to be flexible and adaptable because the diseases that challenge us certainly are not static.

A recent trend that concerns me is the growth of drug resistant bacteria. Today it is easy to forget that prior to the development of antibiotics in the 1940s a child's ear infection could be a frightening and fatal experience. I well remember patients with serious complications and death caused by the lack of antibiotics. If drugs we have depended on for decades are compromised, we may return to a time when even routine infections could be dangerous. As both a grandfather and a physician, I would hate to see that happen.

There is an element of good news in this picture. If some of the synthetic drugs we have developed are no longer as dependable as they once were, studies have shown that the botanical substances these drugs are based on are still effective in treating disease. I have never claimed to be an expert on botany or ecology, but current trends suggest that we need to do more. We need to conserve the plants that may contain the medicines of the future and more importantly we need to learn what local healers seem to understand about the pharmacologic properties and uses of these medicines.

Reduced health care costs is an important by-product of the work we are doing at the Koop Institute. Our students know that the physician of the future must be a health educator first and foremost. Today, the challenge is to treat the patient once he or she has gone to the hospital. Tomorrow, the challenge will be to keep the patient out of the hospital in the beginning.

Preventive medicine means education, empowerment, and personal responsibility. Many patients want alternatives to invasive medical procedures and long stays in the hospital. Physicians can conserve time and resources by teaching patients how to reduce their risk of cancer, heart disease, and other life–threatening diseases. As our students know, the most inexpensive treatment is to keep the patient from becoming sick in the first place. Demand reduction in the health care system is the most immediate cost saving effort.

I think that alternative/complementary therapies may potentially be an important part of this overall educational process. One must have an open mind about complementary therapies and understand belief systems that emphasize the mind-body connection. At a time when many Americans complain of stress, make poor nutritional choices, and are increasingly concerned about environmentally induced illnesses these messages could hardly be more timely.

Many people are confused about alternative medicine, and I do not blame them. For many Americans alternative therapies represent a *new* discovery, but in truth, many of these traditions are hundreds or thousands of years old and have been used by millions of people worldwide. To ease the uncomfortableness of the word *alternative* one must realize that while treatments may look like alternatives to us, they have long been part of the medical mainstream in their cultures of origin.

When I worked in Washington as Surgeon General for eight years, President Reagan had an important credo in his approach to foreign policy: "Trust but verify!" So it is with complementary and alternative medicine. So many people have relied on these approaches for so long that they may have something of value to offer. Let us begin the necessary research so that we could have substantive answers in the near future.

One reason such research is worth doing is that eighty percent of the world's people depend on these alternative approaches as their primary medical care. For years, we have attempted to export Western medicine to the developing world. The sad truth is that the people we are attempting to help simply cannot afford it. I have doubts about how much longer we can afford some of it ourselves. It is possible that a decade from now, we may be more ready to ask the peoples of the developing world to share their wisdom with us.

During the nineteenth century American medicine was an eclectic pursuit where a number of competing ideas and approaches thrived. Doctors were able to draw on elements from different traditions in attempting to make people well. Perhaps there is more to this older model of American medicine than we in the twentieth century have been willing to examine. My experience with physicians has convinced me that they are healers first. As such, they are willing to use any ethical approach or treatment that has been proven to work. However, in the opinion of most doctors, there is not yet enough information on the value of complementary and alternative medicine. I would like to see us undertake the study and research that could provide definitive answers to prudent questions about the usefulness of complementary and alternative medicine for society at large.

C. Everett Koop, MD, ScD
Former Surgeon General of the United States
Senior Scholar, The Koop Institute at Dartmouth,
Hanover, New Hampshire

Preface

Fundamentals of Complementary and Alternative Medicine provides the reader with a basis of knowledge about systems of medical thought and practice referred to today in the United States as complementary and alternative medicine. The book's approach is to present medical, health, and science students and practitioners, as well as other interested individuals with the intellectual foundations and tools to understand and make sense of these various fields that demonstrate great diversity and yet can be unified around certain themes. To provide a useful introduction to these topics, the book is carefully organized with subjects presented in the order in which they should be read for a progressive, comprehensive overview and understanding of the material.

Alternative/complementary medicine, natural medicine, and the use of natural products represent a classic consumer movement and a current social phenomenon of significant dimensions. Students, practitioners, and patients/consumers need a common language for understanding this movement.

Physicians and patients are becoming increasingly involved in *alternatives* driven by the perceived need for health care reform, the desire to move toward a wellness orientation in medical practice, and an intellectual interest and curiosity about the ability of what well–established ancient and historic medical systems continue to offer us today.

In sum, this book presents the contemporary complementary and alternative medical approaches that come from observations within, around and beyond the current Western, biomedical paradigm. The approaches discussed expand our view of the possibilities for light, time, touch, sensation, energy, and mind to enter into health and medicine. The ultimate goal is a synthesis of mind-body medicine, its relation to the emerging field of psychoneuroimmunology, and a possible model for a final common pathway among complementary and alternative medical systems.

Marc S. Micozzi, MD, PhD

Thanks to the team at Churchill Livingstone—Dr. William Marovitz, Inta Ozols, Kamely Dahir, Carol Corcoran, Lara Evangelista, and Bets Radley—who worked with me to publish this book in a timely way.

Contents

Marc S. Micozzi, M.D., Ph.D., is Executive Director of the College of Physicians of Philadelphia and Adjunct Professor of Physical Medicine in the Department of Rehabilitation Medicine, University of Pennsylvania. Previously, he was founding Director and Distinguished Scientist at the National Museum of Health and Medicine, Washington, D.C., and Senior Investigator at the National Cancer Institute, National Institutes of Health, Bethesda, Maryland. As a physician, epidemiologist and anthropologist, he has been involved broadly with complementary medical systems worldwide and is committed to seeking and developing intellectual standards and better understanding in this field. He serves as series editor for a library of texts in complementary medicine and as senior editorial advisor for texts in manual medicine by Churchill Livingstone publishers.

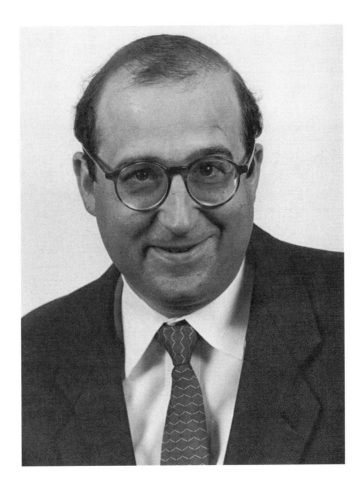

The Basis and Contexts of Complementary and Alternative Medicine

This section provides an introduction to the whole topic of complementary and alternative medicine, its themes and terminology, and the various contexts relative to its proper interpretation. The chapters provide a social and cultural recontextualization of complementary and alternative medicine. The ubiquitous use of plants and natural products among alternatives is reviewed through underlying themes from both the social and biological sciences. The social history of the use of complementary and alternative medicine is provided through a review of the concept of "vitalism" in intellectual and medical discourse, which is important to understanding the common themes of bioenergy and self-healing among complementary and alternative medical systems.

1

Characteristics of Complementary and Alternative Medicine

Marc S. Micozzi

The different medical systems subsumed under the category *alternative/complementary* are large and diverse, but these systems have some common ground in their views of health and healing. I call this overall philosophy *a new ecology of health*, sustainable medicine, or *medicine for a small planet*.

Role of Science

Allopathic medicine is considered the "scientific" healing art, while the alternatives are considered "non-scientific." However, perhaps what is needed is not *less science*, but *more sciences* in the study of alternative/complementary medicine. Some of the central ideas of biomedicine are very powerful, but are becoming intellectually stale. The study of dead tissue cells, components, and chemicals to understand life processes, and the quest for "magic bullets" to combat disease are based upon a reductionist, materialist view of health and healing. We have made tremendous advances over the past hundred years by applying these concepts to medicine. However, the resulting biomedical system is not always able to account for and use many observations in the realms of clinical and personal experience, natural law, and human spirituality.

Contemporary biomedicine is a scientific paradigm with a particular history, as much influenced by social history as it is by scientific laws. In the laudable effort to make medicine scientific, we have emphasized that knowledge about the world—including nature and human nature—must be pursued by the following criteria: (1) objectivism—the observer is separate from the observed, (2) reductionism—complex phenomena are explainable in terms of simpler, component phenomena, (3) positivism—all information can be derived from physically measurable data, (4) determinism—phenomena can be predicted from a knowledge of scientific law and initial conditions. We all know that this is not the only way of "knowing" things but it has become the twentieth century test to determine whether such knowledge is "scientific."

In fact, science simply requires empiricism—making and testing models of reality by what can be observed, guided by certain values and based upon certain metaphysical assumptions. Science itself is not reality but a sys-

(Continues)

tem of human knowledge. Scientists often detect differences between metaphysical reality and the scientific models constructed through human intellectual activity. These new thoughts about the nature of medicine do not represent a "new science" so much as they represent a new philosophy.

Therefore, the aforementioned criteria are not always applicable. In the science of physics, objectivism is ultimately not possible at the fundamental level due to the Heisenberg uncertainty principle, which states that the act of observing phenomena necessarily influences the behavior of the phenomena being observed. Contemporary biological and ecological science has produced a wealth of observations about interactions between living organisms and their environments in transactional, multidirectional, and synergic ways that are not ultimately subject to reductionist explanations. For positivism and determinism to provide a complete explanation, we must assume that science has all the physical and intellectual tools to ask the right questions. However, the questions we ask are based upon the history of science itself as part of the history of human intellectual enquiry.

Contemporary biomedicine conceptually uses Newtonian physics and pre-Darwinian biology. Newtonian physics explains and can reproduce many observations on the mechanics of everyday experience. Contemporary quantum physics (quantum mechanics) recognizes aspects of reality beyond Newtonian mechanics, such as matter-energy duality, "unified fields" of energy and matter, and wave functions (see Chapter 14). Quantum physics and contemporary biology-ecology may be needed to understand alternatives. Nuclear medicine uses the technology of contemporary physics but does not yet incorporate the concepts of quantum physics in its fundamental approach to patient health. Contemporary medicine does measure the body's energy using electrocardiography, electroencephalography, and electromyography for diagnostic purposes, but it does not enlist the body's energy for the purpose of healing.

The biological science of contemporary medicine is essentially pre-Darwinian in that it emphasizes typology rather than individuality and variation. Each patient is defined as a clinical entity by a diagnosis, with treatment prescribed accordingly. The modern understanding of the human genome does not make this approach to biomedical science less pre-Darwinian. Both the fundamentals of inheritance (Mendel) and natural selection (Darwin and Alfred Russel Wallace) were elucidated long before the discovery of the structure of the gene itself. Although modern biology-ecology continues to explore the phenomena of how living systems interact at the level of the whole—which cannot be seen under a microscope or in a test tube—molecular genetics continues to dissect the human genome.

It may seem outrageously complex to construct a medical system based upon the concepts of modern physics and biology-ecology, while maintaining a unique diagnostic and therapeutic approach to each individual. This would indeed be complex if not for the fact that the body is its own entity, a part of nature, and each body has inate ability to heal itself.

> If biomedicine cannot explain scientific observations of alternatives, then the biomedical paradigm will be revised.

One way of studying and understanding alternative medicine is to view it in light of contemporary physics and biology-ecology, and to focus not just on the subtle manipulations of the alternative practitioners but on the physiologic response of the body. When homeopathy or acupuncture is observed to result in a physiologic or clinical response that cannot be explained by the biomedical model, it is not the role of the scientist to deny this reality, but rather to modify our explanatory models to account for it. In this way, science itself progresses. In the end, there is only one reality. Alternative medical systems, which are relatively old in terms of human intellectual history, always have been trying to describe, understand, and work with the same reality of health and healing as biomedicine. Furthermore, while contemporary biomedicine utilizes new technologies in the service of relatively old ideas about health and healing, alternative methods employ old technologies whose fundamental character may reflect new scientific ideas on physical and biological nature.

Science must account for all of what is observed, not just part of it. That is why physics has moved beyond Newtonian mechanics—biology beyond typology. Is it possible for a biomedical model to be constructed for which its validity includes observations from alternative medicine? Although it may be necessary to wait for new insights from physics and biology to understand alternatives in terms of biomedicine, clinical pragmatism dictates that successful therapeutic methods should not be withheld while mechanisms are being elucidated—or debated. We live in a world filled with opportunities to observe the practice of alternatives. It only remains to apply scientific standards to their study. In the meantime, patients are now waiting for mainstream physicians to understand the mechanisms of alternatives. And also in the meantime, we can come to understand the underlying intellectual content and history of alternatives as complete systems of thought and practice.

A Note About Nomenclature

The word alternative, or the term *alternative/complementary* medicine, now seems to be culturally encoded in the English language. Workers at Harvard Medical School have provided a basis for a functional definition of the term:

"Alternative medicine refers to those practices explicitly used for the purpose of medical intervention, health promotion or disease prevention which are not routinely taught at U.S. medical schools nor routinely underwritten by third-party payers within the existing U.S. health care system."

The Harvard definition seems to be a diagnosis of exclusion, meaning that alternative medicine is everything not being presently promoted in mainstream medicine. This definition may remind us of a popular song from the 1960's called, "the element song,"

(Continues)

which offers a complete listing of all the different elements of the periodic table (set to the tune of "I am the very model of a modern Major General" from Gilbert and Sullivan's *The Pirates of Penzance*). It ends with words to this effect: "These are the many elements we've heard about at Harvard. And if we haven't heard of them, they haven't been disco-vard." I have likened the recent "discovery" of alternative medicine to Columbus' discovery of the Americas. Although his voyage was a great feat that expanded the intellectual frontiers of Europe, Columbus could not really discover a world already known to millions of indigenous peoples who employed complex systems of social organization and subsistence activities. Likewise, the definitional statement that alternatives are not "within the existing US health care system" is a curious observation for the millions of Americans who routinely use them today.

Wellness

The alternative/complementary systems generally emphasize what might be called wellness by the mainstream medical system. The goal of preventing disease is shared by alternative and mainstream medicine alike. In the mainstream medical model, this involves using drugs and surgery to prevent disease in those who are only at risk, rather than reserving these powerful methodologies for the treatment of disease. I have called this trend the medicalization of prevention. One can continue to engage in risky lifestyle behaviors, while medicine provides "magic bullets" to prevent diseases that it cannot treat. Wellness in the context of complementary medicine is more than the prevention of disease. It is a focus on engaging the inner resources of each individual as an active and conscious participant in the maintenance of his or her own health. By the same token, the property of being healthy is not conferred upon an individual solely by an outside agency or entity, but results from the balance of internal resources with the external natural and social environment.

This latter point relates to the alternative approach that relies on the abilities of the individual to get well and stay healthy.

Self-Healing

The body heals itself. This might seem to be an obvious statement, since we are well aware that wounds heal and cells routinely replace themselves. Nonetheless, this is a profound concept among alternatives because self-healing is the basis of *all* healing. External manipulations simply mobilize the body's inner healing resources. Instead of wondering why the body's cells are sick, we ask why the body is not replacing its sick cells with healthy ones? The ability to be well or be sick is largely tied to inner resources, and the external environment—social and physical—impacts on the body's ability.

What is the evidence for self-healing? The long and common history of clinical observations of the "placebo" effect, or the "laying on of hands." To paraphrase Jung: summoned or unsummoned, self-healing will be there. It is so powerful, that biomedical methodology mainly designs double-blind, controlled clinical trials to see what percentage of benefit can be added by powerful drugs to the healing encounter.

Bioenergy

A related concept is that the body has energy (see Chapter 3). Accordingly, as a living entity, the body is an energetic system. Disruptions in the balance and flow of energy cause illness, and the body's response to energetic imbalance leads to perceptible disease. Since the body heals itself, the body can also make itself sick. Restoring, or facilitating the body to restore its own balance, restores health. The symptoms of a cold, flu, or allergy are caused by the body's efforts to rid itself of the offending agent. For example, by raising the body's temperature, a fever reduces bacterial reproduction, and sneezing physically expels offending agents (see Chapter 5).

Pathologists know that there are only so many ways that cells can look sick, because cellular reactions have a defined repertoire for manifesting the body's disease. We have also learned a great deal over the past one hundred years by correlating the appearance of dead tissue cells under the microscope with clinical diagnosis and prognosis. However, studying dead tissue cells for clinical significance does not allow direct observation of the dynamic energy of living cells, systems, organisms, and communities. While correlation of the appearance of stained tissue cells under a microscope to clinical conditions is a very powerful concept in medicine, alternatives appear to provide a path to study the energy of living systems for health and healing (see Chapter 4).

Nutrition and Natural Products

The reliance on nutrition and natural products is fundamental to alternatives, and does not play merely a supportive or adjunctive role. Nutrients and natural products are taken into the body and incorporated in the most literal sense. They provide the body with energy in the form of calories, and with the material resources to stay healthy and get well.

Since the basic plan of the body, as a physical entity and as an energy system, evolves and exists in an ecological context, what the body needs it gets from the environment in which it grew. Lao Tzu states that "what is deeply rooted in nature cannot be uprooted." The human organism is designed to obtain nutrients from natural food sources present in the natural environment; and the body is best suited to obtain nutrients in their natural forms (see Chapter 8).

Plants

Plants are an important part of nature relative to health and a dominant part of the nature in which humans evolved. In addition to producing the oxygen that we breathe, they are seen as sources of nutrients, medicines (such as phytochemicals), essential oils (volatiles for inhalation and/or transdermal absorption), and by some systems, as sources of vibrational energy. Many systems see the use of plants as sources of nutrients in continuity with their use as sources of medicine, paralleling contemporary biomedical guidelines for nutrition as disease prevention.

Individuality

The emphasis of alternatives is on the whole person as a unique individual with his or her own inner resources. Therefore, the concepts of normalization, standardization, and generalization are more difficult to apply to research and clinical practice by comparison to the allopathic method. Some believe that alternatives restore the role of the individual client and practitioner to the practice of medicine; the biomedical emphasis on standardization of training and practice to ensure quality may leave something lost in translation back to restoring the health of the individual (see Chapter 5).

> The focus on the whole person as a unique individual provides new challenges to the scientific measurement of the healing encounter. Mobilizing the resources of each individual to stay healthy and get well also provides new opportunities to move health care toward a model of wellness and toward new models for helping solve our current health care crisis, which is largely driven by costs.

If the body heals itself, has its own energy, and is uniquely individual, then the focus is not on the healer but on the healed. Although this concept may be humbling to the practitioner as heroic healer, it is liberating to realize that in the end each person heals him or herself. If the healer is not the sole source of health and healing, there is room for humility, as well as room for both patient and practitioner to participate in the interaction.

For the purposes of this book, I offer my own functional definition of alternative medicine which (to further these purposes), here is called complementary medical systems. Complementary medical systems are characterized by a developed body of intel-

lectual work that underlies the conceptualization of health and its precepts; that has been sustained over many generations by many practitioners in many communities; that represents an orderly, rational, conscious system of knowledge and thought about health and medicine; that relates more broadly to a way of life (or "lifestyle"); and that has been widely observed to have definable results as practiced.

Although the term *holistic* has been applied to the approach to the "body as person" among alternative medical systems, I apply holism to the medical system itself as a complete system of thought and practice (what I have elsewhere called health beliefs and behaviors). This system of knowledge is therefore shared by patients and practitioners—the active, conscious engagement of "patients" is relative to the focus on *self-healing* and *individuality* that are among the common characteristics of these system.

In this regard, it might be considered that we are trying to document here the classic practice of alternative/complementary medical systems. In trying to build a bridge between a well-developed system of allopathic medicine with complementary medical systems, it is necessary to have strong foundations on both sides of this bridge. It is, of course, not possible to apply these criteria to the work of single individual alternative practitioners who have unilaterally developed their own unique techniques over one or two generations (what might be called unusual); just as it is not possible to build a bridge to nowhere. My definition is meant to apply to systems of thought and not just techniques of practice. Often there is an underlying philosophy of individual practitioners surrounding new techniques they have developed. Or new techniques may be subsumed under existing systems of practice.

Eclecticism itself is a historical form of alternative medicine that drew from among different traditions and was popular in the United States in the last century. In such a system, treatment is determined by the needs of each individual patient, not just by what one given system has to offer. Today, a chiropractor might practice in an Ayurveda clinic, osteopaths might practice in allopathic clinics, and chiropractors or allopaths might use acupuncture. *Naturopathy,* in some ways the most recent of homegrown alternatives from the Euroamerican tradition, consciously employs a variety of traditions ranging from acupuncture to herbal medicine. I have termed naturopathy as *neo-eclecticism* with the underlying philosophy that the body heals itself using resources found in nature (see Chapter 12).

In the end a given system develops in answer to human needs. Alternatives vary widely, but their characteristics cluster around the self-healing capabilities of the human organism and the ability (and reliance) of the human organism to use resources present in nature. What is constant and at the center of such alternative systems is the individual human being. Therefore, if the focus is not on the medical system itself but on being at the center, there is really only one system.

A final point about alternatives: In a way, perhaps particular to the United States, it implies the importance of individuality and choice. In an era when the active engagement of the individual in his or her own health is a paramount goal, the importance of individuality and of choice could not be more salient.

2

Cultural Context of Complementary and Alternative Medicine Systems

Claire Monod Cassidy

There are a great many health care systems in the world. All share the goals of alleviating the suffering of the sick, promoting health, and protecting the wider society from illness.

Despite this underlying universality, systems differ profoundly. They differ in degree of expansion into the world, so that some systems are practiced only locally, as among a single rainforest tribe, while others have spread to every corner of the globe. They differ in degree of technology, from systems that require none at all, to others that can barely function in the absence of electricity and perfect sanitation. Most importantly, they differ in their perceptions of the sick and well human body, and in how they deliver health care.

These similarities and differences among health care systems have been systematically studied for over 100 years. As a result we can now discuss both why so many systems exist and how differences among them matter. Basically, systems arise and persist because each one serves a need. Moreover, patients report satisfaction with care—no matter what kind—if that care is delivered in a manner that meshes with their cultural expectations. The form health care takes is first and fundamentally a matter of sociocultural interpretation. In other words, the

"truth" that guides any health care system is relative and is learned.

This point, although implied by the very existence of numerous health care systems, surprises us—particularly in North America, where we have hoped and assumed that we have had only one real health care system since early in this century. This hope has been couched in language that still argues for the primacy of scientific medicine, including the claim that BIOMEDICINE is scientific. But as the voices of other types of practitioners gain strength, and as the world's cultural diversity increasingly bears in upon American culture, it becomes clear that most of what we know, even scientific fact, is culturally modeled. We remain unaware of this situation most of the time because our cultural assumptions are learned at an early age and are embedded within us to the point that we take them for granted. Only when they are challenged—as they will be by the material in this text—do we become aware of them. Once aware, we can choose either to expand our thinking or to defend the status quo.

> *Biomedicine* is the formal name for the health care system in which the primary practi-
> *(Continues)*

tioners earn the degree of MD; it also is called allopathy. These names emphasize aspects of this system's explanatory model. Other names are flavored by cultural politics, and emphasize biomedicine's expanded or dominant position. Examples include: western, cosmopolitan, modern, orthodox, and conventional. In this chapter all health care practices, including biomedicine, are treated as alternatives, meaning that all are options available to users. They are complementary to the extent that they can be and are used together.

This chapter offers an opportunity to expand thinking through a series of conceptual models that contextualize the variety of health care systems. It considers three questions:

1. What are the many health care realities?
2. How do they resemble each other?
3. What are the implications of the differences?

Reality, Interpretation, and Relativity

A psychiatrist once told me about a Mormon woman who came to him deeply distressed because, 20 years and four children into her second marriage, she realized that she would be spending eternity with her first husband, a man who had died 6 months after their wedding. Mormon couples can be married both for this life and for "eternity," and she and her first husband had chosen to be linked in both ways. Now her first husband was a stranger to her, and she desperately wanted to spend the afterlife with her present husband and children. To his credit, the psychiatrist realized that he could not help this patient. He called a Mormon colleague who quickly linked the patient with a Bishop of the Mormon church. In a single visit, the bishop helped the woman straighten out her fears about the afterlife.

Why could the first psychiatrist not help the patient himself? He did not share her reality model. Instead of telling her not to be so silly, he took a logical and compassionate step, and linked the sick

woman with health care workers who did share her reality model.

Another example: On a chilly wet day, a young woman laughingly pointed out her red tights and red boots to me, saying, "I always wear red on my feet on days like this, to keep me cooking from below up." Was this an amusing poesy shared on an elevator? A sign of psychosis? Certainly, this remark did not make sense from within the biomedical model. But an acupuncturist would understand that the cold element, water, is chased by the hot element, Fire, and the symbolic color of fire is red. A similar behavior pattern would be recognized by practitioners of Ayurveda, the traditional medicine of India, or Curanderismo, the folk medicine tradition of Mexico, Central America, and many Hispanic people in the United States. It also survives in mainstream America when a mother boots up her kids on rainy days to keep them warm and prevent colds.*

These stories provide small illustrations of the statement that the form health care takes is first and fundamentally a matter of interpretation. The wide variety of lifeways shows that humans have found many different ways to answer the same life questions. We can enjoy these differences much as we enjoy a good conversation, or we can grapple with their meanings and implications. Those involved in delivering health care must grapple with them.

Unfortunately, the same derisive tone that labels the interpretation of personal experience as merely superstition is also found in comparisons of medical belief systems. If one is modern then others are, by inference, outmoded; if one is based on fact then others must be laced with superstition. In this way, biomedicine is seen as somehow more true than any alternative system could possibly be. . . . Such a view . . . fails to consider the internal logic of other ex-

(Continues)

---

* That the remark makes sense within the logic of humoral models does not mean that practitioners would say the red boots work, that is, that they themselves, or their color specifically, prevented the young woman from being invaded by cold damp. To determine whether an action is instrumental requires an entirely different level of analysis.

> planatory models. But most health systems are logical and rational systems of thought if the underlying assumptions are known; this does not necessarily mean that these assumptions are correct, only that they can be viewed as having been reached by the coherent use of reason (Snow 1993).

As noted above, this can be difficult if we do not even know why we are reacting with laughter, anger, or defensiveness. The process of socialization—into our culture as children, and into our profession as adults—provides us with truths and logical structures that hang together and answer life's questions well. We even learn to deal with the ambiguities and inconsistencies of what we have learned: We may not notice that we believe two mutually incompatible things before breakfast until someone who has a different perspective points it out to us. Even then, why should we question our own truths, or pay other truths heed? Strange answers make no sense, and provide no guidance or comfort. It is tempting to think that others are irrational or ignorant:

> Mothers may not believe this, but colds are *not* caused by standing in drafts, going without a hat, or getting feet wet. They occur when one sneezing, coughing child shares germs with another (Sears 1991).

The fact that there are numerous cogent *models* of reality is not trivial to Western thinkers. In this cultural region, battles have been fought and lives lost in defense of the ideal of a singular reality (Ames 1993). Earlier in our history, the search for this reality was mainly expressed in religious terms, but for the last 150 years or more, many have believed that science holds the key. By this logic, health care practices that are not considered scientific are not as trustworthy because they are not seeking the singular reality.

This situation helps explain why the psychiatric example above might be shrugged off. Laypeople are known to have beliefs, and clinicians must deal with them. The point of this discussion is that *every-one* has beliefs, and *all* realities are constructed; the facts of science are as culturally contextualized as those of law, theology, or social manners. Scientific fact is only as stable as the logic that produced it and the systems that apply it. Thus, science itself is rapidly experiencing a paradigm shift. Plasma physics operates by a different logic and perceives reality very differently from Newtonian physics; population biology is quite a different kettle of fish from Linnean systematics (see Chapters 1, 4, and 14).

The curious thing about modular reality is that you are likely to find exactly what you expect. The observer is not separate from the observed (see Heisenberg Principle, Chapter 1). Expectations are based on assumptions and the application of logic. When the assumptive base changes, so does the logic, and, as a result, the appropriate response. Consider, for example, streptococcal pharyngitis. According to biomedicine, the *streptococcal bacterium* causes the sore throat. Logically, one could treat with antibiotics to destroy that bacterium. However, some 20 percent of the population carries this germ in their throats without developing an illness (Greenwood & Nunn 1994). Indeed, only a minority of people who are exposed to the sore throat develop it. Thus other factors must be involved; the presence of bacterium may be necessary, but it is not sufficient. Health care systems such as homeopathy understand this concept, and focus more attention on the other factors—the reacting body, the person—than on infectious microorganisms. Care is aimed at strengthening the person, rather than at destroying bacteria.

But surely, people use universal definitions for such material body parts as the heart or blood? No, not quite. Although everyone might agree that the heart is a pulsating organ located in the center of the chest, its energetic and spiritual capabilities are debated. Biomedical thinkers describe the heart as a pump, using a material and mechanical metaphor. Once, even doctors thought of it as the seat of the soul, a memory our society revisits in many romantic songs. This idea still is active in Chinese medical thought. In that anatomy, the physical heart beats, while the energetic heart fills the role of sovereign ruler from whom emanate directing influence and clear insight (Porkert 1974) for all other organs. In

Chinese anatomy, the heart even has a special protector, an organ unknown in biomedical anatomy.

In biomedicine, blood is a living red substance that contains red and white cells, and carries food, enzymes, hormones, and oxygen; it is complex and constantly renews itself. In popular Jamaican thought, however, blood does not renew itself. Its purity (a social rather than medical concept) determines one's success in life (Sobo 1993). Following this logic, many Jamaicans are loath to give or receive blood for transfusions.

Cultural Relativity

In each of the examples above a reader might ask, who's right? But that is not the most useful question because all answers are right from within the logic of the model-in-use. Rightness also is modular, or relative.

A much more useful question is: how does this model serve its users? To be able to ask this question demands that one stand back dispassionately from one's own beliefs and models and recognize them as constructed, and not exclusively correct. To ask this question is to practice *cultural relativity*.

Cultural relativity is a technique for dealing with the many ways in which people explain themselves. It tells practitioners and researchers to remain in a fairly neutral, nonjudgmental stance, *knowing the values of people without adopting or rejecting them* (Kaplan 1984). From this position, a clinician, researcher, or student can observe their own perceptions and those of others, and understand how these interpretations serve users' lives. They can avoid becoming mired in determining which method is true, since nothing is really true when all realities are constructed.

On the other hand, ideas can be true in certain contexts or situations, that is, they make sense to their users. Therefore, the observer must learn to synthesize his or her position with those of others, so as to design an effective response strategy. For example, if people think of penicillin as a cooling drug, and therefore hesitate to use it to treat a "cold" illness such as pneumonia, the practitioner is to neutralize the "cold" of penicillin by suggesting that the patient take the medicine along with a food perceived as "hot" (Harwood 1977). Or, as in the first example cited above, the clinician can refer a patient

to a practitioner whose reality model more closely resembles that of the patient.

The practice of cultural relativity is pivotal to the study of alternative medicine, because each alternative system of medicine provides a different set of ideas about the body, disease, and medical reality. Readers will find it much easier to absorb and use this material if they can willingly—even playfully—step aside from their current beliefs and appreciations, to let in new ones.

The Behavioral Field of Health Care

What belongs under the rubric of health care? Once we know we can examine which components are addressed by which particular health care system, for no single system addresses the whole.

The Field of Health Care from Ego's Point of View

Imagine that each person is immersed in a potential field of health care that instructs how to prevent illness, treat illness, and, more positively, enhance wellness. Figure 2-1 depicts this idea as three triangles (shown as non-overlapping, although in reality, they do overlap, at least partially). The three triangles are embedded in a semi-circle labeled historical, cultural, and social environment which reminds us that all health care is delivered within a context of experience, belief, and expectation that is not always obvious to us.

The central triangle deals with health care as it is delivered to groups of people, the right and left triangles with health care that is received primarily by individuals or families. The small circle in the center represents a person, Ego*, to whom all the contents of the field are available. Lines at the bottom of the drawing mark the health condition, from increasing health (left) to decreasing health (right). The central triangle covers prevention, that is, the avoidance of sickness without seeking high-level wellness.

Each triangle is divided into three sections. The

---

*Ego is used in the anthropologic/geneologic sense, that is, the person from whose point of view the figure is to be understood. It is not used in the common psychiatric sense, that is the "I" that deals with reality.

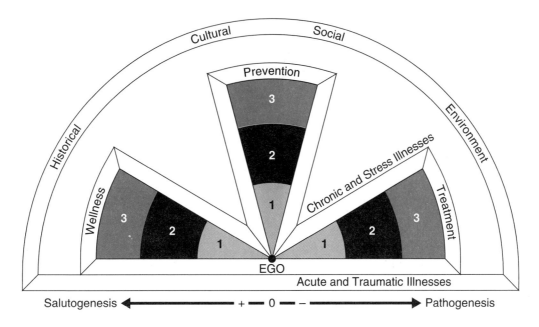

1 Self-care

2 Lower intensity specialist care

3 Higher intensity specialist care

Figure 2-1. The behavioral field of health care from the perspective of an individual.

light blue section represents the forms of health care that Ego can seek and deliver without the intervention of a specialist. Some examples include praying, exercising, brushing teeth, bathing, drinking fruit juice, cleaning house, paying utility bills for receipt of electricity and pure water, taking dietary supplements, washing and bandaging minor wounds, and taking an analgesic or sleeping to treat a headache.

The black area represents a degree of complexity or severity that requires specialist intervention. Most health care needs fall at this level, and most health care systems deliver the majority of care at this level. At this level of wellness, we might find Ego seeking help with finding appropriate work, consulting a dietary specialist, taking a parenting class, or learning meditation techniques. Under treatment, we would find Ego seeking help for traumas, discomforts, or malfunctions that have not responded to home remedies or that Ego recognizes as requiring the attention of a specialist. This section also includes ongo-

ing care and control of chronic conditions and handicaps. Prevention at this level involves preventive dental care, screening tests, and vaccinations, and community prevention activities such as pure food and drug controls and pollution prevention—activities of which Ego is generally unaware and over which he or she has little control.

The dark blue section represents a high degree of complexity and intensity that few specialists emphasize, and that Ego calls upon rarely. This level of treatment deals with extreme illnesses, malformations, and trauma, including care that is delivered in emergency rooms, operating rooms, and intensive care units. This level in the prevention triangle deals with responses to major catastrophes such as epidemics and earthquakes. In the wellness triangle it deals with an issue that is not easily expressed in English, and is generally described in terms with psychological and spiritual overtones, such as "self-actualization," "enlightenment," or "awakening."

Note that the cost of health care rises from level 1 to 3, attaining the highest cost in the prevention and treatment triangles at level 3, but paradoxically potentially the lowest cost at wellness level 3.

Now having drawn and laid out this concept in a linear form, I must critique it. The alert reader already will be asking such questions as: What if Ego has diabetes and is taking all kinds of proactive steps to increase wellness, despite his or her condition? What about healing communities that increase wellness for terminally ill patients? Where do healthy, pregnant women belong on this figure? These are appropriate criticisms: distinctions between the sections are not as precise in real life. A healthy woman who seeks a midwife's care during delivery might belong in wellness section 2, while one who delivers in a hospital with medical intervention belongs in treatment section 2—not because she is sick, but because her pregnancy is being treated as if it were an illness, as it is for most American women in the latter half of the twentieth century. Only in the last few years has the situation been recognized and some effort toward demedicalizing it been made.

The Field of Health Care From the Point of View of the Variant Practices or Systems

Activities included in the wellness triangle in Figure 2-1 range from those that are widely accepted in our society, such as diet and exercise, to behaviors such as praying that many do not classify as health-related. Why include them here?

The dominant biomedical system's materialist effort to segregate medicine from religion grew out of the secularist urge to embrace science at the turn of the century; this concept is artificial, and is not shared by most of the world's health care systems. Indeed, most systems accept the reality of the non-material aspects of the body-person.

Sister Erma Allen once told me of having healed a small boy who had cut his head; she had silently said the [bloodstopping] verse over and over while at the same time applying ice to the wound. I asked how she knew that it was not the *ice* that had stopped the bleeding.

(Continues)

After a pause she reprimanded me gently, 'God sewed it with *His* needle, darlin' (Snow 1993).

The fact that biomedicine prefers materialist explanations also implies that it does not deliver care in all parts of the triangles. Indeed this also is true for all other systems. Each emphasizes a distinctive viewpoint (explanatory model) and develops expertise in just some of the potential areas of health care. For example, biomedicine has had great success in treating acute illness and trauma. Its control of technology also allows for remarkable success in extending life, and in producing pharmaceuticals and technology to address the physical and physiological components of chronic conditions. Simultaneously, however, biomedicine has been criticized for its relatively ineffective care of many chronic conditions, and for repeated inefficiencies in human kindness and humane development, areas which tend to escape its materialist model.

Other systems, notably the so-called holistic systems, integrate human development into their usual care patterns. These systems also control technologies and techniques that address physical and physiologic functioning. Patients praise these systems for their care of chronic conditions, and for their efforts to enhance wellness, which include weaning patients from excessive dependence on health care specialists.

Figure 2-2 portrays these different approaches. Note that neither the biomedical system nor the Chinese medical system deals much with prevention on a mass scale. That is the prerogative of different specialists, especially of public health specialists.

Two vital points emerge from the field discussion and will recur throughout this chapter.

1. No one health care system addresses the whole field.
2. All health care systems address a considerable part of it.

No one system is best for everything, and existing systems overlap considerably in what they offer. There is a temptation to argue that societies ought to achieve economies of scale by making sure only the best survive. However, considering our discussion of cultural relativity, it is impossible to define

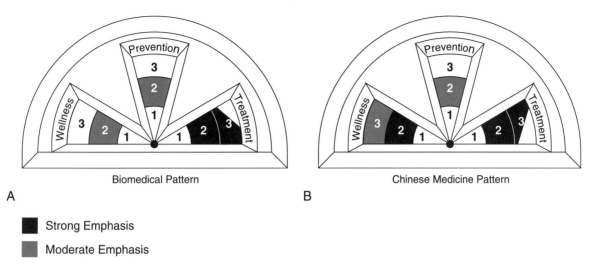

A Biomedical Pattern

B Chinese Medicine Pattern

■ Strong Emphasis

■ Moderate Emphasis

Figure 2-2. The behavioral field of health care, highlighting the components addressed by two particular health care systems. **(A)** Biomedical, **(B)** Chinese medicine.

the "best" in a manner that satisfies everyone. Logic demands that we determine who will be served well by which system, and why. We will return to this issue after discussing some of the important ways in which health care systems differ.

The Cultural Concept of the Health Care System

A cultural medical system is a complex of beliefs, models, and linked activities that providers and users consider useful in bettering health or well-being, and in relieving stress and disease.

Components of A Health Care System:

- A developed theory of the body-person, known as the explanatory model (Kleinman 1980). This theory includes the causes of malfunction, as well as ap-
(Continues)

propriate ways to address this malfunction.
- Plans to educate and train new practitioners, through apprenticeship and/or schooling.
- A health care sub-system that delivers care to the needy.
- Associated means of producing substances or technologies necessary to delivery and educational sub-systems.
- Professional organizations of practitioners who monitor each other's practices and promote the system to potential users.
- A legal mandate that provides for the official recognition of practitioners and maintains a minimum standard of quality.
- A social mandate that informally reveals levels of community acceptance, as by frequency of use, willingness to pay, and stereotypes about practitioners, among other markers.

This definition makes it clear that a health care system is complex and multilayered. Even simple systems, such as those limited in scope to one self-defined ethnic group are difficult for one person to master or describe. Larger systems are correspondingly more complex, encompassing a wide range of viewpoints, numerous subspecialties, and distinctive styles of practice. Biomedicine includes specialties ranging from the intensely material practice of surgery to the far more relational specialties of family medicine and psychiatry. Biomedical complexity is compounded by the fact that it is practiced rather differently in different countries.

> Even the best simultaneous translator is going to have trouble dealing with the fact that *peptic ulcer* and *bronchitis* do not mean the same things in Britain that they do in the United States; that the U.S. *appendectomy* becomes the British *appendicectomy*; that the French tendency to exaggerate means there are never headaches in France, only migraines, and that the French often refer to real migraines as 'liver crises'; that the German language has no word for chest pain, forcing the German patient to talk of heart pain, and that when a German doctor says 'cardiac insufficiency' he may simply mean that the patient is tired. . . . How can [bio]medicine, which is commonly supposed to be a science, . . . be so different in four countries whose peoples are so similar genetically? The answer is that while [bio]medicine benefits from a certain amount of scientific input, culture intervenes at every step of the way (Payer 1988).

This complexity is equally true of Chinese medicine, which embraces many styles, including traditional Chinese medicine, Five Element style, Japanese, Korean, and French styles. Even community-based, or folk systems may have different specialties. Lakota (Sioux) people distinguish medicine men and women who emphasize herbal treatment from holy men and women who practice shamanically (Hultkrantz 1985). The Dineh (Navajo) recognize three types of diagnosticians and Singers who work with rituals, herbs, and the psychosocial body to deliver health care (Morgan 1977).

At a very much smaller scale than the system or

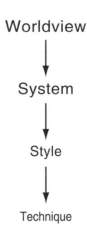

Figure 2-3. Scales of complexity in understanding health care.

the style is the technique of health care (Fig. 2-3). A technique is comparatively simple; it might be single therapy, and often can be practiced without being linked to an explanatory model, detailed training, or professional oversight. Some practitioners specialize in offering single therapies, such as bee sting injections, colonic irrigations, biofeedback, specific dietary supplements, or Swedish massage.

Single therapy practitioners can provide *symptomatic relief* to their patients, but they cannot provide *systematic care*, that is, care guided by a well-developed model of how the body-person works, how the malfunction arose, and how the technique can help. Indeed, the expansive power and persistence of health care systems correlate with the effectiveness of their explanatory models and linked therapeutic modalities.

Systems Embedded in Larger Constructs

But where do explanatory models come from? As noted earlier, health care systems are embedded in the sociocultural system surrounding them. This provides not only access to natural resources, but also ideas, assumptions, and patterns of logic. All these are reflected in explanatory models and health care delivery formats. In formal terms, health care systems are guided by the worldview principles of their society. The larger and more heterogeneous the surrounding society, the wider the range of health care ideas that society can encompass.

Nevertheless, certain worldviews tend to predominate. In the United States and Europe, the hierarchic, or reductionistic, worldview dominates. This worldview model emphasizes hierarchies of value, (judgmentalism) a tendency to be judgmental, competition, forcefulness, and materialism (Cassidy 1994). Biomedicine reflects these patterns in its concern for the expertise of the practitioner over that of the layperson/patient; its tendency to magnify the importance of some specialties or diseases over others (cardiology over pediatrics, cancer over asthma); its preference for treatment modalities that cause obvious reactions in the physical body; and its focus on end-stage physical malfunction, while generally ignoring less developed conditions, and rejecting nonmaterial explanations of cause.

> [Cartesian] assumptions permeate Western society and form the modus operandi of conventional medicine. They have led to our belief in rationalism, causality, objectivity, and the separation of [bio]medicine and psychiatry. The assumptions work very well in acute emergency situations, but are limited when illness becomes chronic. . . . Cartesian thinking can be classified broadly as yang, and its inferred opposite as yin. Chinese philosophic thought can therefore be seen to be inclusive of Western thought, while Western thought has no way of incorporating Chinese holistic thinking (Greenwood & Null 1994).

Other Western health care systems literally originated in reaction to biomedicine (allopathy), including homeopathy, osteopathy, naturopathy, chiropractic and Christian Science. Others have been imported from the East, like Chinese medicine and Ayurveda. All argue (not always convincingly) that their approaches to care are more egalitarian, less judgmental, and gentler than biomedicine. Several offer nonmaterialist explanations of cause and care. In making such arguments, these systems are calling upon another worldview currently held in the United States, namely, the relational (ecological or holistic) worldview. This worldview sees all things as connected in a network of relationships, and deals with how people, things, and energy interact and how these interactions can better the whole. Re-

flected into health care this idea means that practitioners model health in terms of achieving balance, and patients are seen to have expertise, different from that of the practitioner, but expertise nonetheless. Thus practitioner and patient form a partnership, and patients take some responsibility for their own care and development.

Professionalized and Community-Based Systems

These terms distinguish between systems that serve large, heterogeneous patient populations, and smaller, more localized systems that serve culturally homogeneous populations.

A professionalized system tends to be found in an urban setting, is taught in schools with the aid of written texts, and demands formal, usually legal, criteria for practice (Foster & Anderson 1978). Students enter the system by choice, and are approved via entrance examinations. They become practitioners upon completing a designated plan of study, passing more examinations, and often, being licensed by the state or nation. Health care typically is delivered on a one practitioner-to-one patient basis, in locales that have been set aside to this purpose, such as offices, clinics, and hospitals. Practitioners form membership organizations dedicated to policing their respective specialties and presenting them in a positive light to outsiders. The dominant health care systems of modern nations always are professionalized systems. Examples include Ayurveda, biomedicine, Chinese medicine, chiropractic, homeopathy, osteopathy, and Unani (the traditional system of Pakistan and neighboring Muslim nations).

Community-based systems, also known as folk or tribal systems, are less expanded than professionalized systems, though they may have equally complex explanatory models, and equally lengthy histories. Found in both urban and rural settings, training is often by apprenticeship. People enter training sometimes by inheritance, but most often by receiving a call from the unseen world indicating that he or she has the special capacity necessary to become a healer. Training ends when the teacher considers the student to be ready to practice. Rather than written examinations, students are tested by practicing medicine under guidance; essentially, the community itself determines if a student is "good enough." Care is often offered in people's homes, and community-based healers often practice on a part-time basis. Some folk healers form professional associations, with the same goals as professionalized doctors. Examples of community-based systems include Alcoholics Anonymous and similar urban self-help groups, Curanderismo (among the most expanded of folk systems), rootwork (an African-derived system used by some African-Americans), and traditional health care in native American and Euroamerican rural groups.

> For details about community-based systems in North America, consult extended studies such as *Herbal and Magical Medicine* (Kirkland, Mathews, Sullivan & Baldwin 1992), *Walkin' Over Medicine* (Snow 1993), *Ritual Healing in Suburban America* (McGuire 1994), *Cry of the Eagle, Encounters with a Cree Healer* (Young, Ingram, Swartz 1989), *Black Elk, the Sacred Ways of a Lakota* (Black Elk & Lyon 1990), *American Folk Medicine* (Hand 1976), *Powwowing in Union Country* (Reimansnyder 1989), *This Other Kind of Doctors* (Terrell 1990), *Susto: A Folk Illness* (Rubel, O'Nell, Ardon 1984), *Masters of the Ordinary* (Scott 1993), *Ethnic Medicine in the Southwest* (Spicer 1979), *Healing Traditions* (O'Connor 1995).

There is a third type, often called popular health care. Popular health care is not organized systematically; rather, it consists of simple techniques associated with the care of particular conditions. Examples include using cranberry juice for bladder infections, chicken soup for colds, and hot toddies for sore throats. Much of what is published in general-reader magazines or discussed on talk shows is popular medicine. It is typically presented using biomedical terminology, and is often simplified biomedicine.

Distinctions of complexity among health care systems are not absolute. For example, most professionalized systems continue to insist on considerable hands-on training, similar to apprenticeships. Some folk systems, especially urbanized ones, train practitioners in schools and do not expect students to have received a call to practice; these practitioners often earn their living through full-time health care work.

Language Issues

Distinctions made in this section deal with differences of scale. A system is remarkably more complex than a technique, or a single therapy; a professionalized system is expanded further than a community-based system. Failing to understand this point can lead to confusion. For example one writer claims that: 'Subjects were presented with a list of 32 alternative therapies' (Furnham 1992). The list includes practices of completely different scale, from systems that take years to learn (acupuncture, homeopathy, and anthroposophical medicine) to techniques that one receives as a gift (dowsing) or can learn in a few weeks (reflexology, iridology). The worst form of confusing scalars occurs when someone directly compares a technique and a system, does not account for differences of complexity, and concludes that the system failed.

One must be aware of terms that lend themselves to scalar confusion. The single term *acupuncture* can refer to a system, an approach, or simply a needling technique. Which does a given writer or speaker mean? Massage can mean a single technique, or it can refer to a rapidly professionalizing and systematizing practice. Some people use the term medicine to refer exclusively to biomedicine; for most, however, medicine is a term that encompasses all the ways in which people deliver health care.

Another confusing term is *traditional*. Biomedical publications often refer to their own practice as traditional medicine, categorizing all other practices by a term such as *alternative*. However, when biomedicine is referred to as modern medicine, its worldwide nature is being contrasted with the indigenous systems of non-Western societies which are then called traditional. Of course, systems other than biomedicine are used worldwide so all major systems are sometimes classified as the "Great Tradition" systems and other systems are, in contrast, little tradition or folk systems.

In summary, it is most effective to refer to health care systems by their specific names, and to clearly distinguish the scale of which one wishes to speak or write.

Modalities of Health Care

Whatever the other aspects of their character, all health care systems and techniques care for people

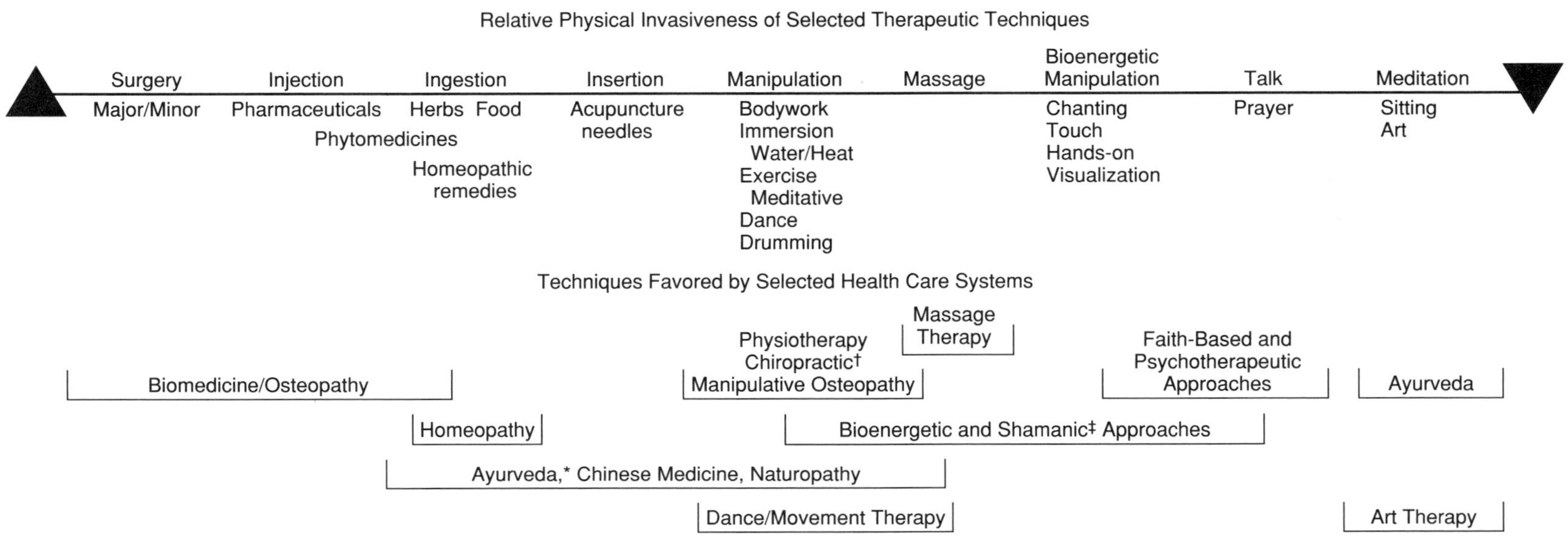

Relative Physical Invasiveness of Selected Therapeutic Techniques

Surgery	Injection	Ingestion	Insertion	Manipulation	Massage	Bioenergetic Manipulation	Talk	Meditation
Major/Minor	Pharmaceuticals Phytomedicines	Herbs Food Homeopathic remedies	Acupuncture needles	Bodywork Immersion Water/Heat Exercise Meditative Dance Drumming		Chanting Touch Hands-on Visualization	Prayer	Sitting Art

Techniques Favored by Selected Health Care Systems

Massage Therapy

Faith-Based and Psychotherapeutic Approaches

Ayurveda

Biomedicine/Osteopathy

Physiotherapy
Chiropractic†
Manipulative Osteopathy

Bioenergetic and Shamanic‡ Approaches

Art Therapy

Homeopathy

Ayurveda,* Chinese Medicine, Naturopathy

Dance/Movement Therapy

* Ayurveda also provides minor surgery.
† Some chiropractors offer dietary management, acupuncture needling, etc.
‡ Many shamanic practitioners also provide herbs.

Figure 2-4. Relative physical invasiveness of selected therapeutic techniques.

by trying to change some aspect of their functioning. Common interventions include surgery, pharmaceutical injection or ingestion, biologicals or botanicals, needling, dietary management, manipulation, massage, meditative exercises, dancing, music therapy, art therapy, water and heat treatments, bioenergetic manipulation (touch therapy), talk therapy, shamanic journeying, sitting meditation, and prayer.

Most health care systems employ several of these modalities. A community-based system like Curanderismo uses dietary manipulation, herbs, first aid techniques, and shamanic techniques to treat a wide range of physical, psychosocial, and spiritual malfunctions. Ayurveda offers surgery, a variety of water treatments from purges to baths, numerous biologic and herbal remedies, dietary management, and both sitting and moving forms of meditation.

Some modalities are more invasive than others. Some enter the physical body by cutting, pricking, or ingesting, and others do not break even this barrier. The second break is between those that touch the surface of the body and others that work with energetic or spiritual levels of the body that can be accessed without touching the skin. Even among those that break into the body there are differing degrees of intensity: replacing a hip is more intrusive than removing a cataract. Pharmaceutical drugs generally are more toxic than phytomedicines (semi-purified plant medicines), which are in turn more forceful than herbs. Forcefulness does not connote effectiveness: mild and gentle modalities can be as effective as intrusive ones, if properly administered.

Figure 2-4 sorts the modalities along a line indicating the level of invasiveness into the physical body. Sorting from intensely to lightly invasive procedures correlates with a movement from materialist to nonmaterialist views of the body-person. Also, actual health care systems roughly correlate with certain areas of the line, further evidence that each system emphasizes certain parts of, but not the entire spectrum of health care options.

Explanatory Models

We have discussed how health care systems intervene, but we have yet to understand the "madness" behind each method. Each system has its own explanatory model that summarizes the perceptions, assumptions, beliefs, theories, and facts that guide the logic of health care delivery. To develop the idea of the explanatory model, we will explore how different systems perceive the body-person and sickness and disease, their preferred causal explanations, and the preferred relationship between patients and practitioner.

Concepts of the Body-Person

There is not one human body, not one anatomy, not one physiology, but many. To understand any system, we must understand its concept of the body. Figure

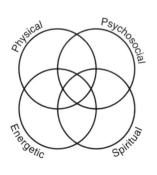

The Four Bodies

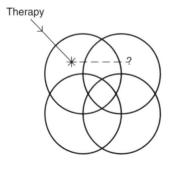

Therapeutic Goal Assumption of Materialist Systems

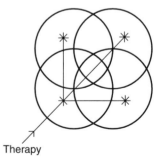

Therapeutic Goal Assumption of Nonmaterialist Systems

Figure 2-5. The four bodies addressed by health care.

2-5 depicts the body-person as four intersecting circles. The figure is simplified, for even within each of the circles there are many ways in which systems can phrase their material, energetic, spiritual, or social perceptions of the body.

The biomedical model of the body-person focuses on the physical body, concerning itself with the structure of its tissues and the movement and transformation of chemicals within cells. Classical chiropractic and osteopathic* models of the body are equally materialistic, emphasizing connections and communications between bones, nerves, and muscles and the rest of the physical body.

Homeopathy views the physical body as having three significant layers, and the body-person as having three distinct aspects (Vithoulkas 1980). Each of these layers and aspects is imbued with *vital spirit* or *vital energy*, and this energy is the ultimate focus of health care delivery. Acupuncture analyzes the physical body in terms of the flow of energy through pathways, or *meridians*, which have not yet been shown to have material counterparts. The energy that flows through and animates the material body is called *ch'i (qi, ki)*, and closely resembles the homeopathic concept of vital spirit, or the Ayurvedic concept of *prana*.

Biofield or bioenergetic therapies intervene in bodies outside the physical body that are sometimes spoken of as emanations and that can be perceived as *auras*. Different specialists perceive and name auras somewhat differently. Wirkus, using bioscience terminology, writes of the thermal, electromagnetic, and acoustic fields (Wirkus 1993), while Brennan, employing esoteric science terminology, labels the same three auras the etheric, astral, and mental bodies (Brennan 1988).

Spiritual and shamanic healers also work with nonmaterial and normally invisible bodies. Most of these healers believe that these spiritual forces imbue the physical body, although some say they extend beyond it, and some say that parts can travel (as during sleep), be removed (exorcism), or lost (Eliade 1964, Ingerman 1991).

Psychotherapists and shamanic healers typically

---

* Osteopathy originated as a manipulative system. Today, only a minority of practitioners maintain this tradition; the remainder practice biomedicine (allopathy) or a combination.

work with the psychosocial body, that is, the 'person' who lives within the other bodies and interacts with the world outside. Terms for this being include "mind" and "emotions," as well as technical terms that each subspecialty uses to showcase its particular explanatory model.

The several bodies are not, of course, separate: only one body-person stands before the practitioner seeking help. But who can say where the physical body, with its ongoing chemical and electrical changes, merges into the energetic body, and where the latter extends into the spiritual body? All are immersed in the psychosocial body; what a person believes markedly affects how he or she will respond to illness and to treatment, or what he or she will deliver in the way of health care.

As illustrated in Figure 2-5, with the exception of heavily materialist models that perceive themselves as treating the physical body and only reluctantly acknowledge the psychosocial body, all health care systems argue that there are both material and nonmaterial aspects to the body. Intervention in one area will affect all others. When a Five Element acupuncturist needles a patient who is having an asthma attack, he or she enters the energetic body and moves energy. In addition, he or she expects the physical, psychosocial, and spiritual bodies to respond: the bronchial tubes will dilate, and pain, anxiety, and fear will dissipate. These changes do not occur coincidentally; according to this system's explanatory model, all the aspects of the body can work at ease when energy flows smoothly.

Concepts of Sickness, Disease, and Imbalance

Though often used generically, the term sickness formally refers to an experience of discomfort or malfunction. Disease and imbalance, however, are abstracted concepts. Thus, a person suffers illness or sickness, and a practitioner assigns meaning to this experience by diagnosing and explaining what has happened. The answers provided by the practitioner are guided by the explanatory model of his or her health care system. Cultural learning also guides the expression of the patient's illness and the practitioner's diagnostic values, so much so that even the pain people feel and report is related to such learned aspects of being as gender and ethnicity (Bates et al. 1995).

A system's preferred malfunction concept is closely linked to its perception of the body-person, particularly, whether a system tends to perceive cause as primarily external or internal (Cassidy 1982, 1995; Fabrega 1974; Foster & Anderson 1978, Murdock 1980). Most health care systems accept that both occur, although most also prefer to emphasize either the invader or the responding organism. External models argue that malfunctions attack from outside the body-person, invading and destroying. Internal models argue that something must first go wrong internally, thereby allowing outer influences to penetrate where they could not have before. These conceptual differences affect each system's views of patient and practitioner. External theorists see the patient as passive and the practitioner as authority, while internal ideology interprets the patient as responsible and the practitioner as partner to that responsibility.

Disease

The concept of disease is preferred by external models. The body-person is relatively passive, while the surrounding environment is teaming with danger. Body-persons are thought to respond similarly to invaders, that is, one person with mumps, leukemia, or pneumonia experiences it much as others do. If people are similar and the environment is dangerous, emphasis is placed on the actions of the invader, and every different type of invader creates a different disease. These assumptive patterns lead to the possible existence of many different diseases, and a major function of practitioners is to distinguish among them, or diagnose. Their second job is to remove, destroy, or immobilize invaders, thereby curing the patient.

This model has long been preferred by biomedicine and has yielded familiar metaphors. Tumor cells and microorganisms that have been awaiting their chance in reservoirs invade human victims. The body wages war, and surgeons and doctors are warriors in white, battling the invaders.* Diseases that

fit this classic model have distinctive symptoms and signs, single causes, and respond to specific therapies. Treatment results in cure. To emphasize the separation between ailments and patients, the former often are called *disease entities*.

Only a minority of the disease entities defined by biomedicine fits the invasion model. Chronic, degenerative, and stress-related disorders frustrate the system because they do not have specifiable boundaries, single causes, or predictable outcomes. Indeed, they force biomedicine to consider explanations that fall outside the usual framework: that the body-person is not passive, but plays some part in the genesis of disease; that many (often unspecifiable) factors must interact before disease arises; that some of these factors might be psychosocial; and that the practitioner's role is less to prescribe than to educate. The area of biomedicine that best reflects this opening state of mind is that of "lifestyle" diseases, or conditions that arise from and can be ameliorated by changes in how people behave and believe. Interestingly, even this door has not opened too widely: the majority of lifestyle discussions still focus on ameliorative factors that address the physical body, such as diet and exercise. Biomedical practitioners who recommend visualization or meditation are likely to consider themselves avant-garde.

Chiropractic and osteopathy share biomedicine's mechanistic view of disease. In these systems, misalignment within the musculoskeletal system can cause malfunctions in other parts of the physical body. The explanatory model states that if the core misalignment can be alleviated, the distant malfunctions will resolve. The cause of misalignment is usually external—a fall, a twist, a jolt, or habitually poor posture—and sometimes internal—that poor posture is related to poor self-image. Patient instructions tend to take a physical form, such as modifications of diet and exercise.

Imbalance

A larger number of health care systems emphasize internal models of disorder and speak of imbalance rather than disease. Their therapeutic goal is to return the person to a state of balance. These systems often name conditions according to their process within the person: for example, in Chinese medicine, *rising liver fire* describes a person's condition momentarily or repeatedly, but is not a freestanding

---

* Similar metaphors are used to describe the need for exorcism: invasion by an evil entity demands a spiritual battle to defeat it. Faith-based systems that use exorcism therapeutically also use external models of disease causation.

and categorical concept like the biomedical disease entity hepatitis.

Balance can be perturbed by external invaders or by interruptions in the smooth working of the internal milieu. However, external causes cannot harm a body-person who is well. Health care therefore tends to the self-protective abilities of the body-person, maintaining and strengthening them. This is not curing, but healing; the practitioner's goal is not to battle the invader or to fix the patient, but rather to prune, weed, and plant within the patient, enabling him or her to grow a vibrant internal garden in which all aspects of his/her body-person coexist with the vagaries of the external environment.

Treatment within internal-cause systems is individualistic, because the logic of this model is such that each person has a unique history and constitution that affects how he or she will respond to the myriad circumstances of life. The practitioner examines the current condition of the patient, relates it to his or her social and medical history, and then selects therapy based on the entire assessment.

Diet, exercise, rest, and other physical interventions might be prescribed, but these recommendations usually are offered in formats that also address the spiritual and energetic bodies, such as yoga, t'ai chi, or Qigong or moving meditations might be recommended for exercise. The person might be advised to develop his or her spiritual/emotional bodies via creative skills such as art, dance, and chanting. Or the patient may be encouraged to minimize his vulnerability to psychic attack via meditation, shamanic journeying, or prayer. The client may be counselled to modify diet not only as to nutrient content, but also as to seasonal appropriateness and essential (as opposed to literal) temperature.

Constitutional Types

The disease entity and imbalance models represent ideals. Practitioners recognize that neither model works all of the time. Thus biomedicine recognizes conditions such as syndromes or chronic diseases have multiple linked causes, not all of which can be specified. Similarly, internal-cause systems recognize that individuality is not absolute, for people do present commonalities or patterned responses to similar challenges.

In fact, many health care systems have developed sophisticated models to link certain constitutional

types with the probability of their developing particular illnesses. In the European/Middle Eastern system that preceded biomedicine, people were categorized as melancholic, phlegmatic, sanguine, or choleric. Though today's biomedical practitioners may view these concepts with an indulgent smile, the underlying idea is by no means absent in modern biomedicine: earlier in this century, bioscientists attempted to link physical and psychosocial diseases with the endomorphic, mesomorphic, and ectomorphic types (Sheldon 1949). Today, there is much interest in Type A personalities, which are said to be prone to heart disease, and Type C, prone to cancer. Constitutional typologies are well developed in the Ayurvedic system (the *doshas* of *pitta, vata, kapha*), and in some styles of Chinese medicine (the five "central foci" of Worsley-style Five Element acupuncture). The old European categories survive in the "hotcold" systems of Latin America and the Philippines.

Figure 2-6 summarizes the data of this section on a linear model. The disease entities model of biomedicine forms one extreme on a continuum, with the process-related imbalance models at the other end. At the mid-point are patterned responses, including constitutional types. At the end featuring diseases, the individual person essentially has been deleted from the argument "one person suffers much like others so focus on identifying the disease", while at the other extreme, the person is the final focus and arbiter of interpretation "in this individual these symptoms mean x, which I know from experience of him/her . . . they may mean y in another individual"). In the middle are positions that share both interpretive energies: "Certain characteristics make it more likely that he or she will experience these symptoms, so perhaps I can reduce my diagnostic chore."

Language Issues

Biomedical disease entities have become standard vocabulary, but these diseases (not the symptoms) are only real to people who use the biomedical model. Practitioners of other systems may use these terms out of familiarity, to communicate with patients or granting agencies, or to complete insurance claim forms, but within their own system of health care, these labels have no real cogency. Acupuncturists, for example, treat what their patients and referring physicians call "depression," but the concept

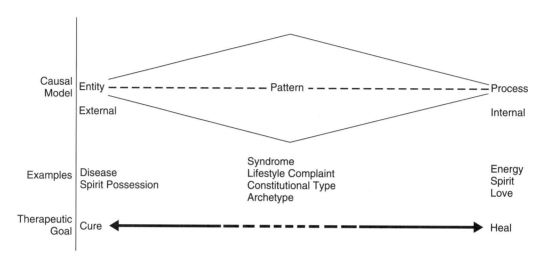

Figure 2-6. Three major approaches to interpreting symptoms.

does not exist in Chinese medicine. In the Five Element model, there are at least five different ways people can express what biomedicine labels depression. Thus, two patients with the same biomedical diagnosis of depression might receive quite different herbal or needle therapies from a Chinese medicine practitioner.

Practitioners and scientists must be careful in their use of biomedical terminology, not assuming it is sufficient to describe what is understood by other systems. Specialists should describe the symptomatology, and then, if they wish, affix a biomedical label while clearly stating that the biomedical label may not reflect the way of knowing of another system. This can serve because symptoms are recognized everywhere; it is the interpretations that differ. By focusing on symptoms the malfunction labels of the other systems would begin to take on the kind of reality that now is owned only by the biomedical labels. The medical conversation would become more accurate and broader.

Concepts of Deep Cause

External and internal causative factors mentioned so far can be understood as proximate causes of malfunction. With the issue of deep cause, we contemplate why *this* person at *this* time or in *this* place has become ill in *this* way. We want to consider sociocultural answers, not epidemiologic ones. We will explore the issue first by returning to our discussion of the body-person and considering the develop-

mental nature of sickness, and second by considering the intentional component of sickness.

The Developmental Nature of Sickness

An ancient chicken-and-egg philosophic argument questions whether the physical body comes first, giving rise to nonmaterial constructs such as emotions and mind, or if mind (spirit, soul) comes first and animates the physical body. Materialist models prefer the first argument, while nonmaterialist models favor the second.

This choice affects both the theory and politics of health care. One can only deliver care in a fashion that does not conflict with one's beliefs. If one accepts as real only what one can see, hear, or measure with machines, then delivering care to the nonmaterial bodies is, at the very least, puzzling. Efforts to test nonmaterialist systems include designing machinery to "prove" the nonmaterial bodies exist, such as using electrical point locators to find acupuncture points and meridians, or kirlian photography to find auras. Materialists suspect nonmaterialist practitioners of misleading their patients or of achieving effects primarily by activating the placebo response. Cynics also argue that nonmaterialist practitioners have their greatest successes in the care of functional, or psychosomatic, diseases. Such diseases are disvalued in materialist systems precisely because they lack specific material signs such as germs, malfunctioning genes, tumor cells, abnormal metabolic values, or broken bones. Those who suffer from functional conditions are suspected of not being really sick.

Nonmaterialist thinkers consider malfunction in the nonmaterial aspects of the body to be as real as physical malfunction. All patient complaints signal true distress; the diagnostic concern is not with triaging between the real and the imaginary, but with identifying what aspect of the person will respond most efficaciously to treatment.

Many such systems employ a developmental model of malfunction in which sickness starts in the nonmaterial bodies, and is expressed in the physical body only later. They fault materialist systems for paying attention only to end-stage malfunction, and failing to treat conditions before they become entrenched. They further argue that a focus on the material level alone provides only symptomatic relief and ignores deep cause, allowing underlying malfunctions to remain unaddressed. Nonmaterialist systems assume that care can modify all parts of the body-person. Some also claim that as the person heals, they cycle backwards through layers of long-buried symptomatology, until, finally, they express the oldest symptoms, release them, and are well. This pattern is called the "law of cure."

> From the adjoining room she heard friends, who could not see her, discussing some of the slanderous stories being circulated about her. Rachel was crushed. When she [arrived home] one of the servants thought she looked as if she had been shot through the heart. Questioned about why she looked so dejected, she started to sob and then to cry uncontrollably as she poured out her experiences of the day. . . . Several days later Rachel suffered a heart attack (Huber 1990).

To give an example, a child might experience a spiritual trauma such as loss of intimacy. Afterwards this child develops eczema. Later still, the child develops allergies and asthma. Untreated, the original spiritual wound, or deep cause, has been magnified, and becomes overt and disabling. Appropriate treatment of the asthma not only will relieve wheezing, but might instigate a recrudescence of eczema and grief. Depending on the system, these results may be expected to occur in sequence, or simultaneously.

Thus, by the logic of internal-cause systems, it is advantageous to treat complaints before malfunction is manifested physically. Even nonmaterial complaints are real, because any suffering affects the whole body-person.

Systems that employ only nonmaterial therapies such as bioenergetic healing, psychotherapy, and shamanism, focus care on the nonmaterial aspects of the person, but expect that the physical body will respond. However, many systems employ a combination of material and nonmaterial therapeutic modalities. The techniques themselves often have a layered character; needling acupuncture points have specific physical and specific spiritual and emotional effects. For example, the same is true of herbal remedies and bodywork. Patients are cared for by the material, energetic, and spiritual actions of the specific therapies, and it is assumed that their physical, mental, emotional, spiritual, and energetic bodies all will respond and change.

Nonmaterialist models also view the person as having an active role in creating and treating his own condition. The role of practitioner is reformulated from authority to facilitator, from "the one who does the curing" to "the one who helps the person heal himself." As treatment is administered, such practitioners encourage patients to consider what attitudes of mind or spirit may have played a part in their illness, and to explore new, life-enhancing ways of believing and behaving—wellness training. The goals of nonmaterialist health care are to care for the nonsomatic aspects of the patient so completely that the somatic aspect rarely suffers.

Unfortunately, in the hands of some practitioners, the focus on patient responsibility becomes excessive and patients feel guilt about their sickness. The materialist emphasis on the patient as the victim of disease can be equally harmful, resulting in patients who feel helpless to change themselves or learn health-enhancing behaviors.

The Intentional Component of Sickness

Practitioners discuss proximate and deep causes of sickness; medical social scientists recognize another cross-cutting domain of causality and contrast—naturalistic and personalistic explanatory approaches. According to the naturalistic approach, the causes of sickness are found in the natural world and lack intention; they cause malfunction by unintentionally ending up in the wrong place. Sickness is considered a normal experience of life, natural and inevitable. The personalistic approach, however, maintains that some form of intention is present, and sickness is considered to be an unnatural result of attracting the attention of the wrong energies, or a response to one's own misbehavior or misperception (Foster & Anderson 1978).

When a person says he has lung cancer, and attributes it to 30 years of smoking, they speak in a naturalistic mode. But if they complain of having been inveigled into smoking, or that this habit is an expression of weak character, they are moving in a personalistic direction. If they attribute their cancer to the corrective or punitive actions of a spiritual entity such as God, they speak fully in the personalistic mode.

These tendencies coexist in most health care systems, though one or the other usually is emphasized. Professionalized health care systems generally prefer such naturalistic explanations as microorganisms, malformations, toxins, age-related degeneration, winds, hot and cold, or damp and dry. But within these systems, some practitioners recognize, even specialize in the personalistic approach. In biomedicine, psychiatry and psychology emphasize this structure, usually attributing malfunction to troubles in the psychosocial body rather than in the spiritual or energetic bodies; in other major systems, practitioners deal with expressions of self-distrust or the results of psychic attacks much as they deal with physical conditions.

Faith-based systems are primarily personalistic in approach. They ask patients to confess ways in which they have angered God, who may have retaliated by sending disease. Some also recognize invasion by evil spiritual entities, and offer exorcism as a treatment. Prayer is offered to alleviate pain and prevent sickness; some faith-based systems also practice the "laying on of hands."

"But she seems to be an intelligent woman," one family-practitioner kept repeating as he
(Continues)

told me of the woman who had refused the surgical removal of uterine fibroids. What he viewed as a completely medical (and secular) situation his patient took to be a tangible sign of divine displeasure . . . God would heal her if it would be his will; no scalpels necessary (Snow 1993).

Shamanic systems combine naturalistic and personalistic approaches. Natural events, such as experiencing a severe emotional or physical shock or fright, may cause parts of the soul to be lost. The shaman recognizes the situation from the symptomatology, and takes a spiritual journey to retrieve the soul parts. Again, a person with an insufficient degree of psychic protection may be psychically attacked by someone else, either purposefully, during an argument, or even by being looked at with envious eyes. The shaman's task is to heal the psychospiritual wound, and then help the patient to develop stronger personal protective skills. (Shamans also serve communities by mediating arguments, changing weather, and treating physical illness with herbs and psychospiritual support.)

Notice that the naturalistic/personalistic frame cuts across the materialist/nonmaterialist frame. Naturalistic explanations often deal with causes which are nonmaterial, like temperature changes or wind invasions. Similarly, personalistic explanations can be materialist; some people see, hear, or feel entities such as ghosts or spirits, and material objects can store nonmaterial energies and can be used to heal or harm. But most importantly, even when the system and practitioner prefer naturalistic explanations, patients regularly demand to know "why me, Lord?" and offer answers couched in the personalistic framework.

Concepts of the Practitioner-Patient Relationship

Systems that prefer external causative models characteristically view the body-person as passive, a victim, and, logically enough, interpret the practitioner as active, the one who cures. By contrast, systems that prefer internal causative models view the body-person as active, and as already capable of healing. The job of the practitioner is to facilitate the discovery of this capacity, and develop it. The patient in this model has life expertise, and the practitioner must use his or her specialized expertise in partnership with the patient.

Of course, some patients will be passive no matter what is asked of them, and equally, some always will demand a say in their care. The biomedical literature discusses, this issue under the rubrics of external and internal locus of control. However, the point made in this chapter is that not just practitioners, not just patients, but entire systems are modeled to emphasize one style of caregiving. Systems that want patients to be passive find active patients frustrating, irritating, and intrusive; systems that want patients to be active find passive patients unresponsive, helpless, and in denial.

A lucid practitioner might be able to match his or her style to the patient's needs, providing either authoritarian or relational (patient-centered) care to fit the situation. But practitioners, too, have preferences and personal styles that cannot be modified easily. Students might even select health care practices that fit their personal styles.

Making Sense of All the Variability

The chapter began with the claim that health care systems vary in many ways, and that the variety can be analyzed with the help of conceptual models. How can this information be applied in a world in which patients use many health care modalities, and in which practitioners are advised to understand and sympathize?

This section explores this question by discussing an example that compares biomedicine and Chinese medicine. We have developed a conceptual map that allows any system to be rapidly compared with another. We will end by summarizing what makes biomedicine unusual, yet convinced that it is normative.

A Comparison of Care in Two Medical Systems

As discussed, biomedicine prefers reductionistic, categorical explanatory models, while Chinese medicine prefers relational, process-related explanatory models (for more detail see Beinfield & Korngold 1991, Kaptchuk 1983, Lock & Gordon 1988, Stein 1990). Both are heterogeneous systems, so that relational tendencies can be found in biomedicine and categorical tendencies exist in Chinese medicine.

How different do these preferences really make these two systems?

Similarities of Biomedicine and Chinese Medicine

- Both aim to provide comprehensive health care, which includes health-enhancing, preventive, reproductive, acute and chronic illness, and trauma care.
- Both prefer to deliver care in specific locales such as clinics or hospitals, and in practitioner to patient dyads; group-based and home- or community-based practices are viewed as possible but nonmodal.
- Both prefer naturalistic explanations of malfunction, arguing that impersonal forces are the main sources of ill health. However, if sometimes reluctantly, both also recognize that personalistic explanations sometimes make sense.
- Both subsume a wide range of practices or specialties. While specialties within internal medicine represent the intensively reductionistic naturalistic components of biomedicine, psychiatry veers toward personalistic explanatory models, and immunotherapy, clinical ecology, and approaches emphasizing lifestyle intervention use a relational flavor. Again, while Five Element acupuncture aims to be primarily relational and holistic in outlook, the post-1949 traditional Chinese medicine style veers toward the reductionistic model and borrows many ideas from biomedicine.

Differences of Biomedicine and Chinese Medicine

- Both want to deliver comprehensive health care, but neither actually does it

(Continues)

(see Figure 2-2). Biomedicine focuses on trauma, acute illness, and end-stage chronic disease intervention. While prevention is discussed as part of biomedical care, wellness is a concept that may not always be stressed. Chinese medicine emphasizes wellness and preventive care, treats chronic and acute illness conditions, but pays little attention to trauma.

- Biomedicine emphasizes materialist explanations, while Chinese medicine emphasizes nonmaterialist explanation based on a distinctive concept of ch'i (qi, vital energy). Indeed, their views of anatomy and physiology, and their favored bodily metaphors (machinery and warring vs gardening) are distinctly different.
- Biomedicine emphasizes the physical body as the locus for intervention, recognizes but remains uncomfortable with the concept of the psychosocial body, and largely denies the existence of the energetic and spiritual bodies. By contrast, Chinese medicine uses the energetic body as the locus for intervention, and assumes that interventions at that level will redound upon all the other bodies.
- Biomedicine sees human beings as biologically similar; therefore, diseases will present similarly and can be treated similarly. Chinese medicine sees each human being as unique, assumes that even if symptoms appear to be similar, the deep cause might be dissimilar; and thus, care should be delivered individualistically
- Biomedicine has defined an immense universe of distinct disease entities, assumes they will present similarly in most people, focuses much energy on diagno-

(Continues)

sis, and defines success as cure. Controlling or palliating symptoms are considered lesser successes, and death is commonly thought of as a failure. Chinese medicine focuses on the flow of energy within the body and between the patient and the cosmos. Ill health arises when this flow is disrupted, impeded, or when there is insufficient energy. Since there are many ways in which this can happen, the practitioner spends much time assessing the character of the flow, both by hearing the patient's story and by listening in to the energetic body (for example, taking the pulses). Imbalance is viewed as commonplace and natural, and there is little to cure, instead, the practitioner hopes to maintain or improve the coherence of the body-person, that is, heal the person. Death is also deemed natural; the dying patient can use acupuncture to ease pain and to achieve a final energetic balance.

Conceptual Mapping of Health Care Systems

It is possible to map differences among health care systems to allow these similarities and differences to be rapidly grasped and applied. Figure 2-2 maps the systems in terms of individual needs; Figure 2-7 redraws Figure 2-2 in terms of the conceptual models explored in this chapter.

Figure 2-7 shows a matrix, with the categorical (reductionistic) vs relational (process-related) worldview represented on the horizontal axis, and the naturalistic to personalistic causal model on the vertical axis. A third axis (not shown) might appropriately deal with delivery issues, especially whether care is delivered to individuals or to communities.

Using this map, we can—hypothetically—locate virtually any system of health care in such a way as to rapidly compare it with another system. And knowing more about the terrain of systematic health care differences makes it easier to understand and use the insights from other systems of health care. Practitioners can use information to design research,

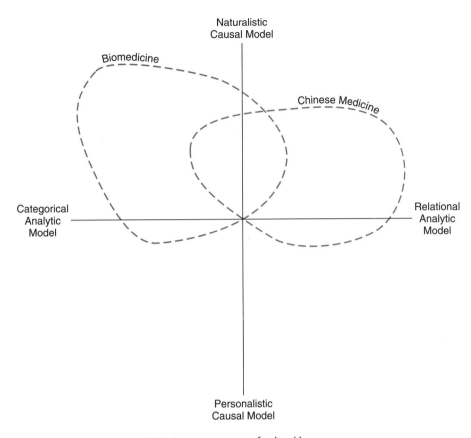

Figure 2-7. A cognitive map for health care systems.

to make themselves and their patients aware of their own prejudices, and to listen more openly to the users of different health care systems.

Figure 2-7 only maps the two systems cited in our example; readers are encouraged to map others as they learn about them in this text. Note that each of the two systems mapped, however, covers a wide area. Biomedicine, while clearly within the realm of categorical naturalistic thinking, spills over the horizontal line into personalistic models (psychology, psychiatry), and over the vertical line into relational territory (family practice, aspects of immunology, lifestyle arguments). In fact, biomedical practice overlaps the Chinese medicine outline at the center of the figure.

The map also shows that in terms of preferred worldview, Chinese medicine is opposite that of biomedicine. On the other hand, it is similar to biomedicine in its general preference for naturalistic causal explanations. These twin characteristics map it into the upper right quadrant. Note again, however, the wide range of practice under the umbrella of Chinese medicine. The more symptomatic and categorical styles of practice map left toward the reductionistic quadrant, and the traditional shamanistic components of Chinese medicine map below the horizontal line.

We are reminded by this map that no single health care system serves the whole field, and that systems differ but also share similarities.

Biomedicine's Findings of the Other Systems to Be Unconventional

Though not drawn onto the map, the other health care systems tend to cluster more centrally or to the right of the center, on both sides of the horizontal axis. Thus the mapping exercise also provides a visual clue as to why biomedicine, from its perch in the upper left quadrant, might find the other systems unconventional. They are non-modal when judged from biomedicine's position. Of course, biomedicine is equally unconventional when viewed from the positions of the majority of systems. From a worldwide viewpoint biomedicine is unusual in the following ways:

1. Its intense attachment to materialist interpretive models.
2. Its focus on the physical body, almost to the exclusion of other possibilities.
3. Its focus on the disease, often to the virtual exclusion of the person.
4. Its vast development of disease types.
5. Its highly technologic delivery system.
6. The invasiveness of its care modalities.
7. Its emphasis on acute disease, trauma, and end-stage malfunction, with relatively little focus on prevention or wellness.
8. Its high cost.

Despite these oddities, biomedicine considers itself conventional and other systems "alternative." How did this situation come about, and why is it not surprising to most people? Why is it hard for people to consider biomedicine as just one more alternative.

Health care is not free of culture or politics. In the United States, we are accustomed to thinking of biomedicine as the best because it is the most expansive, being practiced in every country in the world, though acupuncture and homeopathy run close seconds. It also has the largest educational, legal, and economic mandate. Finally, its explanatory model fits the dominant European and North American worldview paradigm—categorical or reductionistic—most closely.

As part of the expression of this worldview, many say biomedicine is the most scientific. This argument is a very slippery one and must be examined carefully.

Science is a particular method for gathering information and constructing knowledge. In contrast to other systems such as theology, which allows for revelation and law, which allows for precedence, science demands that information be sought in the natural world and that interpretations be tested for accuracy. This is extremely unusual; it means that a person's opinion or mere observation and consequent certitude are not enough to make his or her position acceptable to scientists. Instead, the person must show that he or she has gathered data systematically and accounted for potential biases, and then must submit his or her interpretations to others for examination and retesting. Furthermore, the researcher is enjoined to be a relativist; that is, not to fall in love with his or her interpretations, but to hold them always as models of reality, approximations. This provides remarkable training in humbleness, and to be frank, not very many achieve it.

Role of Science

Euroamerican society in particular has developed science to be the believable knowledge method, the knowledge orthodoxy of the late nineteenth and the twentieth centuries. The determination with which Westerners cling to their cultural preference concerning the power of science approaches a religious fervor. Biomedicine gradually took on the cloak of scientism with the rise of clinical medicine in the early nineteenth century, moving toward a laboratory-based experimental model by the late nineteenth century. Although the experiment is only one way to gather valid data using scientific method, this became accepted as the "scientific" approach; by the early twentieth century American biomedicine already contrasted itself to other systems by claiming to be experimental, hence uniquely scientific. Given that the other major systems are generally not experimental—they depend on well-developed clinical observation skills and experience guided by their explanatory models—it becomes clear why a system that perceives itself as scientific can consider nonscientific systems as inferior in our cultural milieu.

The biomedical model assumes diseases to be fully accounted for by deviations from the norm of measurable biologic (somatic) variables. It leaves no room within its framework for the social, psychological, and behavioral dimen-

(Continues)

sions of illness. . . . The biomedical model has thus become a cultural imperative, its limitations easily overlooked. In brief, it has now acquired the status of dogma. In science, a model is revised or abandoned when it fails to account adequately for all the data. A dogma, on the other hand, requires that discrepant data be forced to fit the model or be excluded (Engel 1977).

But is biomedicine really scientific, if judged from the perspective of science, rather than cultural preference? Recent studies suggest that only 30 percent of what biomedicine achieves has been tested adequately (Altman 1994, Andersen 1990). A full 70 percent of practice uses the same well-developed clinical observation skills and experience guided by explanatory model that powers the other health care systems.

Those who can stand back dispassionately—that is, those who really do think like scientists—understand that a great deal of the argument over which systems are modal or alternative is really an argument over cultural turf. As such, victory in this argument serves the usual political purpose of maintaining power by insisting upon the virtue of one's own values, often by attacking the perceptions of one's rivals; these are political, not scientific, acts.

The Importance of Viewing Health Care As a Matter of Cultural Modeling

That health care is a matter of cultural modeling rather than scientific truth matters to practitioners whose goals really are to relieve suffering. It also matters to those who wish to be scientific in their thoughts and choices. Differences must be dealt with. So, pragmatically, we end by asking: Who do the differences serve? How do the differences serve?

Users of Alternative Medicine

Demand for nonbiomedical health care in Europe and North America is at a peak that has not been met for about 150 years. Surveys of users of alternative medicine tell similar stories: people want to feel cared for, and biomedicine's emphasis on laboratory

medicine, factoring the person out of the diagnostic and treatment equation, invasive treatments including high levels of painful side effects,* rushed delivery of care, and immensely high cost, all connote an uncaring system, and are making biomedicine unattractive to increasing numbers of people.

Who are these people? Surveys indicate that the users of the major nonbiomedical systems are mainly urban, female, well-educated, with middle to high incomes, (Cassileth et al 1984, Eisenberg et al 1993, McGuire 1994). These people are in excellent positions to judge the quality of the care they receive from the variety of practitioners that they consult. This point matters because mainstream practitioners and researchers often attack nonbiomedical health care by saying that the users are being misled, either purposefully by the practitioners, or by their own desires, distress, and ignorance.

The defensive, politically-motivated arguments of biomedical practitioners are being increasingly weakened by three facts:

1. Studies show that where health care is obviously pluralistic, laypeople are astute at matching systems with complaints (Young 1981).
2. On the whole, patients report satisfaction with alternative health care (Emad 1994, Hare 1993, Workshop on Alternative Medicine 1994, O'Connor 1995).
3. Rapidly accumulating results of scientific research on alternative treatments show that they often are as effective or more effective than biomedical treatments of identical conditions, or that they provide valuable complementary effects when biomedicine is in use (Benor 1993, Byrd 1988, Jacobs 1994, Jobst 1995, Reilly 1994, Workshop on Alternative Medicine 1994, O'Connor 1995).

The Constituency for Alternative Medicine

Current biomedical discussion on the best use of nonbiomedical alternatives focuses either on annexing particular techniques (for example, jetti-

---

* Approximately 20 percent of illnesses that lead to hospitalization are iatrogenic, that is, caused by the biomedical care itself (Greenwood & Nunn 1994).

soning the systemic embedding of the treatments in explanatory models) or on using the alternatives adjunctively (for example, recommending acupuncture as adjunctive therapy to minimize the side effects of chemotherapy). Readers are now prepared to interpret these proposals as expressions of a biomedical perspective that claims its health care reality is superior to all others.

Of course, the situation looks a little different from the viewpoints of alternative practitioners as well as from the perspective of potential patients, many of whom are glad that modern health care provides a menu of alternatives to choose from.

Who would benefit if the U.S. national health care system was organized such that several alternatives were widely available and people learned about them from childhood?

Beneficiaries of Widely Available Alternative Health Care Systems in the United States

- Those who have a high need for affiliation, and who therefore want a relational style of health care.
- Those who wish to alleviate symptoms gently or with fewer side effects.
- Those who will not take hopeless for an answer.
- Those who would wish to prevent disease or enhance wellness.
- Those who interpret the body-person as having more than a physical aspect, and who want to be able to address the energetic, psychosocial, and spiritual bodies when receiving or delivering health care.
- Those who are concerned with the end-stage focus and invasiveness of typical biomedical care.

Note that this discussion assumes that there is space for all forms of health care. This should be true in a democratic society, and, it is true in the sense that all the systems already exist and serve people. The drive behind current research is to discover what services each system can provide, and to compare their effectiveness in providing these services. Interestingly, this drive will fail if it is expressed solely in terms of conditions or complaints, which is only half of the equation. The other half consists of the people who are to receive the care. There always will be a range of desires and needs; some patients will always prefer care that is technological and has rapid overt effects, while others always will prefer care that is relational, gentle, and virtually contemplative.

It is to be hoped that the worlds' people will become more skilled at utilizing all our health care resources and options, to make it possible for everyone—practitioners and people—to know enough about their options to successfully triage care in a manner that maximizes patient satisfaction and health, while minimizing suffering, iatrogenic disease, and cost.

It remains for you to consider your own goals for practice. Where do you fall on the various continua discussed in this chapter? Are you satisfied with the care that you deliver, or would you like to modify some rough spots? How can the alternative systems help you do so? How can they help your current or future patients?

Summary

This chapter introduces concepts that are fundamental to understanding values and issues in the practice of health care, and provides a sociocultural context and models that will be useful in understanding the practices described in subsequent chapters.

We began by stating that the form health care takes is fundamentally a matter of sociocultural interpretation. As we end it should be clear that health care systems differ in important ways and no one system provides all the answers, or even the best answers for all users or circumstances. Differences among systems are not random, but are driven and logically organized by underlying assumptive patterns that are revealed in explanatory models, therapeutic modalities, and styles of practice.

These differences are *not* unbridgeable; the concepts developed in this chapter should allow most practitioners and researchers to approach even strange ideas with new appreciation, as well as provide them with tools that allow for better communication and understanding. After all, the deepest and most common goal of all health care systems is to relieve pain and prevent suffering.

Acknowledgments

Special thanks to Haig Ignatius, MD, MAc, and Marc Micozzi, MD, PhD, for their generous reading of this chapter in its draft stages. Continuing thanks to many colleagues whose deep thinking about medical philosophical and practice issues guides and sustains my own explorations. Thanks too, to my husband and daughter whose love and support is most precious.

References

Altman D. 1994. The Scandal of Poor Medical Research. BMJ 308:283–284

Ames R. 1993. Sun-Tzu: The Art of Warfare. Ballantine Books. New York

Andersen B. 1990. Methodological Errors in Medical Research. Blackwell Scientific Publications, Oxford

Bates MS, Rankin-Hill L, Sanchez-Ayendez M, Mendez-Bryan R. 1995. A cross-cultural comparison of adaptation to chronic pain among Anglo-Americans and native Puerto Ricans. Med Anthropol 16(2):141–173

Beinfield H, Korngold E. 1991. Between Heaven and Earth, A Guide to Chinese Medicine. Ballantine Books, New York

Benor D. 1993. Healing Research: Holistic Energy Medicine and Spirituality. Helix Verlag GmbH, Munich

Black Elk W, Lyon WS. 1990. Black Elk, The Sacred Ways of a Lakota. Harper & Row, San Francisco

Brennan B. 1988. Hands of Light, A Guide to Healing Through the Human Energy Field. Bantam Books, Toronto

Byrd RC. 1988. Positive therapeutic effects of intercessory prayer in a coronary care unit population. South Med J 81:826–829

Cassidy CM. 1995. Social science theory and methods in the study of alternative and complementary medicine. J Altern Comple Med 1:19–40

Cassidy CM. 1994. Unraveling the ball of string: reality, paradigms, and the study of alternative medicine. Adv J Mind-Body Health 10:3–31

Cassidy CM. 1982. Protein-energy malnutrition as a culture-bound syndrome. Cult Med Psychiatry 6:325–345

Cassileth B, Lusk E, Strouse R, Bodenheimer B. 1984. Contemporary unorthodox treatments in cancer medicine, a study of patients, treatments and practitioners. Ann Intern Med 101:105–112

Eisenberg D, Kessler R, Foster C, Norlock F, Culkins D, Delbanco R. 1993. Unconventional medicine in the United States. N Engl J Med 328:246–252

Eliade M. 1964. Shamanism, Archaic Techniques of Ecstasy. Princeton University Press, Princeton, New Jersey

Emad M. 1994. 'Does acupuncture hurt?': Ethnographic evidence of shifts in psychobiological experiences of pain. Proc Soc Acupunct Res 2:129–140

Engel G. 1977. The need for a new medical model challenge for biomedicine. Science 196(4286):129–136

Fabrega H. 1974. Disease and Social Behavior: An Interdisciplinary Perspective. MIT Press, Cambridge, Massachusetts

Foster G, Anderson B. 1978. Medical Anthropology. John Wiley & Sons, New York

Furnham A. 1992. Why people choose complementary medicine, in Andritsky W (ed). Yearbook of Cross-cultural Medicine and Psychotherapy, pp. 165–198

Greenwood M, Nunn P. 1994. Paradox and Healing, Medicine, Mythology and Transformation, 3rd ed. Paradox Publ, Victoria British Columbia

Hand WD (ed.). 1976. American Folk Medicine: A Symposium. University of California Press, Berkeley, California

Hare M. 1993. The emergence of an urban U.S. Chinese medicine. Med Anthropol Q 7:30–49

Harwood A. 1971. The hot-cold theory of disease: implications for treatment of Puerto Rican patients. JAMA 216:1153–1158

Huber P. 1990. Presidential candidate's wife accused of bigamy. Old News 1:5, Marietta, Pennsylvania

Hultkrantz A. 1985. The shaman and the medicine man. Soc Sci Med 20:511–515

Ingerman S. 1991. Soul Retrieval, Mending the Fragmented Self. Harper Collins, San Francisco

Jacobs J, Jimenez LM, Gloyd SS, et al. 1994. Treatment of acute childhood diarrhea with homeopathic medicine: A randomized clinical trial in Nicaragua. Pediatrics 93(5):719–725

Jobst KA. 1995. A critical analysis of acupuncture in pulmonary disease: Efficacy and safety of the acupuncture needle. J Altern Comple Med 1:57–85

Kaplan A. 1984. Philosophy of science in anthropology. Annu Rev Anthropol 13:25–39

Kaptchuk T. 1983. The Web That Has No Weaver. Understanding Chinese Medicine. Congdon & Weed. New York

Kirkland J, Mathews HF, Sullivan III CW, Baldwin K,

(eds.) Herbal and Magical Medicine: Traditional Healing Today. 1992. Duke University Press, Durham, North Carolina

Kleinman A. 1980. Patients and Healers in the Context of Culture. University of California Press, Berkeley, California

Lock M, Gordon DR (eds). 1988. Biomedicine Examined. Kluwer Academic Publishers. Dordrecht

McGuire MB. 1994. Ritual Healing in Suburban America. Rutgers University Press, New Brunswick, New Jersey

Morgan W. 1977 (1931). Navajo treatment of sickness: diagnosticians, in Landy D (ed), Culture, Disease and Healing, Studies in Medical Anthropology. Macmillan Publ Co., New York, pp. 163–168

Murdock GP. 1980. Theories of Illness, A World Survey. University of Pittsburgh Press. Pittsburgh, Pennsylvania

O'Connor BB. 1995. Healing Traditions, Alternative Medicine and the Health Professions. University of Pennsylvania Press. Philadelphia

Payer L. 1988. Medicine and Culture, Varieties of Treatment in the United States, England, West Germany, and France. Penguin Books, New York

Porkert M. 1974. Theoretical Foundations of Chinese Medicine: Systems of Correspondence. The MIT Press, Cambridge, Massachusetts

Reilly D, Taylor MA, Bettie N, et al. 1994. Is evidence for homeopathy reproducible? Lancet 344(8937): 1601–1606

Reimansnyder BL. 1989 (1982). Powwowing in Union County, A Study of Pennsylvania German Folk Medicine in Context. AMS Press Inc., New York

Rubel A, O'Nell CW, Ardon RC. 1984. Susto: A Folk Illness. University of California Press, Berkeley, California

Scott AW. 1993. Masters of the Ordinary: Integrating Personal Experience and Vernacular Knowledge in Alcoholics Anonymous. Dissertation. Michigan Microfilms, Ann Arbor, Michigan

Sears W. 1991. Sick enough to stay home? Redbook, September

Sheldon WH, Hartl EM, McDermott E. 1949. Varieties of Delinquent Youth, An Introduction to Constitutional Psychiatry. Harper and Brothers, New York

Snow LF. 1993. Walkin' Over Medicine. Westview Press, Boulder, Colorado

Sobo EJ. 1993. One Blood, The Jamaican Body. State University of New York Press, Albany, New York

Spicer EH (ed). 1979. Ethnic Medicine in the Southwest. University of Arizona Press, Tucson, Arizona

Stein HF. 1990. American Medicine as Culture. Westview Press. Boulder, Colorado

Terrell SJ. 1990. This Other Kind of Doctors: Traditional Medical Systems in Black Neighborhoods in Austin TX. AMS Press Inc., New York

Vithoulkas G. 1980. The Science of Homeopathy. Grove Press, New York

Wirkus M. 1993. Mietek Wirkus: School of bioenergy, the healing art. Newsletter of the International Society for the Study of Subtle Energies and Energy Balance 4(2): 8–10

Workshop on Alternative Medicine (Chantilly VA) 1994. *Alternative Medicine: Expanding Medical Horizons, Report to the National Institutes of Health on Alternative Medical Systems and Practices in the United States.* NIH Publ 94-066, Government Printing Office, Washington DC

Young D, Ingram G, Swartz L. 1989. Cry of the Eagle, Encounters with a Cree Healer. University of Toronto Press, Toronto

Young JC. 1981. Medical Choice in a Mexican Village. Rutgers University Press, New Brunswick, New Jersey

3
Historical Context of the Concept of Vitalism in Complementary and Alternative Medicine

Ted J. Kaptchuk

Practitioners of most alternative healing believe that one source of their intervention is a kind of "vital energy" their system uses still not appreciated by conventional biomedical science. Subtle health-promoting influences pervade the alternative healing world. Health is accessible through gentle technologies that activate, evoke, or redirect universal beneficent healing influences. The universe is thought to provide an endless influx of forces that can help to "put things right." Health is harmony in the cosmic energy; illness is cured by reordering the protective forces. A person threatened by disorder and disease is guaranteed a response from fundamentally benign, lawful, coherent, potent, and even meaningful powers. One can almost speak of a faucet that pours out healing juice. Homeopathy connects with the "spiritual vital force" (Hahnemann 1980); chiropractic calls it "innate" or "universal intelligence" (Palmer 1910); psychic healing manipulates "auric," "psi," or psionic powers (Moore 1977, Reyner 1982); believers in New Thought are restored by correct "Mind" (Braden 1987); acupuncture utilizes "qi" (Eisenberg 1987);

Ayurvedic medicine and yoga teachers are in touch with "prana" (Lad 1984); and naturopaths invoke the "vis medicatrix naturae" (Turner 1990). Unseen powers are said to permeate the universe and have a profound effect on human beings undetectable by scientific instruments. This chapter delineates this concept of alternative medicine by tracing the historical development of the idea of vital energy. Individual alternative healing practices are described in terms of their fundamental propositions and the ontological status that they confer on the vital principle.

History: The Rise and Fall of the Mainstream Vitalist Principle

Vitalism is the proposition that more is needed to explain life than just physical or mechanical laws. It is less archaic than recent advocates or detractors of alternative medicines claim, and has its origins not within alternative health care systems themselves, but within the elite universities of eighteenth and nineteenth century Europe. This doctrine arose in the west as a response to the mechanistic thesis and atomistic physiochemical reductionism of the scientific revolution (Lain Entralgo 1948).

In order to understand the new science and the vitalist formulation, review of the previously dominant Aristotelian worldview is helpful. In the Aristotelian universe, unlike the new scientific world, there was no such thing as totally inert matter changing because of external forces. Aristotelian physical matter had inherent tendencies, intentionality, and teleological properties. Things happened in the material universe because of latent tendencies that unfolded: fire's goal was to ascend, earth's was to descend. The future exerted a compulsion on the present. The organic universe was the model for the inorganic universe; the acorn both embodied and obeyed its future potential as an oak tree. The material realm was a continuum of the organic realm, but at a reduced level of complexity.

In terms of human beings, this sense of continuation persists. Medieval biology could not conceive of an extreme dichotomy of soma (body) and psyche (mind), much less their separate existence (Gilson 1940, cf. Hartman 1977). This would have conflicted with theology (Kemp 1990). Psyche had no reality apart from soma. A human being's material body overlapped and interpenetrated and was given actuality and form by a subtle substratum of souls. Each soul organized the soma into a distinct hierarchy of function and awareness. Somehow, pneuma, a mediator of the same eternal essence as the celestial bodies, allowed for both an embodied and mindful integrity of psyche and soma (Hall 1975). Pneuma served as a common denominator of all phenomena and allowed all forms of being—from human to minerals—to maintain their cohesiveness and growth, and to transform into other forms of being.

These medieval notions were replaced by the new science. Rather than conceiving nature as an organic being that matured through self-development, seventeenth-century scientists viewed nature as a machine whose parts only moved in response to other parts. Volition, intentions, cognition, and mental states were relegated to peripheral or epiphenominal status in biology; some scientists even came to believe that all life could be explained in mechanical and physiochemical terms (Ledermann 1989).

For some doctors and scientists, explaining life as

an intricate system of levers, pulleys, or bubbling and fermenting microchemical flasks was inadequate. They criticized the new philosophy as excessively mechanical, material, and simple and argued that life was determined by more than the laws of the inanimate world. These physicians and biologists tried to animate the newly constituted passive matter of science with a vitalist hypothesis to explain the feeling and thought behind organic and human life (Roger 1986). The most important figure in this effort was the chemist-physician George Ernest Stahl (1659–1734), whose prominent university status at Halle was enhanced by his former position as physician to Fredrich Wilhelm I(Rather 1961). He proposed the *anima,* or "sensitive soul," to fill the perceived void in the new science. Anima was the agency that made life distinct from lifeless matter. Stahlian animism was undoubtedly influenced by the earlier 'archeus' of Paracelus (1493–1541) and van Hemont (1577–1644), two pre-Cartesian chemist-physician-mystics of the Nordic renaissance who were involved in an entirely different dialogue (Lain Entralgo 1948). Francois Boissier de Sauvages (1706–1767) introduced the anima into the teaching of Montpellier, one of Europe's oldest and most important medical schools, but he preferred using the word "soul" for this animating life-force. His student, Paul Joseph Barthez (1734–1806), whose credentials included having been Napoleon's physician, felt that both words were too occult and old-fashioned and, in 1778, introduced the phrase *principe vitale* or *vital principle* (Haigh 1975, Wheeler 1939). The vitalist hypothesis could not totally obliterate the newly created Cartesian chasm of an inert matter (res extensa) and a mind (res cognitans)—it conceded too much to the new physics. But the power relationship had been reversed; in life, primary agency was no longer physiochemical or mechanical, but rather a benevolent power with a self-directive healing power.

Unbound by the precise and quantifiable laws of physics and chemistry, the vitalism argument, by its very nature, quickly fractured into many interpretations. Some physicians took a phenomenal position and saw the vital principle to be a regulative principle (Lipman 1967). Others took a realist position and postulated that a constitutive part animated matter; this approach is much more important to alternative healing (Benton 1975). Realist theories took various forms: from various shades of incorporeal and spirit agency; to diverse mental powers; to different kinds of distinctive forces analogous and on the same plane of reality as conventional electromagnetism, but still not scientifically measurable (Larson 1979, Toulmin & Goodfield 1962).

In the nineteenth century, the mechanistic physical chemical view gained complete ascendancy in biology and medicine. From Wohler's synthesis of organic material in 1828, to Atwater and Rosa's demonstration in 1897 that the laws of thermodynamics apply to life as well as inorganic matter, there was a gradual elimination of any need to believe in a vital principle or life force to explain perceived inadequacies of physicochemical explanations (Needham 1955). Vitalism's main argument was the opponent's weakness; vitalism had to retreat before each new scientific discovery. This weakened vitalism migrated to the alternative medical worldview that was being created in the nineteenth century, where it was welcomed and eventually merged with other important forms of vitalism.

Mesmeric Vital Energy

At the time that vitalism was being developed in elite academia and just before it received an official name, the Viennese physician Anton Mesmer (1734–1815) uncovered what he believed to be the real vital energy. In 1775, Mesmer discovered that the source of a popular religious exorcist's powers was not divine intervention, but rather a vital force. The cures were due to "animal magnetism," a subtle fluid that pervades the universe and is analogous to gravitation (Ellenberger 1970). Mesmer declared that the scientific evidence of the new vital force is the healing influx; harmony with the cosmic fluid is health. All disease was due to an unequal distribution or blockage of this fluid; healing is the restoration of equilibrium and healers can manipulate this fluid to cure patients (Mesmer 1980). An influx of subtle fluids from the celestial bodies is the substantive basis of all life and health, and later even morality (Darton 1968).

Mesmer relocated to Paris and his popularity quickly generated controversy. In 1784, King Louis XIV, through the Royal French Academy of Science, appointed a prestigious investigatory commission including ambassador Benjamin Franklin, chemist

Antoine Lavoisier, and physician-inventor, J. I. Guillotin. Mesmer demanded clinical outcome comparisons. Instead, the blue ribbon panel wanted to investigate mechanism. In a series of some of medicine's earliest controlled, blinded trials, the panel discovered that healing occurred whenever subjects believed they were being mesmerized and no effect occurred if subjects were ignorant of magnetic passes. The commision sentenced mesmerism to the medical fringe, where it became a critical component of alternative medical thought (Fuller 1982).

Mesmer's followers quickly split into denominations. Mesmerists divided between those who understood the force as a physical agency and others who detected a more incorporeal power. A lower mesmeric interpretation made the force analogous to a physical electromagnetic vibration that resembled more recognized scientific energies. A higher mesmeric interpretation, that quickly fused with earlier mystical and occult traditions, saw the force as ethereal and reduced the physical agency to an epiphenomena of no consequence. In addition to healing, the force had abilities for clairvoyant medical diagnosis, telepathy, and became a scientific vehicle to contact spiritual forces or spiritual beings (Darton 1968). Between the poles of lower and higher mesmerism were various intermediate versions, each spawning a complex lineage; all shared the distinctive mesmeric view that life's agency and healing potential can be found in a vital energy or presence distinct from the ordinary mechanical forces. Mesmerism became the inspiration for many unconventional therapies.

Lower Mesmerism and Psychic Healing

Tracing the history of mesmerism can be difficult because many of Mesmer's descendants often changed their names, like other new arrivals on Ellis Island, to avoid the stigma associated with the term mesmerism since its excommunication from official science. New designations could be helpful, however. If an earlier vital energy was discredited, new forces could be discovered to take its place. For example, Robert Hare (1781–1858), a chemist at the University of Pennsylvania and the inventor of the oxyhydrogen blowpipe, was an early convert to mesmerism. In 1856, he developed a spirit-scope to measure mesmeric and spiritual presences, and also coined the scientific-sounding term *psychic force* in

1856 (Moore 1977, McClenon 1984). In 1935, Joseph Bank Rhine (1885–1980), who spent most of his career at Duke University trying to shift psychical research from the seance room to the laboratory, adopted the more respectable "parapsychology" from German (McVaught and Mauskupf 1976, Moore 1977). In 1947, Robert Thouless (1894–1984), a British psychologist and parapsychologist at Cambridge, thought psi phenomena or psionic energy was a noncommittal label for paranormal energetics (Moore 1977). Historically, theosophists preferred the word *auric* or *astral* force (Campbell 1980, Coddington 1990), while modern researchers have recently chosen the phrase *subtle energy.* These name substitutions indicate the lower mesmeric concern for keeping vital energy on a par with other more physically established forces as the primary agency for life.

Lower mesmeric forms of healing energy are easily recognized in the contemporary alternative therapies that speak of an electromagnetic dimension which can become depleted or unbalanced . . . [causing] the blockage of energy flow, requiring physical or spiritual cleaning in order for healing to occur (Glick 1988). Alternative therapies—such as therapeutic touch (Krieger et al 1979), laying on of hand (Vlamis 1978), polarity (Vlamis 1978), paranormal healing (Rose 1954), and the countless individual psychic, auric, and psionic healers—while often unaware of their heritage, all bear the characteristic mesmeric style of manipulating unseen and refined forces that evade biomedical detection. The proof of the force is healing, and secondary evidence can be sensations of heat, tingling, or vibratory motions (Fuller 1989). Curiously, despite the suspicions—and even hostility—of colleagues, some conventional researchers hover on the edge of this type of healing and continue to scientifically investigate the phenomenon (Beutler et al 1988, Benor 1990).

Higher Mesmerism and Channelling

The trance states of higher mesmeric traditions were used to contact noncorporeal realities. Healing dispensations, medical diagnosis, or medical advice were a common product of "tuning-in," as was clairvoyance, spirit sightings, levitations, ectoplasmic emissions, table turning, spirit tapping, and spirit photographs. This higher trance phenomena quickly merged with earlier occult and theurgic movements (such as neo-Platonism, Renaissance occult and kabbla, pre-Christian religions, theurgic traditions, and Swedenborgianism [Galbreath 1971]), creating a mass phenomenon in the nineteenth century (Oppenheim 1988, Braude 1989). This spiritualist movement was later reincarnated in various theosophical and occult movements in today's New Age scene (Melton 1988, Beckford 1984). Such contemporary phenomena as "experiencing the healing powers of interplanetary Brotherhoods and curing their medical ailments by soul travel to different planes of reality" (Levin & Coreil 1988) are all direct descendants of higher mesmerism. Alternative healing methods and associations such as Spiritual Frontiers Fellowship Edgar Cayce's Association for Research and Enlightenment (Carter 1972), Great White Brotherhood and modalities such as past lives therapy (Netherton & Shiffrin 1978) are involved with a panoply of spiritual beings that are detectable by mesmeric trances, currently spoken of as altered states of consciousness, channeling, higher states of awareness, or transmissions from spiritually evolved beings. These are rarely organized as healing professions and routinely exceed the limits of healing practices, becoming instead alternative or emergent religions.

Electric Devices and Crystals

Electrical devices and crystals that emit or harmonize energies for healing are important first cousins of mesmerism. Luigi Galvani's (1737–1798) experiments, which caused the severed legs of frogs to jump as if alive, coincided with Mesmer's own research. This discovery of animal electricity, or electrical body fluid, was considered to be analogous or identical with animal magnetism and all mysterious vital forces (Sutton 1981). Electrical machines and gadgets with healing properties were ubiquitous in the nineteenth century (Marvin 1988) and continued into the twentieth century. Contemporary radionic machines, magnetic beds, transcranial electrostimulators, neuromagnetic vibrators, and electromagnetic chairs all bear the imprint of their preceding mesmeric electrical cousins (Schaller & Caroll 1976, Easthope 1986). Important scientific research has been generated by scientists interested in low-frequency electromagnetic devices despite the stigma of an association with charlatanism (Macklin 1993).

Crystal healing, a form of lithotherapeutics, has ancient roots distinct from mesmerism (Forbes 1972). In the last two hundred years, however, it has repositioned itself to become part of the vital energy family. In the 1840s and 1850s, Baron Charles von Reichenbach [1788–1869], the discoverer of kerosene, also managed to detect a refined and definitive mesmeric energy in crystals. He gave it the scientifically oriented name of *odic force*. Modern crystal healers continue this merged tradition and speak of crystals as "able to tap the energies of the universe," and be an especially potent "focus of healing energy" (Fuller 1989).

Mind Cure

Mind cure, or the healing systems that consider thoughts or deep feeling to be the primary arbitrator of health, are an important offshoot of mesmerism. The discovery of the mind as the ultimate unseen force of healing is related directly to Phineas P. Quimby (1802–1866). Quimby first worked as a magnetizer or magnetic healer (reconstituted names for a mesmerist) in Portland, Maine. He decided that healing was not so much animal magnetism or an esoteric energy, but rather, results from changes in the mind. The force was not a physical force, but a mental state. Mesmer's fluid was really Mind, and everything was controlled by Mind, with a capital M. Disease is what follows the disturbance of the mind or spiritual matter (Dresser 1969).

Quimby began the New Thought movement that believes disease is wrong thinking. Change the thought and you have health (Judah 1967). Divine Mind, Divine Truth, and Love are primary agency, not the physical world. Physical reality is clay in the hands of the Mind. New Thought and positive thinking all derive from Mind Cure, as do such metaphysical groups as Unity Church of Christianity, United Church of Religious Science, and International Divine Science (Braden 1963). New and more contemporary forms of this approach to healing are constantly being offered. For example, "A Course on Miracles" (Perry 1987), "prosperity consciousness" (Cole-Whittaker 1983, Chopra 1993), and Living Love (Cornucopia) (Keyes 1989), are all based on the same premise. And beyond any organization, this notion of "what you think is what is real" infuses important sectors of the modern alternative health community, resonating through history in uncanny ways. For example, the words Quimby wrote in 1859 could easily have been taken from Bernie Siegal's best-selling alternative healing book *Love, Medicine and Miracles* (Siegel 1986): love is the true answer to our desire . . . it contains nothing but true knowledge and love, no sorrow, nor pain, nor grief, nor shame nor fear (Dresser 1969). Love or True Mind heals all.

Mind Cure often advocated "entering the silence" to make Mind impressions, self-love or autosuggestion imprint more effectively (Fuller 1982, Meyers 1965). Almost a hundred years ago, William James (1842–1910) described a phenomena that still is current when he said that the mind-cure principles are beginning so to pervade . . . . One hears of the "Gospel of Relaxation" of the "Don't Worry Movement" or people who repeat to themselves "Youth, health, vigor" (James 1961). Mind Cure's meditation, relaxation, and breathing techniques (which partially derive from somnambulistic or mesmeric trance states [cf. Davis 1885]) were some of the indigenous western practices that prepared the way for Asian style meditations that are so influential in the alternative health movement (see below).

Christian Science

Quimby's most famous legacy to unconventional healing is through his student and patient who later became known under the name Mary Baker Eddy (1821–1919). She went on to establish Christian Science, radically declaring that all disease, pain, misfortune, and evil are illusion. Knowing Divine Truth and Divine Science allow perception of the underlying perfection. Divine Mind is the only reality. Rigid, doctrinaire, exclusive, and sectarian, Mrs. Eddy denied any relationship with Mind Cure, mesmerism, or alternative healing, but her venomous denunciations of Quimby and malicious animal magnetism revealed her origins only too clearly, and assured Christian Science a place in the history of vital energy (Schoepflin 1988, Fox 1984, Feldman 1963).

Chiropractic, Osteopathy and Massage

Mesmeric vital energy took a very somatic and even mechanical twist in the creation of chiropractic, the largest contemporary alternative health care profession in North America, licensed in 50 states (Wardwell 1992). Discovered in 1895 by D. D. Palmer (1845–1913), chiropractic's origin is a unique marriage of the indigenous healing craft of bonesetting (Cooter 1987, Schiotz & Cyriax 1975) and the American tradition of mesmeric healing (Beck 1982). For 10 years before his discovery of chiropractic, Palmer worked as a magnetic healer. Like Quimby, he occasionally employed hand passes and magnetic rubbings of the spine (Fuller 1982). In an intuitive flash, (or, some say, clairvoyant communication [Beck 1982]), he realized that "putting down your hands" worked better than an esoteric "laying on of hands." Mechanical adjustment was more precise than magnetic activity administered from a distance. Yet, even 20 years after abandoning his magnetic clinical work, Palmer's mesmeric heritage are readily evident in his writings: Disease is a manifestation of too much or not enough energy. Energy is liberated force; in the living being it is known as vital force . . . It is an intelligent force, which I saw fit to name Innate, usually known as spirit (Beck 1991).

Disease is disruption in what Palmer calls *innate intelligence.* The nervous system is the conduit for this force. By aligning the spine, one frees the nerves so that this force can move without interference and produce healing. The vital energy is guided and shaped by the structure of the body. The noncorporeal agency of life is housed in the nerves and guarded by the spinal vertebra. Chiropractic and spinal manipulation, despite its alternative associations, recently has generated considerable interest from researchers, both in terms of basic science (Goldstein 1975), controlled clinical trials (Shekelle et al 1992, Anderson et al 1992), and comparative health care outcome trials (Meade et al 1990). Official government reports, such as the Manga Report in Canada (Manga et al 1993) and a recommendation from the Agency for Health Care Policy and Research (Bigos et al 1994), of chiropractic for acute low back pain, have blurred the demarcation between alternative and mainstream medicine and encouraged wider acceptance of chiropractic.

Osteopathy, chiropractic's older cousin, was developed by Andrew Still (1828–1917), who was also a magnetic healer for many years. In 1874, he discovered that misaligned bones impeded the flow of fluids and blood, and he developed the system of osteopathy. In addition to having episodes of clairvoyance and channelling, Still also had connections to metaphysical, Mind Cure, and spiritualist groups (Gevitz 1988, Terrett 1991). Obviously, osteopathy has taken a different trajectory from chiropractic. By breeding out its mesmeric influence, it has become practically indistinguishable from mainstream medicine (Baer 1987, Gevitz 1982).

Massage is one of the earliest and most pervasive forms of healing (Sigerist 1961). Yet in the last hundred years, many unconventional massage therapies have increasingly found their rationale in vital energy theory. Many styles of massage therapies exist (Knapp & Antonucci 1990) with different theories and therapeutic goals including rolfing (Rolf 1977), reflexology (Carter 1969), Aston-Patterning (Low 1988), Hellerwork, and shiatsu (Namikoshi 1969). The multiplicity of forms, the fact that anyone can give a massage, and constant introduction of new methods has hampered the regulation, licensing, and professional development that is analogous to chiropractic. Nonetheless, "bodywork" provides an extensive and important network of much energy work (Good & Good 1981).

Homeopathy

While mesmerism dominated the vital energy tradition, the mainstream vitalist hypothesis also continued to survive and remained operational in the alternative medical world. Often this survival was made possible by an explicit or implicit strategic union with mesmerism. Homeopathy is the most important system of medicine to derive from this tradition.

For a considerable period of time during the last century, homeopathy was the most serious challenge to conventional medicine (Rothstein 1985), and currently is enjoying a serious revival (Kaufman 1988). Discovered by Samuel Hahnemann (1755–1843), homeopathy espouses the belief that whatever symptom-complex a substance can cause in a healthy person, infinitesimally small amounts of the same substance can cure diseases with the same symptom configuration. The small dosage has the capacity to evoke the spiritual, self-acting (automatic) vital force, everywhere present in his organism. (Hahnemann 1980) *Sililia similibus curentur*—like cures like. The tiny dosage enhances the spiritual essence of the bodily response to disease. The alchemical homeopathic remedy was to rescue the insufficient self-help mechanisms of the physical body, and supply a corrective to nature (Neuburger 1933). Hahnemann's idea of vital energy derived from early German romantic sources (via Paracelsus and van Helmont) and the later academic tradition of G. E. Stahl (Coulter 1977). Yet, even from its inception, an alliance with mesmerism was discernible. Hahnemann, himself, described mesmeric healing as a marvelous, priceless gift of God to mankind (Hahnemann 1980). Today, it is virtually impossible to distinguish homeopathy's vital force from other conceptions rooted in mesmerism. Despite its alternative status, however, homeopathy has generated considerable conventional biomedical research and debate (Kliejnen et al 1991a, Hill & Doyon 1990, Linde 1994).

Herbalism and the 'vis matecatrix naturae'

Another energy in alternative medicine is the healing force of nature, which has a long history independent of mesmerism or the vitalist hypothesis (Neuburger 1933). In 1772, William Cullen (1710–1790), a professor of the University of Edinburgh—himself no friend of this approach in medicine, proposed the term *vis matecatrix naturae* to describe this power (Neuburger 1933). Again, like the academic vitalist hypothesis, the natural force became more important in the alternative world, and eventually was indistinguishable from the whole concept of vital energy.

The rise of the market economy and industrialization allowed for nostalgia and a romantic view of nature, which made possible the natural healing movements that date from the early nineteenth century. Alternative healing movements "irregulars" launched crusades to overthrow the orthodox medicine "regulars," who used "contaminated unnatural poisonous" drugs and bleeding (Warner 1987). The

earliest American natural healing movement was Thomsonian herbalism. While the history of herbal medicaments lies deep in antiquity (Wheelwright 1974), but Samuel Thomson (1769–1843), a native of New Hampshire, initiated the first herbal social reform movement in the 1820s and 1830s. Borrowing from indigenous colonial and Indian treatments, Thomsonians substituted herbal purges and soperifics for mainstream minerals, chemicals, and bloodletting. This movement developed into the profession of eclectic medicine, which mounted a challenge to conventional medicine with a systematic herbal approach, its own medical schools (Berman 1951), and eventually, a strong following in Europe (Griggs 1981). Somewhere in this history, herbalism formed an alliance with mesmerism. The two languages fused. Herbalists insisted that treatment must be in harmony with nature and the vital force, and must assist the vital force instead of destroying it (Brown 1985). The last eclectic medical school closed in Ohio in 1939 (Rothstein 1988), and herbalism as a professional system of healing had practically disappeared in the United States, although it survived in Great Britain (Sharma 1992). In the United States, vestiges of the herbal movement remain in popular self-help manuals and the concept of medicinal herbs remains an important symbol for alternative medicine. Some scientific research continues into popular herbal remedies (Johnson et al 1985, Melchart et al 1994, Ernst 1995), but most of the conventional biomedical discussion is in terms of potential adverse effects (Huxtable 1992).

Hydropathy and Naturopathy

Water cure or hydropathy is another healing movement that relied on a natural force. Like herbalism, hydrotherapy has early roots but only became a health reform movement in the nineteenth century (Donegan 1986). It has practically disappeared, except for spas and in physical therapy. Nevertheless, its legacy has important ramifications for contemporary alternative healing.

Originally hydropathy was imported to the United States from Germany in the 1840s as the Priessnitz method, and later reimported in the 1890s as the Kneipp method. In these systems, water was the pure force of healing. Often combined with massage, exercise, and health food, water could purify the body of "morbid matter" (toxins), stimulate nervous energy, and promote natural healing (Cayleff 1988). Quickly, the water cure movement became a catchall for other methods and by 1850, associated with dietary regimens, dress reform, home doctor, and, finally, with all natural methods including herbs, mesmeric energies, electropathy, and manipulation. This natural healing movement took on many forms and names, such as drugless healing, sanipractic, vita-o-pathy, sagliftopathy, panpathy, and physculopathy (Whorton 1986, Fishbein 1932), but the most enduring one is the name associated with Benedict Lust (1872–1945), a water cure therapist who trained under the Bavarian hydropath Father Kneipp.

In 1895, Lust purchased the term *naturopathy* to describe his eclectic water cure system and the term was used publicly for the first time in 1902, in association with Lust's New York-based American School of Naturopathy (Baer 1992, Cody 1985). His naturopathy was a nature cure system, defined as "the art of natural healing and the science of physical and mental regeneration on the basis of self-reform, natural life, clean and normal diet, hydropathy (Priessnitz, Kneipp, Lehmann, and Just systems), osteopathy, chiropractic, naturopathy [sic], electrotherapy, sun and air cult, diet, physiotherapy, physical and mental culture to the exclusion of poisonous drugs and non-adjustable surgery" (Fishbein 1932). Naturopathy, whose eclecticism resembles the current holistic movement, once was common practice in many states during the 1920s and 1930s under the name "drugless practitioner" (Whorton 1986, Gort & Coburn 1988), but now functions legally only in eight states, the stronghold being the Pacific Northwest (Baer 1992). Legal constraint prevents its widespread adoption as a unifying ideology for all natural therapies. Nevertheless, naturopathy is a potent concept in the alternative health movement and sometimes is used as a synonym for alternative health.

Acupuncture and Asian Medical Systems

The vital energy of alternative medicine received a dramatic infusion of credibility and possibility with the introduction of acupuncture and other Asian medicines into the United States in the 1960s, following several unsuccessful introductions (Haller 1973).

The Chinese notion of "qi" (as well as the Indian and Tibetan equivalents) obviously developed before any western Cartesian detachment of mind from matter. Qi was not so much an entity added to lifeless matter, but the state of being—either animate or inanimate (Sivin 1987, Kuriyama 1986, Chiu 1986). It was more akin to pneuma than any other western idea (Needham 1956). Asian medical systems, similar to archaic western systems, relied on heirachies and gradations of organizations to explain differences between organic and inorganic forms of being (Yoke 1985). Qi was characteristic of rocks, plants, and even human rationality. It was the common thread that allowed for "ladders of the soul" that extended from minerals to human life (Yoke 1985).

The qi of acupuncture or the prana of India have been swept in the undertow of western vitalistic ideas. Contemporary western literature generally translates qi as vital energy. Ancient Chinese notions, which defy severing of mind-body, have been discarded from modern Asian medical dialogue (both in Asia and the west) in favor of vital energy. Nonphysician acupuncturists have gained licensing, registration, or certification in 27 states plus the District of Columbia between 1977 and 1993 (McGae 1982, Lytle 1993). Though still small, acupuncture is one of the most rapidly growing health care professions and its success provides an important ideologic boost to alternative health care. The excitement of acupuncture has generated basic scientific investigations (Pomeranz & Stux, 1988), and over 200 controlled clinical biomedical research studies (Riet et al 1990, Kleijnen et al 1991b, Eisenberg 1995).

The Eastern opening also brought new massage (shiatsu, anmo, tui na, acupressure, jin shin jyutsu), new esoteric psychic energies (reiki johrei, qi gong), and countless new forms of meditation to supplement and supplant indigenous American forms. Again, they usually are formulated in nineteenth century vitalist terms (Muira 1989).

Psychological Interventions

Of all the mesmeric forces, the most complex, prolific, and hidden ones lie concealed in psychology, which deals with mind (with a small m). Significant aspects of clinical psychology's origins are connected with attempts to legitimize, mainstream, or find the real source of mesmerism and vital energy. In 1843, James Braid (1795–1860), an English physician, sought to clean up mesmerism's tainted reputation by postulating that its effects were due to a mental force, not a mysterious fluid. He changed its name to hypnosis, after the Greek god for sleep (Kaplan 1974). Hypnosis became a major concern in psychology—depending on perspective, even a legitimate mesmerism—and retains its importance in some areas of conventional medicine (Hall & Crasilneck 1978). Hypnosis was taken seriously by such figures as Jean Martin Charcot (1825–1893) and Hippolyte Bernheim (1840–1919), and is a crucial ingredient of Sigmund Freud's (1856–1939) early development of psychodynamic psychiatry (Ellenberger 1970). Hypnosis became less critical after Freud, becoming simply a porthole to the unconscious. Vital energy transforms into various forms of dynamic tensions that are thought to have potent psychological and physiological consequences. A clinical research agenda has also become a companion for psychotherapies (Strupp & Howard 1992).

Hypnosis and such forms of passive volitional intention as autogenic training and guided imagery also later interact with the academic behavioral psychology developed by I. P. Pavlov (1849–1936), J. B. Watson's (1878–1958) rigorous investigations of classic conditioning, and E. L. Thorndike's (1874–1949) work in operant conditioning (Thorndike 1931). This cross-fertilization of disciplines and ideas eventually contributed to the formation of such modern cognitive behavioral mind-body interventions as biofeedback (Basmajian 1981), modern autogenic training (Linden 1990), visualization and guided imagery (Sheikh 1983), the relaxation response (Benson 1975), and the reexamination of older self-control practices such as meditation (West 1991). These cognitive behavioral interventions, along with the psychosomatic movement, began as academic pursuits, but have become valuable intellectual and clinical resources for alternative medicine. The vital force now can be conceptualized in psychosomatic terms or in the current mind-body framework. These mind-body techniques shift between conventional and nonconventional. They are less on the fringe, almost accepted, and often wholly accepted aspects of vitalist ideology. They are the lowest, most scientific aspects of the mesmeric legacy, a kind of legitimate mesmerism. Because of their university connections, these mind-body interventions have generated much research (Eisenberg et al 1993, Turner & Chapman 1982, Holroyd & Penzien 1990). The vital energy has gone psychological. This has lent significant credibility to alternative medicine. Psychology has been a rich source of new interventions and theory for both conventional and alternative medicine. Occasionally, these efforts have been used to support more outlandish alternative healing ideas, to the discomfort of more scientifically inclined researchers. In any case, the mesmeric force has become a hyphenated mind-body connection between the invisible mind (small m) and the visible body. In the last 50 years, there probably have been more new psychological interventions and names developed—between 250 (Herink 1980) and 400 (Karasu 1986) types, depending who counts and when—than in the entire history of mesmeric forces.

Holistic Medicine

Vital energy and vitalism regrouped and reorganized itself during its post 1960s renaissance. Holism or holistic medicine has become the new family name, coined in order to avoid the tarnished image of older discredited medical ideas. The term originates within conventional medical debates of the early twentieth century over vitalism and reductionism.

Reductionism has been the corollary of the ascendancy of a physiochemical mechanistic viewpoint. The trajectory of reductionism is roughly described by Morgagni's (1761) situation of life-activity and pathology in organs, followed by Bichat's (1800) focus on tissue, leading to Broussais's (1830s) attention to lesions in tissues, to Virchow's (1848) localization in cells, to Koch's (1882) germ theory, all the way to modern dissection of genes. Obviously, this process is complex and not linear (cf. Mendelsohn 1965). Emphasis on a mechanical physiochemical agency leads to progressively smaller analytic pieces. Yet again, within academic medicine, there have been important antidotes to reductionism; organismic tendencies try to counterbalance or prevail over excessive reductionism. Antireductionist tendencies within conventional medicine emphasized homeostasis, predisposition, susceptibility, and psychosocial factors as opposed to those tendencies that emphasized an idea of disease that Tauber calls ontologic autonomous well-circumscribed states (Tauber 1994). A few of the many names associated with non-reductionism within biomedicine include Claude Bernard, Walter Cannon, L. J. Henderson, George Draper, Charles Sherrington, Hans Seyle, Helen Dunbar, George Engels, and Arthur Kleinman (Tracy 1992).

One anti-reductionist position developed in the philosophy of biology was by J. C. Smuts, the Cambridge-educated, South African statesman who, in 1926, coined the word holism (Smuts 1926). Holism was meant to be both antivitalist and antimechanistic, and argued that the entirety of an organism necessarily implied a teleologic purpose that could not be exhaustively explained by the laws governing component parts. The idea and word was appropriated by a few conventional scientists (Needham 1955) and was later used positively by conventional medicine to imply humanistic, psychosocial, or systemic approaches in health care. For example, a December 18, 1948 editorial in the *Journal of the American Medical Association* speaks of the holistic concept as being "an integrated approach to the sick person as a being in a state of mental, moral, and physiological imbalance with his environment" (Editorial 1948). In the 1970s, holistic partially changed its association. A 1979 *New England Journal of Medicine* editorial criticized holistic medicine saying: "patients must be dealt with as whole people. But this worthwhile philosophy is ill served by those who seek quick solutions to all the ills of mankind through the abandonment of science and rationality in favor of mystic cults" (Relman 1979). The word holism is adopted by many unconventional health practitioners, most of whom are seemingly unaware of Smuts or his philosophy (Whorton 1989), causing confusion; holism has become an amorphous label often glibly used or made trivial (Kopelman & Moskop 1981) for any perspective that sees biomedicine as too reductionist and/or materialist. It also has become a generic name for any therapy that does not consider its clinical perspective to be reductionist. And finally, it has become the new family name for any intervention—no matter how reductionist, such as chiropractic or crystals—that is informed, knowingly or unknowingly, by some form of a nineteenth century vitalist perspective. Very recently the word complementary has been introduced often replacing the word holistic, first in the United Kingdom in the 1980s and then in the United States in the 1990s.

Vitalism's Attraction

Vitalism can be attractive. Life is more than chemicals and mechanism. Agency is more than chemistry and physics. Mind, ideas, volition, intentions, spiritual entities, beliefs, innate intelligence, feelings, and mysterious vital forces can all become critical phenomena. The multivalent possibilities of vital energy—its lower, higher, natural, psychological, or supernatural forms—allow practitioners and patients to customize explanations and treatment options. Its very imprecision allows for enormous flexibility and adaptability.

In conventional medicine, it is sometimes too easy for a person to become an irrelevant spectator, overwhelmed by a mechanical world of technology, tests, and surgery. The vitalist perspective, on the other hand, aligns itself with coherent, life-affirming principles. The vitalist universe is not random, detached, or mindless; it is benign, coherent, and extremely hospitable for people. Instead of a medicine whose central issues can seem coldly mechanical and buried in unaccessible physiology, vitalism instinctively invites a person to experience a unifying, transcendent, and reassuring ontological presence. Whatever the outcome of the recent scientific investigations of vitalist medical traditions, vitalism's attractiveness for practitioners and patients is likely to remain a growing presence in health care.

REFERENCES

Anderson R, Meeker WC, Wirick BE, et al. 1992. A meta-analysis of clinical trials of spinal manipulation. J Manipulative Physiol Ther 15

Baer HA. 1987. Divergence and convergence in two systems of manual medicine: osteopathy and chiropractic in the United States. Med Anthro Q 1:2176–193

Baer HA. 1992. The potential rejuvenation of American naturopathy as a consequence of the holistic health movement. Med Anthropol 13:369–383

Basmajian JV, ed. 1981. Biofeedback Principles and Practice for Clinicians. Institute for Psychosomatic Research, New York

Beck BL. 1991. Magnetic healing, spiritualism and chiropractic: Palmer's union of methodologies, 1886–1895. Chiro Hist 11:2, 11–16

Beckford JA. 1984. Holistic imagery and ethics in new religious and healing movements. Social Compass 21 (2-3):259–272

Benor DJ. 1990. Survey of spiritual healing research. Comp Med Res 4:3, 9–33

Benson H. 1975. The Relaxation Response. Morrow, New York

Benton E. 1975. Vitalism in nineteenth-century scientific thought: a typology and reassessment. Stud Hist Phil Sci 5:1

Berman A. 1951. The Thomsonian movement and its relation to American pharmacy and medicine. Bull Hist Med 25:5

Beutler JJ, Attenvelt JT, Schooten SA, et al. 1988. Paranormal healing and hypertension. BMJ 296:1491–1494

Bigos SJ, Bowyer OR, Braen GR, et al. 1994. Clinical Practice Guideline #14. Acute Low Back Problems in Adults. US Department of Health and Human Services, PHS Agency for Health Care Policy and Research. Rockville, Maryland

Braden CS. 1987. Spirits in Rebellion: The Rise and Development of New Thought. Southern Methodist University Press, Dallas

Braude A. 1989. Radical Spirits. Beacon Press, Boston

Brown PS. 1985. The vicissitudes of herbalism in late nineteenth- and early twentieth-century Britain. Med Hist 29:71–92

Campbell BF. 1980. Ancient Wisdom Revived: A History of the Theosophical Movement. University of California Press, Berkeley, California

Carlson CJ. 1979. Holism and reductionism as perspectives in medicine and patient care. West J Med 131:6 466–470

Carter M. 1969. Helping Yourself With Reflexology. Parker, West Nyack, New York

Carter ME. 1972. My Years with Edgar Cayce. Harper & Row, New York

Cayleff SE. 1988. Gender, ideology and the water-cure movement, in Other Healers: Unorthodox Medicine in America. The Johns Hopkins University Press, Baltimore

Chiu ML. 1986. Mind, Body and Illness in Chinese Medical Tradition. Unpublished Ph.D. thesis. Harvard University

Coddington M. 1990. Seekers of the Healing Energy. Healing Arts Press. Rochester, Vermont

Cody G. 1985. History of naturopathic medicine. in Pizzorno JE, Murray MJ, (eds). A Textbook of Natural Medicine. John Bastyr College Publications Seattle

Cole-Whittaker T. 1983. How to Have More in a Have-Not World. Fawcett Crest, New York

Cooter R. 1987. Bopnes of contention? Orthodox medicine and the mystery of the bone-setter's craft in Bynum WF, Porter R (eds). Medical Fringe & Medical Orthodoxy 1750–1850. Croom Helm, London: pp. 158–173

Copra D. 1993. Creating Affluence. New World Press, New York

Coulter HL. 1977. Divided Legacy: A History of the Schism in Medical Thought, Vol II, Wehawaken Books, Washington, D.C.

Darton R. 1968. Mesmerism and the End of the Enlightenment in France. Harvard University Press, Cambridge, Massachusetts

Davis AJ. 1885. The Harbinger of Health. Colby and Rich, Banner Publishing, Boston

Donegan JB. 1986. Hydropathic Highway to Health. Greenwood Press, Westport, Connecticut

Dresser HW (ed). 1969. The Quimby Manuscripts. Citadel Press. Secaucus, New Jersey

Easthope G. 1986. Healers and Alternative Medicine. Gover, Aldershot, England

Editorial. 1948. Holistic Medicine. JAMA. December 18, 1948

Eisenberg D. 1985. Encounters with Qi: Exploring Chinese Medicine. W.W. Norton, New York

Eisenberg D. 1995. Traditional Chinese Medicine. In Alternative Medicine: Implications for Clinical Practice. Harvard Medical School, Department of Continuing Education. Boston

Eisenberg D, Delbanco TL, Berkey CS, et al. 1993. Cognitive behavioral techniques for hypertension: are they effective? Ann Intern Med 118:964–972

Ellenberger HF. 1970. The Discovery of the Unconscious. Basic Books, New York: pp. 53–60

Ernst E. 1995. St. John's wart, an anti-depressant? a systematic, criteria-based review. PhytoMed 2(1):67–71

Feldman AB. 1963. Animal magnetism and the mother of Christian Science. Psychoanal Rev 50:153–160

Fishbein M. 1932. Fads and Quackery in Healing. Blue Ribbon, New York

Forber TR. 1972. Lapis Bufonis: the growth and decline of a medical superstition. Yale J Biol Med 45, 139–149

Fox M. 1984. Conflict to coexistence: Christian Science and medicine. Med Anthro Fall 292–300

Fuller R. 1982. Mesmerism and the American Cure of Souls. University of Pennsylvania Press, Philadelphia

Fuller R. 1989. Alternative Medicine and American Religious Life. Oxford University Press, New York: p. 104

Galbreath R. 1971. The history of modern occultism: A bibliographical survey. J Pop Cult 5:726–754

Gardner M. 1988. Isness is her business: Shirley MacLaine, in Not Necessarily the New Age: Critical Essays, R. Basil ed. Prometheus Books. Buffalo, New York: p. 193

Gevitz N. 1982. The D.O.'s: Osteopathic Medicine in America. The Johns Hopkins University Press, Baltimore

Gevitz, N. 1988. Andrew Taylor Still and the social origins of osteopathy, in, Studies in the History of Alternative Medicine. St. Martin's Press, New York

Gilson E. 1940. The Spirit of Mediaeval Philosophy. Charles Scribner's Sons, New York

Glick DC. 1988. Symbolic, ritual and social dynamics of spiritual healing. Soc Sci Med 27:11, 1197–1206

Goldstein M. 1975. The Research Status of Spinal Manipulative Therapy. U.S. Department of Health, Education and Welfare, PHS, NIH, Bethesda, Maryland

Good BJ, Good MJ. 1981. Alternative health care in one California community. Public Regulation of Health Care Occupations in California, Sacramento

Gort EH, Coburn D. 1986. Naturopathy in Canada: changing relationships to medicine, chiropractic and the state. Soc Sci Med 26:10, 1061–1072

Griggs B. 1981. Green Pharmacy: A History of Herbal Medicine. Jill Norman & Hobhouse, London

Hahnemann S. 1980. Organon of Medicine, Sixth Edition, W. Boericke trans. B. Jain Publishers, New Delhi: p. 97

Haight E. 1975. The roots of the vitalism of Xavier Bichet. Bull Hist Med 49:72–86

Hall JA, Crasilneck HB. 1978. Hypnosis. JAMA 239:8 760–761

Hall TS. 1975. History of General Physiology Vol 1. University of Chicago Press. Chicago

Haller JS. 1973. Acupuncture in nineteenth century western medicine. N Y State J Med, May, 1213–1221

Hartman E. 1977. Substance, Body and Soul: Aristotelian Investigations. Princeton University Press, Princeton, New Jersey

Herink R. ed. 1980. The Psychotherapy Handbook. New American Library, New York

Hill C, Doyon F. 1990. Review of randomized trials of homeopathy. Rev Epidemiol Sante Publique 38: 139–147

Holroyd KA, Penzien DB. 1990. Pharmacological versus non-pharmacological prophylaxis of recurrent migraine headache: a meta-analytic review of clinical trials. Pain, 42:1–13

Huxtable RJ. 1992. The myth of beneficent nature: the risks of herbal preparations. Ann Intern Med 117:2 165–166

James W. 1961. The Varieties of Religious Experience. Collier, New York

Johnson ES, et al. 1985. Efficacy of feverfew as prophylactic treatment of migraince. BMJ 291:569–573

Judah JS. 1967. The History and Philosophy of the Metaphysical Movements in America. Westminster Press, Philadelphia

Kaplan F. 1974. 'The Mesmeric Mania': The early Victorians and animal magnetism. J Hist Ideas 35:4

Karasu TB. 1986. The specificity vs. non-specificity dilemma: towards identifying therapeutic change agents. Am J Psychiatry 14:3–6

Kaufman M. 1971. Homeopathy in America: The Rise and Fall of a Medical Heresy. The Johns Hopkins University Press, Baltimore

Kaufman M. 1988. Homeopathy in America: The Rise and Fall and Persistence of a Medial Heresy. The Johns Hopkins University Press, Baltimore

Kemp S. 1990. Medieval Psychology. Greenwood Press, New York

Keyes K. 1989. Discovering the Secrets of Happiness. Love Line Books, Coos Bay, Oregon

Kleijnen J, Knipschild P, ter Riet G. 1991a Clinical trials of homeopathy. BMJ 302:316–323

Kleijnen J, ter Riet G, Knipschild P. 1991b Acupuncture and asthma: a review of controlled trials. Thorax 46: 799–802

Knapp JE, Antonucci EJ. 1990. A National Study of the Profession of Massage Therapy/Bodywork. Knapp and Associates, Princeton, New Jersey

Kopelman L, Moskop J. 1981. The holistic health movement: A survey and critique. J Med Philosophy May 6 (2) 209–235

Krieger D, Peper E, Ancoli S. 1979. Therapeutic touch: searching for evidence of physiological change. Am J Nur A ril, 660–662

Kuriyama S. 1986. Varieties of Haptic Experience: A Comparative Study of Greek and Chinese Pulse Diagnosis. Unpublished Ph.D. thesis, Harvard University

Lad V. 1984. Ayuraveda. Lotus Press, Sante Fe, New Mexico

Lain Entralgo P. 1948. Sensualism and vitalism in Bichat's 'Anotomie Generale'. J Hist Med 3

Larson JL. 1979. Vital forces: regulative principles or constitutive agents? Isis 70

Ledermann EK. 1989. Philosophy and Medicine. Gower, Aldershot, England

Levin JS, Coreil J. 1986. 'New Age' healing in the U.S. Soc Sci Med 23:9

Linde K, Jonas WB, Melchart D, et al. 1994. Critical review and meta-analysis of serial agitated dilutions in experimental toxicology. Hum Exp Toxicol 13:481–492

Linden W. 1990. Autogenic Training. A Clinical Guide. Guilford Press, New York

Lipman TO. 1967. Vitalism and reductionism in Liebig's physiological thought. Isis 58:167–185

Low J. 1988. The modern body therapies: Aston-Patterning. Massage Magazine. 16:48–55

Lytle CD. 1993. An Overview of Acupuncture. U.S. Department of Health and Human Services, PHS, FDA, Washington, D.C.

Macklin RM. 1993. Magnetic healing, quackery and the debate about the health effects of electromagnetic fields. Ann Intern Med 118:5, 376–383

Manga P, Angus DE, Papadopoulos C, et al. 1993. A Study to Examine the Effectiveness and Cost-Effectiveness of

Chiropractic Management of Low-Back Pain. Pran Managa & Associates, Ottawa

Marvin C. 1988. When Old Technologies Were New: Thinking About Electric Communication in the Late Nineteenth Century, Oxford, New York

Meade TW, Dyer S, Browne W, et al. 1990. Low back pain of mechanical origin: randomized comparison of chiropractic and hospital outpatient treatment. BMJ:300

Melchart D, et al. 1994. Immunodulation with Echinacea—a systematic review of controlled clinical trials. Phytomedicine 1:245–254

Mendelsohn E. 1965. Physical models of physiological concepts: explanation in nineteenth-century biology. Br J Hist Sci 2:7

Meyers D. 1965. The Positive Thinkers: A Study of the American Quest for Health, Wealth, and Personal Power from Mary Baker Eddy to Norman Vincent Peale. Doubleday, Garden City, New Jersey

McClenon J. 1984. Deviant Science: The Case of Parapsychology. University of Pennsylvania Press, Philadelphia

McRae G. 1982. A critical overview of U.S. acupuncture regulation. J Health Polit Policy Law, 1:163–196

McVaugh M, Mauskupf JB. 1976. Rhine's extra-sensory perception and its background in psychial research. Isis. 67:161–89

Melton JG. 1988. A history of the New Age movement, in, B. Basil, ed., Not Necessarily the New Age: Critical Essays. Prometheus Books, Buffalo, New York

Mesmer FA. 1980. Dissertation on the Discovery of Animal Magnetism in, GJ Bloch ed, trans, Mesmerism: A Translation of the Original Medical and Scientific Writings of F.A. Mesmer, M.D. William Kaufmann, Los Altos, California

Miura K. 1989. The revival of qi gong in contemporary China in Taoist Meditation and Longevity Techniques. Center for Chinese Studies, University of Michigan, Ann Arbor, Michigan

Moore RL. 1977. In Search of White Crows: Spiritualism Parapsychology and American Cult. Oxford University Press, New York

Namikoshi T. 1969. Shiatsu. Japan Publications, New York

Needham J. 1955. Mechanistic biology and the religious consciousness in Science, Religion & Reality. George Brazziler, New York

Needham J. 1956. Science & Civilization in China. vol 2. Cambridge University Press, Cambridge

Netherton M. & Shiffrin N. 1978. Past Lives Therapy. William Morrow, New York

Neuburger M. 1933. The Doctrine of the Healing Power of Nature. New York Homeopathic College, New York

Oppenheim J. 1988. The Other World: Spiritualism and Psychical Research in England, 1850–1914. Cambridge University Press, Cambridge

Palmer DD. 1910. Chiropractic Portland Printing House, Portland: p. 691

Pavlov IP. 1928. Lectures on Conditioned Reflexes. International Publishers, New York

Perry R. 1987. An Introduction to a Course in Miracles. Miracle Distribution Center. Fullerton, California

Pomeranz B, Stux G. eds. 1988. Scientific Basis of Acupuncture. Springer-Verlag, Berlin

Rather LJ. 1961. G.E. Stahl's Psychological Physiology. Bull Hist Med 35:27–49

Relman AS. 1979. Holistic Medicine. N Eng J Med 300: 6, 212–313

Reyner JH. 1982. Psionic Medicine. Routledge & Kegan Paul. London

Roger J. 1986. The mechanistic conception of life, in, God and Nature. University of California Press, Berkeley

Rolf IP. 1977. Rolfing: The Integration of Human Structure. Harper & Row, New York

Rose L. 1954. Some aspects of paranormal healing. BMJ 1329–1332 Dec 4

Rothstein WG. 1985. American Physicians in the 19th Century. The Johns Hopkins University Press, Baltimore

Rothstein WG. 1988. The botanical movements and orthodox medicine in Other Healers: Unorthodox Medicine in America. The Johns Hopkins University Press, Baltimore

Schaller WE, Carool CR. 1976. Health, Quackery and the Consumer. W.B. Saunders, Philadelphia

Schotz EH, Cyriax J. 1975. Manipulation: Past and Present. William Heinemann Medical Books, London

Schoepflin RB. 1988. Christian Science Healing in America, in, Other Healers: Unorthodox Medicine in America. The Johns Hopkins University Press, Baltimore

Sharma U. 1992. Complementary Medicine Today: Practitioners and Patients. Tavistock/Routledge, London

Sheikh AA. 1983. Imagery. Current Theory, Research and Application. John Wiley, New York

Shekelle P, Adams AH, Chassin MR, et al. 1992. Spinal manipulation for low-back pain. Ann Intern Med 117: 7

Siegel BS. 1986. Love, Medicine & Miracles. Harper & Row, New York

Sigerist HE. 1961. A History of Medicine. Oxford University Press, New York

Sivin N. 1987. Traditional Medicine in Contemporary China. Center of Chinese Studies, University of Michigan, Ann Arbor, Michigan

Smuts JC. 1926. Holism and Evolution. Macmillan, New York

Strupp HH, Howard KI. 1992. A brief history of psychotherapy research, in, D.K. Frehen, ed, History of Psychotherapy, American Psychological Association, Washington, DC

Sutton G. 1981. Electric medicine and mesmerism. Isis 72, 253:375–392

Tauber AT. 1994. Darwinian aftershocks: repercussions in late twentieth century medicine. J R Soc Med 87:27–31

ter Riet G, Kleijnen, Knipschild P, et al. 1990. Acupuncture and chronic pain: a criteria-based meta-analysis. J Clin Epidemiol 43:1191–1199

Terrett AJ. 1991. The genius of D.D. Palmer: an exploration of the origin of chiropractic in his time. Chir Hist 11:1

Thorndike EL. 1931. Human Learning. Century, New York

Toulmin S, Goodfield J. 1962. The Architecture of Matter. Harper & Row, New York: pp. 322–330

Turner JA, Chapman CR. 1982. Psychological interventions for chronic pain: a critical review. I. Relaxation training and biofeedback. Pain 12:1–21

Tracy SW. 1992. George Draper and the American constitutional medicine, 1916–1946: reinventing the sick man. Bull Hist Med 66:53–89

Turner RW. 1990. Naturopathic Medicine. Northamptonshire, England Wellingborought, p. 21

Vlamis G. 1978. Polarity therapy. Alternatives. 2:4(April) 23–26

Wardwell WI. 1992. Chiropractic: History and Evolution of a New Profession. Mosby Year Book, St. Louis

Warner JH. 1987. Medical sectarianism, therapeutic conflict, and the shaping of orthodox professional identity in antebellum American medicine in, Bynum WF, Porter R (eds). Medical Fringe & Medical Orthodoxy 1750–1850 London: Croom Helm

West AM, ed. 1991. The Psychology of Meditation. Clarendon Press, Oxford

Wheeler R. 1939. Vitalism. H.F. & G Witherby, London

Wheelwright EG. 1974. Medicinal Plants and Their History. Dover, New York

Whorton JC. 1986. Drugless healing in the 1920's: the therapeutic cult of sanipractic Phar Hist 28:14–24

Whorton JC. 1989. The first holistic revolution: alternative medicine in the nineteenth century in Stalker D, Glymour C, eds. Examining Holistic Medicine, Prometheus Books, Buffalo, New York

Yoke HP. 1985. Li, Qi, and Shu: An Introduction to Science and Civilization in China. Hong Kong University Press, Hong Kong

Zefron LJ. 1975. The history of the laying-on of hands in nursing. Nursing For XIV:4, 350–363

4

Contemporary Context of Complementary and Alternative Medicine

Integrated Mind-Body Medicine
Alan D. Watkins

The pursuit of health and the treatment of illness has become a major social activity in the western world. Our society is spending more time and more money on health practices than ever before. For example, the United States now spends more than 12 percent of its gross national product on health care. Within this pursuit of health there is an enormous range of activities, from organ transplantation to meditation. We are changing from a military-industrialized complex to a society dominated by spending on health care and its associated technologies. Fifty years have now passed since the last global war necessitated massive military spending. The fragmentation of the eastern block and the dissolution of the cold war, also has reduced the need for an enormous financial outlay on military projects. Finally, there has been a steady improvement in general health, wealth, and nutrition since the turn of the century. These changes are reflected in the lower infant mortality rates, increased life expectancies, better nutritional standards, and less poverty-related disease in most western societies. Since we are no longer preoccupied with basic survival, we have begun to focus more on the issue of improving the quality and quantity of our lives.

While these fundamental changes in world politics and the world economy have been taking place, there also has been a technologic revolution in science and medicine. At the turn of the century, doctors had very few drugs at their disposal that could alter the course of disease. Physicians were mostly powerless observers of illness, and providing comfort rather than cure. This image presents a sharp contrast to the highly trained specialists of today, who are masters of intervention. Moribund individuals sometimes are literally brought back from the dead, and premature infants with no reasonable hope of independent survival are kept alive to subsequently grow into adults. Lungs unable to breathe are replaced, arteries blocked or fit to burst are bypassed, and cancer cells are sometimes dissolved with toxic chemicals. It is little wonder that many patients perceive modern medicine as omnipotent, and doctors as God-like figures.

Use of Complementary Medicine

Despite the staggering success of allopathic medicine, record numbers of patients are turning to complementary practitioners in the United States (Office of Technology 1990), Europe (Watt 1981, British

49

Medical Association 1986), Australia (Donnelly 1985), and New Zealand (Clinical Oncology Group 1987) for a disparate number of ailments. Several surveys have indicated that between 1986 and 1991 the proportion of the population using complementary medicine in the United Kingdom increased by 70 percent (British Medical Association 1993, Fulder 1985), and have trebled in Holland and France (Van Dijk 1993, Syndicat National de la Pharmace 1993). In 1991, the European over the counter market for homeopathy was £590 million, and for herbal remedies, £1.45 billion (Fisher 1994). Paradoxically, this boom is occurring at the time when allopathic medicine is able to intervene more powerfully than ever before, looking deep into the very fabric of our bodies with magnetic resonance imaging (MRI), and even genetically engineering the DNA inside the nuclei of our cells.

Why are so many people turning to complementary therapy? Do we feel lost in the technology and uncared for by allopathic medicine? Or are we being misled by the pop medicine we encounter in magazines and newspapers into believing that complementary therapies are as effective as allopathic medicine for all our ills? Recent research suggests that far from being ignorant and ill-informed (Charlton 1992), the majority of individuals visiting complementary therapists are, in fact, well educated and affluent (McGuire 1988). So why are so many of these individuals deciding that allopathic medicine cannot deliver what they need?

Biomedical Prowess

There is no doubt that biomedicine is unequalled for the care of many physical ailments, particularly those related to trauma, emergency medicine, and end-stage disease. However, it is less effective in preventing the development of disease, in altering the course of chronic physical disease, and in addressing the mental, emotional, and spiritual needs of an individual. The biomedical model of illness used by allopathic practitioners largely concerns itself with physical disease—the more advanced, the clearer. Biomedicine finds it very difficult to invest time and resources in prevention, partly because prevention is so difficult to measure. If a disease is prevented

by a certain intervention, did that intervention prevent the disease, or did the disease simply not occur as expected?

Allopathic efforts at prevention have focused on screening programs designed to detect early disease such as cervical smear programs, mammography clinics, and cholesterol and blood pressure checks, rather than on primary prevention. The nonspecific symptoms and signs that are the frequent forerunner to many major diseases are given less attention.

Allopathic medicine also struggles with chronic physical disease. Based on the belief that disease, once established, follows an inexorable path of steady deterioration, the allopath seeks to alleviate symptoms for as long as possible, charting the downward progress and deciding when heroic measures are to be called for in a last stand to prevent the patient's demise. In its preoccupation with physical disease, allopathy does not adequately address the mental, emotional, and spiritual needs of its patients. It will address organic mental disease, to which it can give a psychiatric label, but not mental, emotional, or spiritual disease, which is largely viewed as irrelevant or, at best, insoluble and not part of the allopathic practitioner's territory (Charlton 1993). These limitations of allopathic medicine have led many individuals to seek alternative approaches. This chapter examines the basis of allopathic and complementary medical systems, and argues that these approaches are not mutually exclusive on a philosophical, practical, or mechanistic level.

Meaning and Reality

A house is made up of a number of bricks. Science comprises a number of facts. The bricks alone do not make the house a reality any more than facts make science a reality. Both must be held together—in the case of the house, by cement and mortar, and in the case of science, by theory and interpretation. Facts usually are elicited to support a theory, rather than to be independent of it. In this respect, scientific reality is relative. The theories and facts on which health care systems are based, changes across different cultures. Just as there are differences in architectural interpretation, there are differences in factual interpretation. Thus symptoms and signs are interpreted differently, depending on the underlying culture of each society. Allopathic medicine tends to deny the existence of these multiple realities, perceiving itself as the only true reality, and the only reality based on scientific fact. However the briefest study of the history of Western science and medicine reveals that even the facts that allopathy claims as reality are constantly changing.

Evolution of Scientific Medicine

How did allopathic medicine develop its view of a singular reality? In many human societies, health care often was provided by a tribal doctor or shaman. These individuals developed powerful intuitive skills and the ability to enter trance states (often drug-induced), in order to consult with the spirit world. Illness was attributed to the spirits taking away the soul or psyche of the sufferer. The shaman would enter a trance to pursue the soul and to negotiate with the spirits for its return.

Evil spirits also could manifest within a subject's body, and the shaman would exorcise the spirit by inducing a trance or convulsions in the possessed individual using drugs, rituals, or rhythm. Thus, the earliest forms of therapy involved both attention to the psyche, and to the physical body. By the time of the earliest structured civilizations, these two aspects of health care had become separated, with the herbalists becoming the dominant providers of health and the priests and magicians dividing responsibility for spiritualism. Priests were able to consult the gods and magicians used psychic powers to divine health problems from the study of entrails or the throwing of bones. This early separation of spiritual and physical aspects gave birth to the two schools of thinking, namely, the vitalists and the mechanists.

Vitalists believed illness was the result of psychic or spiritual forces, while mechanists believed in more physical explanations. One of the earliest and most influential advocates of the mechanistic school was Hippocrates of Cos. Hippocrates and his followers recognized the natural recuperative powers of the body and did not deny the importance of spiritual energy, but still concentrated on treating illness and identifying specific mechanistic causes for ill health.

They believed that an imbalance in one of the four humors—blood, phlegm, and black or yellow bile—could produce ill health. The concept that an imbalance of humor could predispose toward illness is remarkably similar to the current view of homeostasis, which dominates much of pathophysiology today.

The homeostatic model suggests that disease occurs, for example, when the balance between inflammatory and anti-inflammatory forces is disturbed. This concept is akin to the Chinese notion that ill health is caused by an imbalance in the vital energy, or chi. The Greeks used allopathic remedies to treat imbalances in the humors, and mechanistic medicine gradually became synonymous with the administration of allopathic remedies. Another major figure in the development of western medicine was Galen, the Royal Physician to Marcus Aurelius, in the second century A.D. Galen used all manners of drugs and herbal remedies enthusiastically, often creating bewildering and noxious concoctions. However, Galen recognized the importance of the psyche in physical disease, and his observation that melancholic women were more likely to develop disease of the breast is considered by many to be the earliest western record of the effects of the psyche on the immune system.

Because many remedies offered by mechanistic allopaths were either toxic or ineffectual, the vitalistic approach resurfaced. This re-emergence also was stimulated by the teachings of Jesus and the early Christians. Jesus effected instant cures through the power of faith. Christian healers used the power of a divine force and promoted the manifestation of the spirit within an individual. Such healers relied upon inspiration—literally, the spirit inside themselves—for therapeutic guidance. For several centuries the clergy played an active role in healing the sick. By the middle ages the teachings of the Christian church (particularly the Vatican) became the dominant force in guiding society. They viewed ecclesiastical intervention in cases of possession, convulsions, and trance states as suspect paganism, bordering on witchcraft, and possibly satanic. As a result, the church backed out of its role in healing, and medicine was left to physicians, who were firm followers of the polypharmacy advocated by Galen. Vitalism declined.

The Birth of Reductionism

In the mid-sixteenth century, polemical changes were occurring throughout society. Copernicus put forth his view that the sun, not the earth, was the center of the universe. Versalius contested the common practice of fitting the results of medical research (such as the discoveries made from cadaver dissection) to fit the theories of the day. This was the birth of scientific thinking. Vitalism was somewhat rehabilitated by Paracelsus, who suggested that there was a mechanistic explanation for miracles, namely, the human imagination. Despite this shift to rational thinking, allopathic treatment lagged behind and was still based largely on Galenic principles of polypharmacy, with little recourse to scientific testing.

Desperate attempts to alter body humors were foisted upon those that could afford to pay for it. For example, eyewitness accounts document the sorry last days of Charles II in the grip of some malady. His surgeon responded by removing 16 ounces of blood from his right arm. Not to be outdone, his physician ordered further blood letting and scarification. Having probably rendered the King anemic, his medical attendants then proceeded to dehydrate him with a potent cocktail of emetics and purgatives. Spanish fly, a blistering agent, was then applied to his shaven scalp, and when this failed to produce therapeutic benefit someone ordered a red-hot cautery. For the better part of a week, 14 physicians competed in their abuse of the king until finally, one bright spark arranged for the Oriental Bezoar Stone to be transferred from its normal habitat in the stomach of an eastern goat to its final resting place in the body of King Charles. Before he died, Charles apologized to his physicians for taking such a long time to do so.

Fortunately, by the mid-seventeenth century, reason began to prevail. Thomas Syndenham, whose name was later associated with an inherited form of chorea, suggested that medical training take place at the bedside rather than in university classrooms. Syndenham also suggested that symptoms be separated from the underlying disease, giving birth to the school of Nosologists, who began to classify diseases as Linnaeus was classifying plants.

Descartes' assertion that the mind and body were separate entities encouraged the description of physical diseases that did not involve the mind. By the mid-eighteenth century, Morgani suggested that a patient's symptoms could be traced to physical malfunctions in specific organs. Forty years later, Bichat demonstrated that diseased tissues, not organs, were at fault. The great Virchow completed this reductionist trend in 1850, by showing that specific cells within tissue were responsible for disease. Thus, in the late nineteenth century the plethora of symptoms and signs presented by the patient could be reduced to a cellular malfunction.

This reductionist approach proved extremely effective in increasing scientific understanding of disease. When the complexity of the body was reduced to simple processes, it became possible to measure these processes. Measurement of bodily functions thus became central to scientific medical thinking. Individual experience, which could not be measured, diminished further and the intuitive wisdom of healers was dismissed as anecdotal.

Reductionism reinforced the basic separation of the measurable physical body and the unquantifiable psyche. Since changes in the psyche and spirit could not be easily quantified, they were dismissed as irrelevant or nonexistent. Consequently, the reality described by science was based largely on a physical reality. Illness was explained in terms of measurable physical malfunction and the role of the spirit was diminished substantially.

By the end of the nineteenth century, allopathic practitioners were being taught to elicit a systematic history, search the biochemical and structural integrity of the body for abnormalities, and then reduce all the symptoms and signs of illness to a single diagnostic category.

This biomedical approach produced some early success, particularly in identifying the cause of infectious diseases, which were the major source of ill health in society at the time. However, such advances in scientific thinking had not produced substantial improvement in treatment. The toxic nature of the allopathic remedies of the day spawned the development of less noxious, alternative approaches, such as homeopathy. Thus, complementary approaches to health enjoyed a revival, but they frequently were met with open hostility and derision from the allopathic community (Inglis 1980).

As scientific thinking and methodology became more rigorous, the toxic treatments of the past fell into disuse, more efficacious drugs were discovered and refined, and the gentler, more spiritual complementary therapies were again relegated to the fringe of medical practice. Modern pharmacology fortified the view that psychological factors, such as the placebo response, were irrelevant. The new powerful medicines that had been developed could cure the patient regardless of his or her desires. Allopathic doctors became entrenched even more firmly in their belief that the patient's thoughts, feelings, and emotions were irrelevant to recovery. Promoting an expectation of health using the placebo effect was consequently seen as deceitful, and even unethical.

While western society was developing increasing faith in the biomedical model and the power of pharmacologic intervention, new scientific discoveries also reinforced the biomedical reductionist view that thoughts, feelings, and emotions were irrelevant to health. For example, the immune system and the endocrine system were being shown to be self-regulatory, independent of the functioning of the mind. The view that health was largely a function of the physical body and unrelated to higher cortical function is the model used in allopathic medicine today. The phenomenal successes of high-tech medicine reinforces this reductionist approach. The biomedical reductionist model appears to be the antithesis of the holistic approach used by the majority of complementary medical practitioners (Rosch 1985).

Therapeutic Approaches

Differences between biomedical reductionism and holism are exemplified by their respective approaches to therapy. Biomedicine assumes that all individuals are basically the same, and therefore, solutions to any one particular diagnosis also will be identical. Treatments are aimed at the antagonism of a single pathologic process. By contrast, complementary medicine assumes that all individuals are different; the manifestation of disease depends on the unique characteristics of the individual patient. Therefore, a constellation of therapeutic activities is deemed necessary; these may vary on a daily basis

according to the changing needs of the patient and the changing clinical situation.

These differences also affect research into the efficacy of treatment modalities. Allopathic medicine dissects a therapeutic approach in order to identify a single mechanism that underpins efficacy. It uses the randomized placebo controlled trial (RCT) to aid this dissection, and to determine whether a single therapeutic ingredient is active. Complementary medicine places much greater emphasis on the validity of individual therapeutic experience. Research into complementary medicine is made arduous by the difficulty in designing controls for individualized treatments, but with precision and care, such research is possible (Lewith 1993).

Therapeutic Exclusivity

Are the therapeutic approaches of allopathy and complementary medicine really mutually exclusive? On a practical level, it is possible to integrate complementary medicine into allopathic practice, as has been proven by chiropractic (see Chapter 7). In fact the strong desire to incorporate complementary medicine into allopathic practice is reflected in a 1983 survey that indicated that approximately 80 percent of trainee primary care physicians in the United Kingdom wished to receive training in complementary therapy (Reilly 1983). By 1987, this figure had risen to 92 percent (Reilly 1993). It was reported in 1986 that approximately 30 percent of primary care physicians in two British counties already had received training in complementary therapy (Wharton 1986, Anderson 1986). So, contrary to the stereotypical image of an unqualified practitioner dispensing untested remedies, a large proportion—in some countries, the majority—of those providing complementary therapies are allopathically qualified (Cassileth 1984).

Allopathic and complementary approaches thus can be employed simultaneously in the treatment of disease. Practitioners with training in both allopathic and complementary medicine are well placed to recognize the limitations of both systems. They might be the most suitable practitioners to decide which therapeutic approach, or combination of approaches, best suits the needs of the patient.

Using the skills and knowledge inherent in both systems, he or she is in a position to address the physical, emotional, mental, and spiritual dimensions of health, that is, be truly holistic. In the United Kingdom, the realization that allopathy and complementary medical approaches are not mutually exclusive spawned the birth of the British Holistic Medical Association (BHMA) in the early 1980s. One of its founders, Dr. Patrick Pietroni, has written about the paradigm shift that is occurring within allopathic circles (Pietroni). As allopathic practitioners realize the limits of scientific enquiry, they begin to utilize other systems that address areas with which science struggles. Thus, there is a shift from the reductionist biomedical approach to a holistic approach that incorporates multiple realities and multiple explanations for ill health.

Pietroni also describes models of experimental health centers in the United Kingdom that use this holistic approach. One such health center, situated in the crypt of a London church, incorporates allopathic primary care physicians, osteopaths, psychological counsellors, and spiritual healers. The primary care physician has initial contact with the patient and deals with the presenting problem from a biomedical standpoint, involving complementary practitioners within the practice when appropriate. All allopathic and complementary practitioners meet on a regular basis to communicate about individual patients, ensuring that all their physical, mental, emotional, or spiritual needs are being met.

Pietroni's London practice is by no means the only model of holistic practice in the United Kingdom. In Southampton, on the south coast of England, four primary care physicians run the Center for the Study of Complementary Medicine. The physicians at The Center are trained in a wide variety of complementary medical techniques. Over the last 15 years they have developed a method of predicting the exact number of consultations a particular problem will require, as well as the likelihood of improvement. Each individual might be treated simultaneously with a number of complementary techniques and allopathic remedies depending on their individual characteristics and the presentation of the problem.

Many treatments and therapeutic approaches, initially perceived as complementary, have become incorporated into mainstream allopathic practice. For example, at least 25 percent of all prescriptions written in the United States are for drugs that were originally identified from plants by folklore and herbalists (Reynolds 1991, Farnsworth 1983). Hypnosis, which was dismissed for many years as a deception, is now widely accepted by psychiatrists and clinical psychologists as an invaluable therapeutic tool, particularly in the United States. The undoubted success of chiropractic techniques for back pain have ensured that these techniques will complement allopathic approaches permanently.

Philosophical Exclusivity

Complementary and allopathic therapies also are not mutually exclusive on a philosophical level. Allopathic medicine is often characterized as reductionist and complementary medicine as holistic. It is an oversimplification to suggest that allopathy is entirely reductionist and complementary medicine is entirely holistic. Each type of practice has both elements to varying degrees. Reducing a problem to its component parts does not preclude an analysis of the whole, and it is possible to respond to the patient's needs as well as the needs of the disease at the same time. Allopaths often do try to attend to the mental and emotional domain through a referral to a psychiatrist. Complementary practitioners reduce a symptom complex to its component parts in much the same way as an allopath would do. They may even prescribe a complementary technique in the same way that an allopath would prescribe a pill.

It often is argued that complementary medicine cannot be integrated with allopathic medicine, because it would then be forced into a reductionist mold. For example, in the classical acupuncture practiced by the Chinese, needles are placed according to the unique characteristics of the individual. In the formula acupuncture practiced in the West, needles are placed at the same points in all patients. This formula has been labelled reductionist, and therefore less likely to be effective. But classical acupuncture must, by definition, also use a formula of sorts, or else it would be impossible to know where to place the needles at all.

As highlighted earlier, biomedicine tends to see

itself as a singular reality, with its validity supported by scientific facts. It views much of the evidence for the efficacy of complementary practices as anecdotal. However, there also are numerous anecdotes in the biomedical literature, called case histories, and the study of these case histories has significantly increased our understanding of basic physiologic and pathologic processes. For example, in 1986, two types of T-lymphocytes were identified in mice, and were thought to be crucial to the development of allergic reactions (Mossman 1986). The existence of these subsets in man was fiercely disputed. However, subsequent case histories demonstrated that such cells did exist in man (Field 1993). The scientific literature is full of such examples.

In addition, science often studies the isolated extremes of biologic malfunction to help elucidate the mechanisms of normal biologic function. Thus individuals with rare genetic deficiencies can tell us a great deal about normal cellular function. This method of gathering information from the investigation of rarities is similar to the gathering of information from the few long-term survivors of malignancy who were treated with a complementary technique. In fact the study of isolated genetic deficiencies has flourished in recent years as a result of genetic engineering, which enables scientists to produce large numbers of animals with a single gene defect. The scientific literature is awash with reports on the effects of such isolated deficiencies and their implications for normal function.

Thus, allopathic and complementary medicine can be simultaneously holistic and reductionist, and the philosophical differences are not as broad as some would like to think. Nevertheless, most complementary medical practices may remain unaccepted by allopathic medicine until large scale RCTs investigating their efficacy have been conducted.

Despite repeated calls for such research by the British Medical Association (British Medical Association 1993), The Royal College of Physicians (The Royal College of Physicians 1992), The Royal Society of Medicine (Watt 1988), the European Parliament (March 1994), the House of Representatives (Office of Technology 1990), and the WHO (WHO Global Strategy 1994), few such trials have been performed. Many agencies in control of research funds see com-

plementary therapies as alternative and therefore a threat to orthodoxy. This perception has been fuelled by the antagonistic and divisive opinions of a number of protagonists among both the complementary and allopathic communities. Some allopaths are content to dismiss complementary medicine as ineffectual without any experimental evidence on efficacy from small or large scale RCTs; this kind of pejorative attitude is completely unscientific and is usually voiced by individuals who claim to be scientists themselves on the basis of a purported concern for scientific standards.

Investigations of complementary medicine are further hampered by the perception that complementary approaches lack neurophysiologic or biochemical explanations. Such explanations could be subjected to scientific testing, thereby helping to bring complementary practices into mainstream medical practice. Occasionally, scientific explanations have been found, such as the demonstration that acupuncture relieves pain by stimulating the production of endorphins. As a result, acupuncture gained greater acceptance amongst allopaths, although it still has fallen short of full integration.

Mechanistic Exclusivity

The above discussion makes it apparent that complementary and allopathic medicine are not mutually exclusive on a philosophical or a practical level. The only remaining barrier to the integration of complementary and allopathic practices is the question of mechanism of action. If practices such as healing touch, homeopathy, aromatherapy, ayurveda, curanderismo, or any of the complementary systems are to be integrated, these systems either have to be proven effective by allopathic mechanisms, or allopathy has to accept that they may work via mechanisms that are foreign to the present biomedical model. For example, is there a scientific explanation why a homeopathic remedy works when the original compound has been diluted beyond detectable limits? Or should we accept the suggestion that the original compound has in some way left an energetic imprint on water molecules? In order to determine whether scientific explanations can be found to explain the possible efficacy of complementary practices, it is necessary to examine complementary medical research more closely.

The enormous volume of complementary medical research that has been conducted is astounding. Much of this work has failed to reach allopathic attention because it is rarely published in scientific journals, and journals that do publish such work frequently are not referenced on the main scientific databases. This partly is because much of this research is not rigorously controlled or of high scientific quality (not unlike a great deal of allopathic research).

The lack of scientific controls in complementary medical research does not necessarily invalidate the research findings, it merely makes them less available to generalization. There are many reasons for this lack of scientific rigor. A nearly complete lack of funding has forced research to be limited to small scale trials, making it difficult to demonstrate statistically significant results that can be followed up. In addition, controls for many complementary practices are difficult to design. Finally, many allopathic clinicians and scientists are inhibited from investigating this field because they fear that their work will be dismissed by allopathic colleagues as unscientific and irrelevant.

The recent controversy following the investigation of a potential mechanism of action of homeopathic potencies (Davenas 1988), highlights these dangers only too well. Consequently, much of the complementary medicine research has been conducted by individuals with little training in clinical trial research and scientific method.

The funding difficulties of complementary medicine have been less acute in Europe, particularly the United Kingdom, where there is a stronger tradition for complementary health practices and research. In the last few years, a number of "centers of excellence," based in allopathic teaching hospitals, have evolved. These centers are conducting well-controlled scientific studies on which therapeutic decisions can be made. However, most of this work is still at the stage of determining whether therapeutic efficacy can be established; there has been very little research investigating possible mechanisms of action of complementary therapies. Therefore, we will have

to look to other areas of scientific research to answer the mechanistic questions.

Subjective and Objective Benefit

Many of the studies demonstrating the clinical benefit of complementary techniques have reported improvements in what allopaths would call subjective measures of disease activity. These measures are based on the patient's perception of the disease, and might be a general feeling of well-being, or specific symptoms related to the disease under investigation. Many allopaths dismiss any treatment that has a solely subjective impact. They suggest that such a therapy merely makes the patient feel better, having no real effect on the disease as measured by objective parameters.

This view that only quantifiable objective improvements in disease activity are a valid assessment of therapeutic benefit is inaccurate. Subjective improvements might also be produced by improvements in pathology that are not detectable by currently available tests. Patients may feel better because they *are* better, pathologically.

Furthermore, the subjective assessment of disease activity by the patient and the allopathic doctor usually is what guides clinical practice. For example, if a patient is feeling better, he or she is much more likely to discontinue medication. Similarly, if the patient reports to the doctor that he or she is feeling better then the doctor is equally likely to stop certain medications. Objective benefits might not actually be perceived by the patient. For example, in a study of 82 asthmatics, 15 percent of patients were unable to perceive a 50 percent reduction in their capacity to exhale rapidly (Rubinfeld 1976).

It is rather artificial to classify a therapeutic improvement as either entirely objective or subjective, since clearly objective measures, such as blood pressure, can be influenced by subjective factors. Thus, the subjective well-being of the patient can alter the recorded pressure, and the interpretation of the different sounds heard when measuring a patient's blood pressure also involve a certain degree of subjectivity. In addition, a subjective perception of improved health might result from an objective improvement in pathology (Figure 4-1).

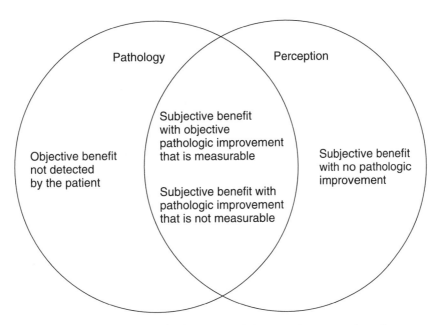

Figure 4-1. Overlap of subjective and objective therapeutic benefit.

Subjective improvement in symptoms, or an increased sense of well-being, are valid therapeutic goals, just like objective improvements. Most of the research to date on complementary therapies demonstrates that benefits are predominantly subjective. It is likely that until complementary therapies are able to show consistent objective benefits, they will not be fully integrated into allopathic medicine. However, studies that have reported objective improvements are usually dismissed on the grounds that they are not scientifically robust, or because there is no mechanistic explanation for how such objective improvements can be brokered.

One possible explanation for how complementary therapies could produce objective benefit is by first producing a subjective benefit. Such subjective, perceptual improvements might promote objective improvements in disease activity. Perception is an evaluative process involving a number of areas of the brain, including the limbic emotional centers. Recent research suggests that higher cortical centers and limbic emotional centers are capable of altering health and disease. The brain communicates with the immune system in a rich flow of hormones, neuropeptides, and cytokines. Thus, perception influences pathology and pathology influences perception (Watkins 1995).

Psychoneuroimmunology

An overwhelming amount of evidence suggests that higher cognitive centers and limbic emotional centers are capable of regulating virtually all aspects of the immune system and, therefore, have a profound effect on health and illness (Ader 1991, Blalock 1994, Reichlin 1993). This area of research is referred to as *psycho-* (from the mind, or psyche) *neuro-* (via the brain or neurons) *immunology* (to the immune system) (PNI). Two mind-body pathways of communication have been identified, namely, autonomic and neuroendocrine. The autonomic nervous system innervates the bone marrow, thymus, spleen, and mucosal surfaces where immune cells develop, mature, and encounter foreign proteins (Felten 1992). Some authors have suggested that the development and aging of both the immune and autonomic nervous systems might be related (Ackerman 1989, Bellinger 1988).

The autonomic innervation of immune tissue is

extremely complex. There are three different arms to the autonomic innervation of immune tissue, namely, the sympathetic, parasympathetic, and non-adrenergic non-cholinergic (NANC). Each neural network communicates with the immune cells directly through the release of chemical messages. These messages range from adrenaline, noradrenaline, and acetylcholine, to small proteins, called neuropeptides, that previously were thought to only occur in the brain. These chemical messages may have an inflammatory or anti-inflammatory effect on the immune tissue. The situation is complicated further by the finding that a specific neuropeptide can be released from sympathetic, parasympathetic, or NANC nerves, and that each type of nerve can store and release both inflammatory and anti-inflammatory chemical messages.

The pattern of chemical message released also may vary over time in a specific tissue, depending on the chronicity of the inflammatory process. Furthermore, there is a very complicated interaction between the autonomic nerves and the immune cells within each immune compartment, and this relation changes, depending on the immune tissue involved. Thus, the nerves may alter the function of the inflammatory cells and the inflammatory cells may alter the function of the nerves (Watkins 1995).

In addition to this direct physical communication between nerves and immune tissue, a second indirect chemical communication channel involves hormone production by the hypothalamus and pituitary gland at the base of the brain. These hormones, which normally regulate the function of other glands in the body, are capable of altering the function of virtually every type of immune cell. Immune cells have surface receptors for virtually all the hormones produced by the brain, including growth hormone, thyroid-stimulating hormone, the sex hormone-releasing hormones, vasopressin, and prolactin, as well as many of the hormones produced by the other endocrine glands in the body (Blalock 1994, Felten et al 1992). They also possess receptors for the natural endorphins and enkephalins produced by the brain, which profoundly affect immune system function, some causing suppression, others causing enhancement of the immune system. The release of many of these hormones is intimately related to thoughts and emotions. Each thought and feeling has a chemical consequence within the brain in terms of the chemical messages passing between brain cells and the hormones produced by the emotional centers. For example, after just five minutes of stress, an animal's hypothalamus produces the signals that eventually promote increased levels of cortisol (Chover-Gonzalez 1993).

The complex control of the immune system by brain hormones and the autonomic nervous system is complicated further by the demonstration that these two pathways profoundly affect each other as well (Terao 1993). Furthermore, the immune system talks back to the brain via the autonomic nervous system and the production of its own chemical signals.

The central nervous system and the immune system function as an integrated whole to maintain a state of healthy balance within the body (Watkins 1995). The immune system communicates information to the brain that the brain cannot perceive, and the brain informs the immune system about cognitive information which the immune cells are unable to detect. Thus, there is now substantial evidence to suggest that thoughts, feeling, emotions, and perceptions do indeed alter immunity (Watkins 1995). Therefore, complementary therapies that alter subjective feelings of well-being might be potentially promoting changes in pathology by activating these brain-immune pathways (Watkins 1994).

Evidence for PNI Mediating the Effects of Complementary Therapies

Thus, the autonomic nervous system and the hormonal system are capable of generating a wide variety of messages that can modulate immune function. Any one of these brain-immune signals might be affected by a complementary therapy. It seems likely that complementary therapies, which rely on a constellation of activities, might affect several brain-immune signals simultaneously. Therefore great care must be taken when designing controls for studies investigating complementary techniques. For example, if acupuncture relieves pain by promoting the local release of endorphins, assessing the analgesic effects of acupuncture by inserting needles into sham acupuncture points may be invalid since sham needles may also stimulate the release of endorphins, thereby producing analgesia in controls and confounding any treatment effect. On the other hand, if acupuncture is effective in asthma by reducing cholinergic tone, then it would be valid to use sham acupuncture points as a control since the release of endorphins would have no significant effect on cholinergic activity and airway calibre.

But what evidence is there that complementary therapies work via the brain-immune pathways outlined above? Very few studies have actually investigated the mechanism of action of complementary therapies. Some data does suggest that the activity of the autonomic nervous system may be altered during chiropractic (Beal 1985, Bouhuys 1963), hypnosis (Neild 1985, DeBeneditts 1994), conditioning (Hatch 1990), and acupuncture (Han 1980, Jian 1985). Other studies have suggested that acupuncture (Kasahara 1992) and spinal manipulation (Vernon 1986) might be mediated by endorphin release.

How do these brain-immune pathways relate to the placebo effect? It has been argued that every therapeutic intervention—whether complementary or allopathic—involves a placebo effect. It frequently is stated that 50 percent of the analgesic effect of painkillers is due to a placebo response. All the same, most allopathic physicians consider it unethical, or even deceitful to actively encourage a placebo response.

This unwillingness to harness an undoubtedly powerful therapeutic effect is largely due to the fact that the placebo effect is unpredictable, unreliable, and mediated by nonspecific mechanisms that are dismissed as unmeasurable and irrelevant. However, it is now clear from PNI research that an expectation of recovery can alter subjective feelings of well-being, and result in autonomic activation as well as the production of pituitary hormones. Thus, there are specific testable pathways by which expectation (the placebo effect) can alter immunity. It is likely that expectation has different effects in different individuals—producing large shifts in autonomic balance and hormonal output in some, and negligible changes in others. This would explain the unpredictability of the placebo response.

The second factor that has inhibited a greater understanding of the placebo response has been the development of the placebo-controlled trial. The effectiveness of newly developed drugs are established by comparison to identical, but therapeutically inactive compounds called placebos. Placebos are employed as if they had no specific effect on the disease in question, rather than a nonspecific effect. Therefore, the enormous clinical benefit that could be produced by a placebo response was undermined by the use of inert placebo medications, thereby reinforcing the view that any therapy harnessing placebo effects was at best ineffective, and at worst unethical. This view, combined with the view that complementary therapies affect only subjective measures of disease activity, have made it possible for allopathic physicians to argue that complementary practices are of limited benefit.

Such arguments are fallacious. The expectation of recovery that promotes a placebo response is quite separate from a subjective improvement, and incidentally, is also different from hope. It is possible to feel subjectively better, without expecting a full recovery. Similarly, it is possible to expect a recovery without feeling better. Complementary therapies cannot be dismissed as mere placebos; they are producing substantial, subjective, and at times, objective clinical benefit unrelated to the placebo effect.

Thus, both expectancy (the placebo response) and subjective feelings of well-being might be produced by the brain-immune pathways identified in PNI research. Complementary therapies may produce clinical benefit by promoting a placebo response, or they may alter subjective feelings of well-being. Alternatively they may directly activate brain-immune pathways without involving expectancy or subjective feelings (Figure 4-2). For example, hypnosis can alter expectancy or subjective feelings, and therefore may be an extremely powerful activator of brain-immune pathways in some individuals. By contrast, acupuncture might directly affect the brain-immune pathways by modulating incoming signals from the immune system to the hypothalamus, without involving the higher centers, expectation, or emotions.

Individuals differ in their responsiveness to different activation stimuli—be they expectancy, subjective sensations, or complementary therapies. This would explain why complementary therapies that are supposedly mediated via placebo mechanisms, according to the allopathic argument, can outperform placebos in a double blind trial (Reilly 1994).

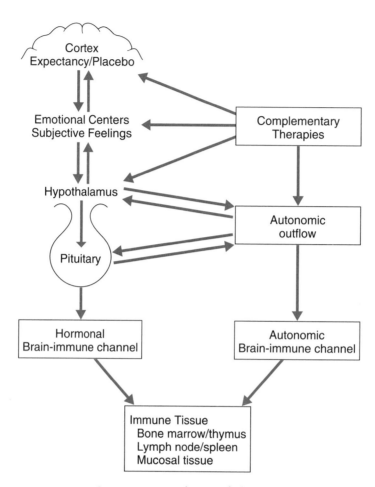

Figure 4-2. Brain-immune pathways of alternative medicine.

It would also explain the need for a constellation of complementary activities to ensure that these pathways were fully activated.

Vital Energy

The importance of energy in health has been recognized for centuries, and by many cultures. Many complementary therapies place great emphasis on the concept of energy. Ayurveda suggests an energetic body exists beneath the physical body, not on a biologic level but on a quantum level. Traditional Chinese medicine is based on the concept that disruption of vital energy can lead to disease. The therapeutic interventions used in traditional Chinese medicine are designed to unblock or move this energy. In fact, encouraging the natural flow of this energy through such practices as Tai Chi Shuan is seen as vital in maintaining health and preventing illness. Acupuncture is claimed to alter the flow of energy around the body through the insertion of needles along the energy meridians.

Such explanations seem, at first glance, to run completely contrary to biomedical explanations, since the energy meridians do not conform to allopathic maps of the nervous or vascular systems. But does this energy also flow through the bodies of patients presenting to allopathic practitioners? Allopathic patients do complain about lack of energy, and most allopathic practitioners have difficulty interpreting such statements. The biomedical model does not appear to have any way of incorporating the concept of energy. Lack of energy usually is taken to indicate physical or mental fatigue. But this change in language does not get the allopath off the hook. A cause for fatigue must still be found. Searches for objective pathology, such as anemia, thyroid dysfunction, or occult cancer usually are fruitless. Unable to find any quantifiable pathology, but pressed to diagnose the cause of fatigue, allopathic practitioners may assert that there is nothing wrong, or allude vaguely to a virus. More recently, chronic fatigue syndrome (myalgic encephalomyelitis) has become a popular diagnosis.

The treatment of such nonspecific diagnoses drains the energy of the allopath himself. It is difficult to prescribe treatment when there is no firm diagnostic label. Most allopaths end up doing nothing, or dispensing some nonspecific advice about fatigue. Brave doctors might suggest some sort of tonic. By contrast, complementary therapies practiced in the west, such as Healing Touch (see Chapter 9) are specifically directed at dealing with the problems of energy. Despite its own limitations, allopathic biomedicine often dismisses such approaches as scientifically untested and unfounded.

Why does western biomedicine struggle with the concept of energy? Energy is a complicated and obtuse subject. There are no accepted ways of measuring—and therefore validating—the level of energy within the human body. As a result, it is impossible to determine whether energy levels change during an illness and whether they change in response to a treatment, although it is clear that the healthy are more energetic than the ill. Finally, the concept of energy is intimately related to spirituality and religion—untangible concepts.

Actually, allopathic medicine does measure a number of energy systems within the body. For example, the energy produced by the heart is recorded by an electrocardiogram (ECG). The electrical energy of the heart is of particular interest (see chapter 1).

The heart is a main source of energy within the body. Electrically it is 40 to 60 times more

(Continues)

powerful than the brain, emitting 2.5 watts of electrical power. The heart trace seen on the ECG is the averaged electrical signal from all the cardiac muscle cells, and this can be recorded anywhere on the body from the top of the skull to the tip of the toes. What happens to this energy when it reaches the body surface? Does it stop abruptly at the skin? Perhaps more importantly, is the energy altered by the tissue through which it passes?

The height of a heart trace certainly is reduced if there is fluid around the heart (a pericardial effusion), or if there is a large amount of fat in the skin. But does disease in other tissues alter this energy in some subtle way? Perhaps the energy detected by practitioners of Healing Touch is the heart's electrical energy just above the skin's surface. It has been suggested that if we walk into a room where two people have just been arguing, even if they now are sitting quietly, the atmosphere we can sense is actually the electrical energy emanating from the hearts of the two individuals.

Heart energy is, of course, not the only type of energy in the body. The Hindu concept of chakras also describes other energy centers within the physical body. But there is no doubt that the heart is the predominant energy source. How is heart energy related to our health? Fascinating answers are being provided by the current detailed analysis of heart energy or heart frequency using modern digital processing computers (Ori 1992, Stein 1994). This hard scientific research has revealed that there are three basic types or patterns of heart energy, and these reflect the activity in the autonomic nervous system (McCraty 1995).

Thus, activity or energy in the nervous system is directly related to energy in the heart. Mental stress and negative emotions, such as anger, increase the energy in the sympathetic nervous system (Sloan 1994, Kamada 1992, Williams 1982), and in contrast, positive emotions such as care and compassion increase the energy

(Continues)

in the parasympathetic nervous system (McCraty 1995). Thus the activity of the brain and the vital energy in the body are connected via the autonomic nervous system. In addition, since the brain and the immune system work as an integrated unit (vide infra) it now becomes possible to see how the brain, the heart, and the immune system are interrelated. Thus, energy and matter come together, and this juncture is explained by scientifically testable pathways and mechanisms.

Conclusion

It is clear that contemporary biomedicine does not have all the answers; neither does complementary medicine. If we can abstain from linear thinking, then we can achieve a breakthrough in understanding. We must put aside the polarised arguments of the allopaths who reduce all individuals to the same, and the complementary advocates who suggest that we are all different. Both systems have something to offer. They are not as mutually exclusive, on a philosophical, practical, or even mechanistic level. The brain, the heart, the immune system, energy, and matter all work together and so must we. The future of medicine is in our hands. If we open our minds, then that future looks very promising indeed.

References

Ackerman KD, Felten SY, Dijkstra CD, et al. 1989. Parallel development of noradrenergic sympathetic innervation and cellular compartmentalisation in the rat spleen. Exp Neurol 103:239–255

Ader R, Felten DL, Cohen N. 1991. Psychoneuroimmunology 2nd Ed. Academic Press, San Diego

Anderson E, Anderson P. 1986. Complementary medicine and the general practitioner (letter). BMJ 293:53

Beal MC. 1985. Viscerosomatic reflexes: a review. J Am Osteopath Assoc 85:786–811

Bellinger DL, Felten SY, Felten DL. 1988. Maintenance of noradrenergic sympathetic innervation in the involuted thymus of the aged Fischer 344 rat. Brain Behav Immun 2:133–150

Blalock JE. 1994. The immune system: Our sixth sense. Immunology 2:8–15

Bouhuys A. 1963. Effects of posture in experimental asthma in man. Am J Med 34:470–476

British Medical Association. 1986. Alternative therapy: report of the Board of Science and Education. London British Medical Association

British Medical Association. 1993. Complementary Medicine: New Approaches to Good Practice. Oxford University Press, Oxford

Cassileth BR, Lusk EJ, Strouse TB, Bodenheimer BJ. 1984. Contemporary unorthodox treatments in cancer medicine: a study of patients, treatments, and practitioners. Ann Intern Med 101:105–112

Charlton BG. 1992. Philosophy of medicine: alternative or science. J R Soc Med 85:436–438

Charlton BG. 1993. The doctor's aim in a pluralistic society: a response to "healing and medicine". J R Soc Med 86:125–126

Chover-Gonzalez AJ, Harbuz MS, Lightman SL. 1993. Effect of adrenalectomy and stress on interleukin-1 beta-mediated activation of hypothalamic corticotropin-releasing factor mRNA. J Neuroimmunol 42:155–160

Clinical Oncology Group. 1987. New Zealand cancer patients and alternative medicine. NZ Med J 100:110–113

Davenas E, Beauvais F, Amara J, et al. 1988. Human basophil degranulation triggered by very dilute antiserum against IgE. Nature 333:816–818

DeBeneditts G, Cigada M, Bianchi A, et al. 1994. Autonomic changes during hypnosis: a heart rate variability power spectrum analysis as a marker of sympatho-vagal balance. Int J Clin Exp Hypnosis XLII (2) 140–152

Donnelly WJ, Spykerboer JE, Thong YH. 1985. Are patients who use alternative medicine dissatisfied with orthodox medicine? Med J Aust 142:439–441

European Parliament Committee on the Environment, Public Health and Consumer Protection. 1994. The state of complementary medicine draft report. Lannoye P. March

Farnsworth NR. 1983. Natural Products and Drug Development. Copenhagen Munksgaard

Felten SY, Felten DL, Olschowka JA. 1992. Noradrenergic and peptidergic innervation of lymphoid organs. Chem Immunol 52:25–48

Field EH, Noelle RJ, Rouse T, et al. 1993. Evidence for excessive Th2 CD4$^+$ subset activity in vivo. J Immunol 151:48–59

Fisher P, Ward A. 1994. Complementary medicines in Europe. Query Journal 309:107–111

Fulder SJ, Munro RE. 1985. Complementary medicine in the United Kingdom: patients, practitioners, and consultations. Lancet Sep 7:2:542–545

Han JS, Tang J, Ren MF, Zhou ZF. 1980. Central neurotransmitters and acupuncture analgesia. Am J Chin Med 8:331–348

Hatch JP, Borcherding S, Norris LK. 1990. Cardiopulmonary adjustments during operant heart rate control. Psychophysiology 27 (6):641–647

Inglis B. 1980. Natural Medicine. Fontana/Collins, Glasgow

Jian M. 1985. Influence of adrenergic antagonist and naloxone on the anti-allergic shock effect of electro-acupuncture in mice. Acupunct Electrother Res 10: 163–167

Kamada T, Shinji S, Kumashiro M, et al. 1992. Power spectral analysis of heart rate variability in type As and type Bs during mental workload. Psychosom Med 54: 462–470

Kasahara T, Wu Y, Sakurai Y, Oguchi K. 1992. Suppressive effects of acupuncture on delayed type hypersensitivity to trinitrochlorobenzene and involvement of opiate receptors. Int J Immunopharmacol 14:661–665

Lewith GT, Aldridge D (eds). 1993. Clinical Research Methodology Within Complementary Medicine. Hodder and Stoughton

L'Homeopathie en 1993. Lyons: Syndicat National de la Pharmacie Homeopathique, 1993. (Quoting CO-FREMCA and IFOP public opinion surveys.)

McCraty R, Atkinson M, Tiller WA, et al. 1995. The effects of emotions on the short term power spectral analysis of heart rate variability. Am J Cardiol (in press)

McCraty R, Atkinson M, Tiller WA, Watkins AD. 1995. The electrophysiological correlates of positive emotions: three patterns of sympathovagal balance in normal subjects. Int J Psychophysiol (submitted)

McGuire MB. 1988. Ritual healing in Suburban America. Rutgers University Press, New Brunswick, NJ

Mossman TR, Cherwinski H, Bond MW, et al. 1986. Two types of murine helper T-cell clones. I: Definition according to profiles of lymphokine activities and secreted proteins. J Immunol 136:2348–2357

Neild JE, Cameron IR. 1985. Bronchoconstriction in response to suggestion: its prevention by an inhaled anticholinergic agent. BMJ 290:674

Office of Technology Assessment. 1990. Unconventional cancer treatments. Washington DC. Government Printing Office, (OTA-H-405)

Ori Z, Monir G, Weiss J, et al. 1992. Heart rate variability. Frequency domain analysis. Cardiol Clin 10:(3)499–537

Pietroni P. The Greening of Medicine. Gollancz Ltd

Reichlin S. 1993. Neuroendocrine-immune interactions. N Eng J Med 1246–1253

Reilly DT. 1983. Young doctors' views on alternative medicine. BMJ 287:337–339

Reilly DT, Taylor MA. 1993. Developing integrated medicine: Report of the Research Council for Complementary Medicine Research Fellowship in Complementary Medicine. 1987–90. RCCM, London

Reilly DT, Taylor MA, Beattie NGM, et al. 1994. Is the evidence for homoeopathy reproducible? Lancet 344: 1601–1606

Reynolds T. 1991. J Natl Cancer Inst 83:594–596

Rosch PJ, Kearney HM. 1985. Holistic medicine and technology: A modern dialectic. Soc Sci Med 21 (12): 1405–1409

The Royal College of Physicians, London. April 1992. Allergy: Conventional and alternative concepts

Rubinfeld AR, Pain MCF. 1976. Perception of asthma. Lancet i 882–884

Sloan RP, Shapiro PA, Bagiella E, et al. 1994. Effect of mental stress throughout the day on cardiac autonomic control. Biol Psychol 37:L 89–99

Stein PK, Bosner MS, Kleiger RE, Conger BM. 1994. Heart rate variability: A measure of cardiac autonomic tone. Am Heart J 127 (5):1376–1381

Terao A, Oikawa M, Saito M. 1993. Cytokine induced changes in hypothalamic norepinephrine turnover: involvement of corticotrophin-releasing hormone and prostaglandins. Brain Res 622:257–261

Van Dijk P. 1993. Geneewijzen in Nederland. Ankh-Hermes, Deventer

Vernon HT, Dhami MSI, Howley TP, Annett R. 1986. Spinal manipulation and beta-endorphin: a controlled study of the effects of a spinal manipulation on plasma beta-endorphin levels in normal males. J Manipulative Physiol Ther 9:115–123

Watkins AD. 1994. The role of alternative therapy in allergic disease. Clin Exp Allergy 24:813–825

Watkins AD. April 1995. Perceptions, Emotions and Immunity: an integrated homoeostatic network. Q J Med 88:283–294

Watt J, Wood C (eds). 1988. Talking Health: conventional and complementary approaches. Royal Society of Medicine, London

Wharton R, Lewith G. 1986. Complementary medicine and the general practitioner. BMJ 292:1498–1500

WHO Global Strategy for Asthma Management. Feb 1994. Draft VI. National Heart, Lung, and Blood Institute, NIH World Health Organisation

Williams R, Lane JD, Kuhn CM, et al. 1982. Type A behaviour and elevated physiological responses to cognitive tasks. Science 212:483–485

Complementary Therapy Systems and Approaches

This section describes the background, context, and clinical approaches of a selective variety of alternative therapeutic systems as they have developed throughout European and American history, and of individual approaches that are suggested from contemporary western research, both within and beyond the biomedical paradigm. Where these systems and approaches can be understood in light of the contemporary biomedical paradigm, this view is examined; where they cannot be, this paradox is pointed out. It is made clear when and how medical systems are embedded in nature/ecology and when they are embedded in technology. In each case, these medical practices are presented as products of history that make sense in terms of that history.

5
Homeopathy

Jennifer Jacobs
Richard Moskowitz

*H*omeopathy is a method of self-healing assisted by small doses of medicinal substances and practiced by licensed physicians and other health care professionals throughout the world. In the United States, homeopathic medicines are protected by federal law, and most are available over the counter.

History

The homeopathic method was developed by Samuel Hahnemann, MD (1755–1843), a German physician, chemist, and author of a well-known textbook on the preparation and use of the contemporary medicines. In a series of experiments from 1790 to 1810, Hahnemann demonstrated the following: (1) medicinal substances elicit a standard array of signs and symptoms in healthy people and (2) the medicine whose symptom-picture most closely resembles the illness being treated is the one most likely to initiate a curative response for that patient (Hahnemann 1833).

Hahnemann understood these experiments to mean that the outward manifestations of illness represent the concerted attempt of an organism to heal itself, and that the corresponding remedy reinforces that attempt in some way. He coined the term *homeopathy* to describe his method of using remedies with the power to resonate with the illness as a whole, in contrast with the more conventional method of opposing symptoms with superior force.

> The word *homeopathy* is derived from the Greek roots *omoios,* meaning "similar" and *pathos,* meaning "feeling." Hahnemann also began using *allopathy* from the Greek *alloios,* meaning "other" to denote the standard practice of using medicines either to counteract symptoms or to produce an action unrelated to symptoms, such as purging, bloodletting, or blistering of the skin.

Although Hippocrates, Celsus, and Paracelsus advocated treatment with similars for some patients, and Stahl in the eighteenth century had proposed giving medicines to healthy people (Hahnemann 1833), Hahnemann understood that the detailed correspondence between the clinical symptomatology of patients and the experimental pathogenesis of remedies indicated a universal law of healing with medicinal substances. He developed a systematic philosophy of medicine and a rigorous methodology for diagnosis and treatment that were and still remain wholly unique in the history of medicine.

With the old model of self-healing effectively supplanted by the modern idea of technological control, the Hahnemannian Law of Similars—*similia similibus curentur,* or "Let likes be cured by likes"—never gained general acceptance in medicine and is even considered implausible to most physicians. Even committed homeopaths regard it as a mystery not yet explained or proven, and Hahnemann taught that it could not be deduced *a priori* or independently of experience and would have to be evaluated, as every other healing practice, by how well it works in the treatment of the sick (Hahnemann 1961).

Theoretical Basis

Essentially a methodology for treating the sick, rather than a set of hypotheses about the nature of health and disease, homeopathy begins and ends as a radical innovation in the experimental investigation of medicinal substances. Its cardinal principles follow logically from the Law of Similars and the conceptual transformations required to accommodate it.

Provings

In 1790, while experimenting with cinchona (Peruvian bark), Hahnemann decided to ingest a therapeutic dose. He soon felt cold, numb, drowsy, thirsty, and anxious, and experienced palpitations, prostration, and aching bones; he recognized these symptoms as those of *ague,* or intermittent fever, the syndrome that was then being treated with cinchona (Bradford 1895). He allowed the dose to wear off before taking a second and a third dose that confirmed his original results.

Stunned by the implications of this finding, Hahnemann devoted the rest of his life to ascertaining the therapeutic properties of medicinal substances by administering them to healthy people—himself, his colleagues, and his students. His *Materia Medica Pura* records the detailed symptomatology of over 90 medicines, a truly monumental achievement that represents 20 years of painstaking labor (Hahnemann 1833,1880).

In these *provings,* as he called them, Hahnemann administered the substance in question to a group of reasonably healthy people in doses sufficient to elicit symptoms without provoking irreversible toxicity, anatomic changes, or organic damage. A unique composite portrait, or symptom-picture, was assembled for each substance, differentiating it from every other. Therefore, a homeopathic remedy is a shorthand for the sum of observable responses of all people who have taken that remedy, a distinctive totality that must be studied as a whole and for its own sake, rather than simply as a weapon against a particular disease or a group of symptoms.

The Homeopathic *Materia Medica*

The Hahnemannian concept of medicinal action remains the most distinctive contribution of homeopathy to medical science, with important implications for pharmacology, ethnobotany, and industrial medicine and toxicology. Without recourse to pathologic models or unconsenting animal subjects, provings offer a purely experimental technique for investigating the medicinal action of any substance whatsoever.

The homeopathic pharmacopeia currently recognizes more than 2,000 remedies, with more being added all the time. Most are of plant origin, including flowers, leaves, roots, barks, fruits, and resins. Although many are poisonous in their crude state (such as aconite, belladonna, digitalis, ergot, hellebore, and nux vomica), others are common medicinal herbs (comfrey, eyebright, mullein, yellow dock); foods and spices (cayenne, garlic, mustard, onion); fragrances, resins, and residues (amber, petroleum, charcoal, kreosote); mushrooms, lichens, and mosses.

Mineral remedies include metals (copper, gold, lead, tin, zinc); metalloids (antimony, arsenic, selenium); salts (calcium sulfate, potassium carbonate, sodium chloride); alkalis; acids (hydrochloric, nitric, phosphoric, sulfuric); elemental substances (carbon, hydrogen, iodine, phosphorus, sulfur); and constituents of the earth's crust (silica, aluminum oxide, ores, rocks, lavas, mineral waters).

Remedies from the animal kingdom include venoms (of jellyfish, insects, spiders, molluscs, crustaceans, fish, amphibians, snakes); secretions (ambergris, cuttlefish ink, musk); milks, hormones, glandular and tissue extracts (sarcodes); and nosodes, or disease products (tuberculosis, gonorrhea, syphilis, abscesses, vaccines).

The investigative method of provings is applicable equally to the study of conventional drugs, unproven folk remedies, toxic or laboratory chemicals, pollutants, and commercial or industrial products (dyes, insecticides, paints, solvents). The homeopathic materia medica is as boundless as the creation of the earth and as inexhaustible as its transformation by human or environmental forces.

Finally, the richness and diversity of the materia medica database increases the likelihood that some degree of medicinal help can be found for most people, while its basic principles are simple enough that even a novice can achieve some results with a small number of remedies. As long as a few commonsense guidelines are observed, the method is perfectly safe for lay people of average intelligence to learn at their own pace, and to use for first aid and for the treatment of common domestic ailments. Considerable study and experience are required, however, to take full advantage of this enormous tool.

The Vital Force

Like acupuncture, herbalism, and other natural methods, homeopathy belongs to the vitalist tradition in medicine, based on the old *vis medicatrix naturae*, the natural healing capacity, and summarized in the aphorisms of Paracelsus.

> The art of healing comes from Nature, not the physician. . . . Every illness has its own remedy within itself. . . . A man could not be born alive and healthy were there not already a Physician hidden in him . . . (Paracelsus 1958).

Underlying these approaches is the following coherent philosophy of ancient lineage (traced elsewhere in this volume) whose precepts still ring true despite modern efforts to ignore or surpass them.

> - Healing is a concerted effort of the entire organism and cannot be achieved by any part in isolation from the whole.
>
> *(Continues)*

> - All healing is essentially self-healing, which is a basic property of all living beings.
> - Healing applies only to individuals and therefore is inherently problematic, even risky, and never reducible to any technique or formula, however scientific its foundation.

Within homeopathy, the fact that curative remedies imitate and therefore resonate with manifested signs and symptoms makes sense. Illness is viewed as the organisms attempt to heal itself. Hahnemann identified the life energy itself (the vital force), as the ultimate source of health and illness alike, ending only with the death of the organism. Whatever we wish to call it, some version of the vital force is required to refer to the obvious bioenergetic integrity of living beings.

The Totality of Symptoms

Just as provings include the full range of symptomatology elicited by each remedy, homeopathy teaches that illness is primarily a disturbance of the vital force, and manifests itself as a totality of physical, mental, and emotional responses that is unique to each patient and cannot be adequately understood as a mere specimen of any disease process. Without including every symptom, or assuming that mental symptoms and physical symptoms instigate each other, the Hahnemannian totality of symptoms simply describes the principal signs and symptoms as they appear in the patient, and is complete as soon as a reasonable sense of the illness as a whole is discernible.

To the practicing homeopath, this composite totality or psychophysical style—far more than any abstract disease category or printout of laboratory abnormalities—furnishes the truest picture of the health and illness of the patient as a whole, as well as of the particular condition for which treatment is being sought.

In practice, the totality of the symptoms demands that the remedy take into account the living experience of the patient, including the full range of thoughts and feelings. It by no means rejects or ignores the technical expertise of the physician, and does not hesitate to make use of pathologic diagnosis or of conventional drugs or surgery. Homeopathy uses the technical language of abnormalities to educate the patient, allowing the patient to retain control and to participate at every step. The diagnosis also is important in predicting patient response to homeopathic treatment, as well as the prognosis.

The totality of symptoms also explains why mental and emotional symptoms sometimes weigh heavily in choosing the remedy. Whereas most physical symptoms refer to a certain part of the body (arm, nose, back, or stomach), psychological states describe how patients feel as a whole (afraid, depressed, happy, confused). The totality of symptoms gives special importance to describing the condition of the patient as a whole.

The Single Remedy

Based on the materia medica, the Hahnemannian method employs one remedy at a time for the whole patient, comparing the totality of symptoms of the individual with those of various remedies until the closest possible match is found. The reason is that single remedies have the capacity to match the totalities with the individuality of each patient. Their power and effectiveness are proportional to the ability of patients to respond to them as a whole by virtue of that resemblance.

On the other hand, its encyclopedic scale insures that the homeopathic materia medica can never be grasped in its entirety; some have tried to abbreviate and simplify it, and competent and reputable physicians use two, three, or more remedies simultaneously. Over the counter combination remedies also are available in many pharmacies and health food stores and are safe and effective if used properly.

The totality of symptoms enables the serious student to accumulate detailed personal experience with remedies and generates much of the excitement while learning how to use them. Administering different remedies to each part of a patient makes it difficult to know which remedy has acted; as such, remedies would have to be selected according to the rough indications of folk medicine or the technical language of abnormalities, much like conventional drug treatment. Under these conditions, what is learned will not yield an experience that can build

on itself or a method that can be taught. The revival of American homeopathy in recent years has been achieved largely on the strength of the single remedy concept. Only the totality of symptoms can display remedies and patients are unique individuals worthy of study for their own sake.

The Minimum Dose

Because homeopathic remedies stimulate an ailing self-healing mechanism, rather than correcting a specific abnormality, large or prolonged doses are seldom required and even might spoil the effect. Homeopaths use the smallest possible doses and only repeat them if necessary, allowing remedies to complete their action without further interference. Indeed, the remedy will not work unless it fits the illness so closely as to render the patient uniquely susceptible to its action. The minuteness of the dose makes it exceedingly unlikely that any untoward or dangerous side effects will occur.

In a series of experiments, Hahnemann discovered that remedies are still effective in concentrations that are too small to be detected chemically, and that mechanical shaking or "succussion" of diluted remedies actually enhances their healing effect in a way that has never been fully understood. Assuming that dilute remedies act by energizing the organism, he theorized that succussion liberates that energy from its chemical bonds and releases it into the solution, thus foreshadowing the discovery of subatomic forces in the twentieth century (Hahnemann 1833, 1961).

Hahnemann's advocacy of infinitesimal doses remains one of the most controversial aspects of his work. No one has explained satisfactorily how medicines diluted beyond the molecular threshold of Avogadro's number could possibly have any effect, let alone a curative one. But the standard argument that the remedies are simply placebos cuts both ways. People do, in fact, heal themselves of serious illnesses without drugs or surgery. With its dilutions now detectable by laser spectroscopy and bioassay (Boiron 1976, Noiret 1976), homeopathy envisions a new bioenergetic science that is still in its infancy.

The Laws of Cure

The totality of symptoms also makes clear why drugs that successfully lower the blood pressure, kill bacteria, or correct physiologic abnormality may leave the patient feeling as bad or worse than before. Judgments about improvement, worsening, and the effectiveness of treatment are difficult to interpret apart from the totality of symptoms, from how patients feel as a whole, and from how they function according to their own individual standards. Perhaps the greatest shortcoming of the biomedical model is its failure to comprehend patients as integrated energy systems and to follow them throughout their lifetime.

Since the era of Hahnemann, classical homeopathy has addressed this critical issue by attempting to track the order in which symptoms and illnesses appear, the grouping of symptoms that appear and disappear together, and the relation of each group to the overall health and functioning of the patient. Constantine Hering proposed four general directions in which symptoms tend to move or redistribute themselves during the recovery process.

Symptom Movement in the Cure and Recovery Process

- From above downwards, from the head toward the feet.
- From inside outwards, from interior to peripheral parts.
- From more vital to less vital organs, from more visceral to less essential structures.
- From the most recent to the oldest, in the reverse order of their appearance in the life history of the patient. (Hering 1865 1875).

Although the fourth principle has proved most reliable for case management, and the relative importance of organs and tissues often is difficult to assess—some approximation of the totality of symptoms over time remains indispensable to the general assessment of the patient as a whole, for clinician and researcher alike.

Methodology

Pharmacy

The Homeopathic Pharmacopoeia of the United States (American Institute of Homeopathy, 1979), is the official standard for the preparation of homeopathic medicines. Crude medicinal substances are made into remedies by serial dilution and succussion in a liquid or solid medium. First crushed and dissolved in a specified volume of 95 percent grain alcohol, crude plant materials are shaken and stored, and the supernatant liquid is kept as the "mother tincture." The same procedure is used for animal products, nosodes, and any other substances that are soluble in alcohol. Metals, ores, and other insoluble remedies are pulverized with mortar and pestle and diluted with lactose, succussing until they become soluble.

Tinctures are further diluted with alcohol or lactose, either 1:10 (the decimal scale, written "X") or 1:100 (the centesimal, written "C"), and succussed vigorously, yielding the 1X or 1C dilution. The process is repeated for the 2X, 3X, 4X (or 2C, 3C, 4C), and on up as desired.

In clinical practice, any dilution may be used, but the most popular for self-care are the 6th, 12th, and 30th (X or C). Higher dilutions for professional work are in the centesimal scale, namely, the 200th, 1000th, 10,000th, and 50,000th, written 200C, 1M, 10M, and 50M, and representing dilutions of 10^{-400}, 10^{-2000}, $10^{-20,000}$, and $10^{-100,000}$, respectively.

The general skepticism about diluted remedies—as expressed by Oliver Wendell Holmes and modern critics—is readily understandable, since even the 12C and 30C are well beyond the Avogadro limit and therefore out of the realm of conventional chemistry entirely (Holmes 1842).

Case-Taking

As in general medicine, seeing patients requires more than simply taking down information or selecting remedies. Allowing patients to tell their story, in its entirety, relieves their burden of pain and suffering, making the homeopathic interview a powerful healing experience in its own right. It even might suggest a path of recovery, allowing remedies to continue the process.

Patients are invited to speak and allowed to continue for as long a time as possible without interruption, while homeopaths ask "What else?" as often as necessary, to elicit more symptoms and to remind the patient that no one disease is being sought, but rather the totality of symptoms. Symptoms are written down verbatim whenever possible, leaving space in the right-hand margin for the homeopath's own observations.

After the patient finishes his or her story and the principal symptoms have been noted, the homeopath must investigate further in order to characterize symptoms in detail. Conventional diagnosis is based on common symptoms such as fever, pain, cough, and bleeding, whereas homeopaths look for unusual or idiosyncratic features that tend to be ignored or discarded by conventional physicians.

Fully-Characterized Symptoms Described in a Homeopathic Interview

- Subjective sensations such as pain, vertigo, fatigue, and anger.
- Localization of symptoms (one-sided, wandering, radiating, circumscribed, or diffuse).
- Modalities, that is, factors by which symptoms are modified (intensified or relieved) according to changes in the time of day, the weather, diet, or emotional state.
- Concomitants, or symptoms that appear simultaneously or in sequence (nausea with headache, fever after chill).

The interview also includes physical examination and laboratory work as needed to establish a diagnosis.

Selecting the Remedy

As the case is taken, symptoms are graded in importance by the extent to which information is freely volunteered and clearly delineated, and by how severely limiting they are to the overall health and well-being of the patient. Homeopathic prescribing lays bare the incredible correspondence that exists between the database of the materia medica and the details of each patient's case record. Each of these great texts continually illuminates the other, but an encyclopedic memory or a computer with a similar capacity would be necessary to allow proper study on use of the wealth of remedies and symptoms properly.

For professional homeopaths to gain access to as many remedies as possible, they need help in proceeding from the clinical totality to a menu of possible remedies that they can study and choose from. This is the purpose of the *repertory*, an index of symptoms and the remedies that either have elicited them in provings or that cured them clinically. By finding the remedies that match the leading symptoms in a case, the search for a cure can be narrowed down.

Whether in the form of a book or computer software, the largest, most comprehensive repertories (Warkentin 1991, Archimed 1993) include all types of symptoms from every anatomical region and physiologic system, as well as mental and emotional symptoms, "generalities" (physical symptoms or modalities attributable to the patient as a whole), and rare symptoms whose very oddity points directly to the remedy. The repertory is only a tool for locating remedies; these remedies must then be studied in the materia medica, and the final selection is based on a total or qualitative fit, more than on any narrow, technical calculation.

Regimen and Precautions

Although they remain stable in the cold and across a wide range of temperatures, dilute remedies are inactivated by direct sunlight and should be stored in a dark, dry place, and shielded from X-rays. Patients are instructed to put nothing in the mouth for at least 30 minutes before and after each dose. Coffee and camphorated products might reverse the effects of the remedy and should be avoided throughout the treatment period, even when no remedies are actually being taken. The use of medicinal herbs, and exposure to mothballs and other aromatic substances also should be curtailed.

Although conventional drugs often interfere and should be avoided when possible, severely ill patients should not stop taking medications. Because of their potentially synergistic effect, acupuncture and chiropractic should not be started concurrently with homeopathic remedies, but if already in progress, may be continued. Relapse might also follow dental work that includes drilling and local anesthesia.

Administration and Dosage

Remedies are dispensed in the form of tablets or pellets of sucrose or lactose that are taken dry on the tongue or dissolved in water. Lower dilutions are preferred in acute situations, because they can be repeated as often as necessary and will be somewhat effective even if only broadly similar to the totality of the case. Higher dilutions are used mostly by professionals for chronic treatment; more care must be taken in their selection, and they should not be repeated while their action is in progress.

In homeopathy, the term dosage refers primarily to the number and frequency of repetitions, which must be tailored to fit the patient very much like the choice of the remedy itself. In both acute and chronic cases, the rule is to stop the remedy once the reaction is apparent, repeating only when the reaction has subsided.

Pros and Cons

There are few, if any, absolute contraindications to homeopathic treatment. Although patients with severely disabling illnesses or chronic drug dependence are difficult to help—by any method—homeopathy at least might be considered before resorting to more drastic measures or after conventional methods have failed. Homeopathic remedies are wonderfully safe, economical, simple to administer, and gentle in their action, with very few serious or prolonged adverse effects. Although subtle at first, the effects of treatment are prompt, thorough, and long-lasting.

On the other hand, homeopathy is far from a panacea for all ills. It is a difficult and exacting art. Even after years of study and practice, a skilled prescriber might need to try several remedies before any benefit is obtained. Some cases might show little or no improvement, despite the most conscientious efforts. Remedies are rather delicate and easily inactivated, so certain precautions must be observed. Finally, we do not understand how dilute remedies act and cannot predict how a patient will respond, or which symptoms will change and in what order. Like all medicine, homeopathy is an art dependent upon the life energy of individual human beings.

Historical Development

Early Controversies

Although his successful treatment and prophylaxis of a scarlet fever epidemic brought fame to homeopathy widely throughout Europe, Hahnemann was ridiculed and persecuted for his heresies until 1822, when he was awarded a stipend to publish his writings (Bradford 1895). In addition to his *Organon of Medicine* and *Materia Medica Pura,* he wrote many technical and expository works, maintained a busy correspondence, and continued to practice and conduct experimental research. Hahnemann died secure in the knowledge that his students were practicing homeopathy throughout Europe and America. Fired by ambition and gifted with intellect, he left a body of work and a methodology that have stood the test of time.

Homeopathy in America

In the latter half of the nineteenth century, the United States became the center of the homeopathy movement and produced some of its greatest masters, whose works still enjoy international use. Several factors contributed to the rapid growth and development of American homeopathy.

The first was the absence of laws or bureaucracy to license the practice of medicine, a tolerant attitude born of the hope to break free from the oppressive social and economic constraints of Europe. When the first school of homeopathy opened in Pennsylvania during the 1830s, American physicians were organized on a voluntary basis, and state legislatures were reluctant to prevent uneducated or lay healers from helping anyone who wanted to use their services (Starr 1982).

The second factor was the great migration of those seeking land and fortune in the west, where doctors were scarce and people were forced to heal themselves and their families. Homeopathy was well suited for self-care, and popular manuals on first aid and the treatment of common domestic ailments began to appear during this period (Hering 1844).

Finally, the concept of the materia medica itself was easily adapted to native American medicine. Introducing dozens of native American herbs into the pharmacopeia, American homeopathy was enriched by the botanical lore of midwives, medicine men, eclectics, and other herbalists whose recipes are still in use today (Hale 1867).

Under these conditions, homeopathy flourished in the United States, inspiring the creation of hospitals, medical schools, and insane asylums that scored notable triumphs that attracted public attention (Coulter 1973). During epidemics of cholera, typhus, and scarlet fever, homeopathy consistently proved its superiority over the punishing treatments then in vogue (Bradford 1900). Physicians practicing this new method quickly rose to social prominence, treating such rich and famous patients as President Lincoln and the members of his Cabinet (Coulter 1973). By the turn of the century, 10 percent of all physicians used homeopathy in their practices (Ullman 1991).

During and after the Civil War, however, the tremendous expansion of American industry transformed the nature of medicine. American homeopathy—with its use of minimal doses at rare intervals—never created a large or profitable industrial base capable of financing large educational or research institutions. Experimental medicine, based on rigorous physicochemical causality, generated such unprecedented technical achievements as anesthesia, antisepsis, surgery, microbiology, vaccines, and antibiotics (Bernard 1957).

The American Medical Association (AMA) and its state societies forbade its members to consult or fraternize with homeopaths (Coulter 1973). Such persecution had little effect until state legislatures began to license physicians and accredit medical schools and the pharmaceutical industry won control of the process (Starr 1982). Thereafter, the AMA invited homeopaths and physicians of all schools to become members in exchange for licensing, creating a monopoly against lay healers, midwives, and herbalists. The Flexner Report, published in 1914, proposed a uniform standard of medical education for all physicians and used the power of accreditation to phase out homeopathic colleges who fell short of these standards (Starr 1982).

The AMA strategy succeeded. By the 1920s, the homeopathic schools either had closed or conformed to the new model, and homeopathy was reduced to a postgraduate specialty for the few physicians who were prepared to swim against the tide. Although some fine homeopathic physicians continued to practice, the movement declined rapidly over the next 40 years. By 1970, homeopathy appeared to be moribund, its teachers aged or dead (Kaufman 1971).

American homeopathy has begun to flourish once more, thanks largely to the rebirth of the self-care movement, the health care crisis, and the overmedicalization that provoked these events (Illich 1976). By eliminating lay healers and aspiring to control every abnormality by purely technical means, American medicine has became a colossus that thrives on great cost and great risk (Moskowitz 1988), generating more iatrogenic illness (Steel 1981) and consuming a greater share of the GNP than anywhere else in the world. Facing crises in health insurance, malpractice litigation, and the doctor–patient relationship (Moskowitz 1988), the public—and now the medical profession itself—have turned to alternatives like those described in this text. Safe, effective, and inexpensive enough to sustain busy practices even without third-party reimbursement, homeopathy has become increasingly popular with young family physicians, whose instant waiting lists approximate the virtually limitless demand for their services. As in frontier days, the renaissance of American homeopathy would not be occurring were it not for the devotion of lay people—not only for self-care, but also for organizing study groups in their communities and teaching these methods to their friends and neighbors.

Research

Hahnemann's system of provings—using individuals to determine the symptoms that a medicine could produce—was the first research in homeopathy. Indeed, the whole field is based on this experimental work, which was unprecedented both in methodology and in scope. Provings are still used on many herbal medicines that have been used by traditional healers for centuries, particularly in Asia and in South America. Proving methodology also is being modernized; statistical methods are utilized to determine the significance of various symptoms.

Modern homeopathic research focuses on three basic questions: (1) Do highly dilute substances affect physical and biological systems? (2) Can homeopathic medicines be proven to be effective clinically? and (3) What is the mechanism of action of homeopathic medicines?

Basic Science Research

Basic scientific research in homeopathy primarily has investigated the chemical and biological activity of highly diluted substances. As discussed previously, Hahnemann found that if the homeopathic remedies were highly diluted to concentrations as low as 10^{-30} to $10^{-20,000}$, there would still be a medicinal effect with minimal side effects. Most scientists reject homeopathic theory because of this extreme dilution of the medicine beyond Avogadro's number of 10^{-24}, beyond which point molecules theoretically cease to exist.

In the mid-1950s, a review of 25 investigations of microdoses was published, citing their effects on such widely variant systems as paramecia, the Schick test, growth of *Aspergillus mycelia,* germination of wheat germ, and blood flow in the ears of rabbits (Stephenson 1955). More recent European laboratory studies have demonstrated the effects of homeopathically prepared microdoses on mouse macrophages (Davenas 1987), arsenic mobilization in the rat (Cazin 1987), bleeding time with aspirin (Doutremepuich 1987), and degranulation of human basophils (Poitevin 1988). There also have been studies that showed the insignificant effects of microdoses, such as on the excretion kinetics of lead in rats (Fisher 1987).

More than 100 studies have researched the effects of high dilutions in the fields of immunology, toxicology, and pharmacology (Belon 1987, Bastide 1994). One of the most intriguing studies revealed that highly dilute preparations of thyroid hormone introduced into an aquarium had a statistically sig-

nificant effect on the climbing behavior of frogs, even when the preparation was completely encased in a glass vial (Endler 1994).

The most well known study of the effects of high dilutions was published in 1988, showing degranulation of human basophils by IgE antibodies diluted as high as 10^{-120} (Davenas 1988). This paper was highly criticized in Europe because it challenged the basic tenets of biomedicine, and its findings were later challenged (Maddox 1988). The controversy over this study continues, with attempts to repeat the experiment reporting success as well as failure (Benveniste 1991).

Clinical Research

Prior to the mid 1980s, little clinical research in homeopathy was published outside of homeopathic journals. The first double-blind experiment published in a peer-review medical journal showed statistically significant results in treating rheumatoid arthritis with individualized prescribing of remedies (Gibson 1980). A later study on arthritis showed no effect using homeopathic treatment (Shipley 1983); however, all of the patients had been given the same medicine, *Rhus-toxicodendron*. This study illustrates the difficulty in doing clinical research in homeopathy. Homeopathic medicines are individualized, by definition, based on the totality of symptoms. Most conventional clinical research involves administering the same medicine to all patients.

Recent clinical trials in Europe have suggested a positive treatment association between homeopathic medicines and the treatment of allergic rhinitis (Reilly 1986), fibrositis (Fisher 1989), influenza (Ferley 1989), and asthma (Reilly 1994). A trial of childhood respiratory illnesses had equivocal results (de Lange de Klerk 1995). The *British Medical Journal* published a meta-analysis of homeopathic clinical trials in 1992, which found that 15 of 22 well-designed studies showed positive results, and concluded that more methodologically rigorous trials should be done to evaluate the efficacy of homeopathic treatment (Kleijnen 1991). A recent study comparing homeopathic treatment with placebo in the treatment of acute childhood diarrhea demonstrated improvement in the homeopathy group (Jacobs 1994).

Mechanism of Action

There is no scientific explanation for the mechanism of action of homeopathic medicines, although there are several theories. Recent developments in quantum physics have led some scientists to suggest that electromagnetic energy in the medicines interact with the body on some level (Delinick 1991). Researchers in physical chemistry have proposed the *memory of water* theory, whereby the structure of the water/alcohol solution is altered by the medicine during the process of dilution and retains its new structure even after the medicine dissolves (Resch 1987). Recent developments in chaos theory support these answers, since a basic tenet of this theory is that very small changes can affect large systems (Shepperd 1994).

Cost-effectiveness and Outcomes

Another relevant area of research in homeopathy is cost-effectiveness and outcomes. In France, the annual cost to the Social Security System for a homeopathic physician is 15 percent less than that of a conventional physician and the price of the average homeopathic medicine is one third that of standard drugs (CNAM 1991). Many believe that outcomes research will prove to be the most important area of homeopathic research over the next five years (Jacobs 1994). Such indicators as overall health status (for which there are several widely accepted scales), patient satisfaction, days missed from school or work, and the cost of treatment are used to compare the outcomes of different types of treatment. This approach would be particularly useful in looking at the homeopathic treatment of chronic illnesses, which do not lend themselves to the double-blind methodology.

Homeopathy Today

The use of homeopathy is increasing rapidly throughout the world, particularly in Europe, Latin America, and Asia. In Germany, 25 percent of all physicians use homeopathy (Ullman 1991); in France, 32 percent of general practice physicians use it (Bouchayer 1990); and in Great Britain, 42 percent of physicians refer patients to homeopaths (Wharton & Lewith 1986). In India, homeopathy is practiced in the national health service, at several hundred homeopathic medical schools, and by more than 100,000 homeopaths (Kishore 1983).

Other developing countries have turned to homeopathy as the cost of conventional, western medicine grows out of reach. In both Argentina and Brazil, several thousand physicians use homeopathy, and Mexico has five medical colleges that provide homeopathic training. South Africa has homeopathic medical colleges in several major cities, and the health ministry in Israel recently approved the importation of homeopathic preparations for sale in pharmacies.

The use of homeopathy by the United States has increased tremendously in the last 20 years. A survey showed that 1 percent of the American population used homeopathy in 1989 (Eisenberg 1993). Sales of homeopathic remedies increased by 1000 percent during the 1980s (Food and Drug Administration 1985), and were reported to be $200 million in 1992, climbing at the rate of 25 percent per year (Swander 1994).

Appropriate Use

Homeopathic remedies are most likely to be successful and to optimize overall health for several types of conditions as described below.

Uses of Homeopathic Remedies

- Functional complaints with little or no tissue damage, such as headache, insomnia, chronic fatigue, and premenstrual syndrome.
- Conditions for which no effective conventional treatment is available, such as viral illnesses, traumatic injuries, surgical wounds, multiple sclerosis, and AIDS.
- Conditions that require chronic use of conventional drugs, such as allergies, recurring infections, arthritis, skin conditions, and digestive problems.

(Continues)

- Conditions for which elective surgery has been proposed, but immediate attention is unnecessary, such as fibroid tumors, gallstones, and hemorrhoids.
- Conditions that have not been cured by conventional treatments, either because of the inappropriateness of the medication, the determined nature of the disease, or patient's noncompliance.

Homeopathy is not appropriate for the treatment of chronic diseases involving advanced tissue damage, such as cirrhosis of the liver or severe cardiovascular disease; for people with prolonged dependence on conventional medication such as corticosteroids, anticonvulsants, and antipsychotics; or as a substitute for appropriate conventional treatments such as emergency surgery or reduction of fractures.

Practice Patterns

A recent survey of American physicians documented interesting differences between those using homeopathic medicines in their practices and those employing more conventional remedies (American Institute of Homeopathy 1992). Physicians using homeopathy saw fewer patients and spent more than twice as much time with each patient, averaging 30 minutes per visit, as opposed to the 12.5 minutes spent with each patient by conventional physicians. In addition, homeopathic physicians ordered half as many diagnostic procedures and laboratory tests than conventional physicians and prescribed fewer standard medications.

This survey also polled the most common diagnoses seen by these physicians. Asthma, headaches, depression, allergies, psychological problems, and skin problems were among the top ten conditions treated most frequently by homeopathic physicians. Conventional physicians, on the other hand, saw more hypertension, upper respiratory tract infections, diabetes, sore throats, bronchitis, back disorders, and acute sprains and strains. These practice patterns suggest that patients seek homeopathic care mostly for chronic conditions that are not managed adequately by conventional medicine. The low number of acute problems seen by homeopaths might be due to patients treating these conditions at home.

References

American Institute of Homeopathy. 1989. The Homeopathic Pharmacopoeia of the United States. Falls Church, Virginia

American Institute of Homeopathy. 1992. Unpublished Survey Data

Archimed, Inc. 1993. RADAR Version 3.0. Namur, Belgium.

Bastide M. 1994. Immunological examples of UHD research. In Endler PC (ed): Ultra High Dilution: Physiology and Physics. Klewer Acad Pub, Dordrecht, Germany

Belon P. 1987. Homeopathy and immunology. Proceedings of the 42nd Congress of the LMHI. Arlington, Virginia, 265–270

Benveniste J, Davenas E, Ducot B, et al. 1991. L'agitation de solutions hautement diluees n'induit pas d'activite specifique. Comptes Rendus Acad Sci Paris 312(II): 461–466

Bernard C. 1957. An Introduction to the Study of Experimental Medicine. Greene HC (transl). Dover, New York, pp. 65–67

Boiron J. 1976. Studies of the Physical Structure of Homeopathic Dilutions Utilizing the Raman Laser Effect Proceedings, 31st Congress of the International Homeopathic Medical League, Athens, pp. 459–474

Bouchayer F. 1990. Alternative medicines: a general approach to the French situation. Complem Med Research 4:4–8

Bradford TL. 1895. The Life and Letters of Samuel Hahnemann. Boericke and Tafel, Philadelphia, pp. 37, 124–126

Bradford TL. 1900. The Logic of Figures, or Comparative Results of Homeopathic and Other Treatments. Boericke and Tafel, Philadelphia, pp. 141–145

Cazin J, Cazin M, Gaborit JL, et al. 1987. A study of the effect of decimal and centesimal dilutions of arsenic on the retention and mobilization of arsenic in the rat. Hum Toxicol 6:315–320

Clarke JH. 1962. Dictionary of Practical Materia Medica, 3 vols., Health Science Press, Rustington, United Kingdom

CNAM. Healthcare professionals in private practice in 1990. Social Security Statistics. CNAM publication no 61, Paris

Coulter H. 1973. Divided Legacy. McGrath, Washington, pp. 140–238, 285–316

Davenas E, Beauvais F, Amara J. 1988. Human basophil degranulation triggered by very dilute antiserum against IgE. Nature 333:816–818

Davenas E, Poitevan B, Benveniste J. 1987. Effect on mouse peritoneal macrophages of orally administered very high dilutions of silica. Eur J Pharmacol 135: 313–319

de Lange de Klerk ESM, Blommers J, Kuik DJ, et al. 1995. Effect of homeopathic medicines on daily burden of symptoms in children with recurrent upper respiratory tract infections. BMJ 309:1329–1332

Delinick AN. 1991. A hypothesis on how homeopathic remedies work on the organism. Berl J Res Homeopath 1:249–253

Doutremepuich C, et al. 1987. Template bleeding time after ingestion of ultra low dosages of acetyl salicylic acid in healthy subjects. Thromb Res 48:501–504

Eisenberg DM, Kessler RC, Foster C, et al. 1993. Unconventional medicine in the United States. N Engl J Med 328:246–252

Endler PC, Pongratz W, Kastberger G, et al. 1994. The effect of highly diluted thyroxine on the climbing activity of frogs. Vet Hum Toxicol 36:56–59

Food and Drug Administration. 1985. Riding the coattails of homeopathy. Food and Drug Administration Consumer. p. 31

Ferley JP, Smirou D, D'Adhemar D, Balducci F. 1989. A controlled evaluation of a homeopathic preparation in the treatment of influenza-like syndromes. Br J Clin Pharmacol 27:329–335

Fisher P. 1987. The influence of the homeopathic remedy Plumbum Metallicum on the excretion kinetics of lead in rats. Hum Toxicol 6:321–324

Fisher P, Greenwood A, Huskisson EC, et al. 1989. Effect of homeopathic treatment on fibrositis (primary fibromyalgia). BMJ 299:365–366

Gibson RG, Gibson SL, MacNeill AD, Buchanan WW. 1980. Homoeopathic therapy in rheumatoid arthritis: evaluation by double-blind clinical therapeutic trial. Br J Clin Pharmacol 9:453–459

Hahnemann S. 1833. Organon of Medicine, 5th Ed., Boericke W. and Dudgeon E. (transl). Roy, Calcutta, pp. 45, 53–70, 269–270

Hahnemann S. 1880. Materia Medica Pura, Dudgeon E. (trans). Hahnemann Publishing Society. Liverpool

Hale EM. 1867. Homeopathic Materia Medica of the New Remedies. Lodge, Detroit

Hering C. 1844. The Homeopathist or Domestic Physician. Philadelphia

Hering C. 1865. Hahnemann's Three Rules Concerning the Rank of Symptoms. *Hahnemannian Monthly* 1:5–12

Hering C. 1875. Analytical Therapeutics. Boericke and Tafel, Philadelphia, p. 24

Hering C. 1891. Guiding Symptoms Hering Estate, Philadelphia

Holmes OW, Sr. 1842. Homeopathy and Its Kindred Delusions. Ticknor, Boston

Illich I. 1976. Medical Nemesis. Pantheon, New York

Jacobs J, Jiménez LM, Gloyd SS, et al. 1994. Treatment of acute childhood diarrhea with homeopathic medicine: a randomized clinical trial in Nicaragua. Pediatrics 93: 719–725

Jacobs J. 1994. Future directions in homeopathic research. J Am Inst Homeopat 87:155–159

Kaufman M. 1971. Homeopathy in America: the Rise and Fall of a Medical Heresy. Johns Hopkins, Baltimore

Kishore J. 1983. Homeopathy: the Indian experience. World Health Forum 4:105–107

Kleijnen J, Knipschild P, ter Riet G. 1991. Clinical trials of homoeopathy. BMJ 302:316–323

Maddox J, Randi J, Stewart J. 1988. "High-dilution" experiments a delusion. Lancet 334:287–290

Moskowitz R. 1988. Some Thoughts on the Malpractice Crisis. Br Homeopat J 77:17

Noiret R. 1976. Activity of Several Homeopathic Dilutions of Copper Sulfate in Different Microbial Species, Proceedings, 31st Congress of the International Homeopathic Medical League, Athens, pp. 137–147

Paracelsus PATB. 1958. Selected Writings, Guterman N. (transl). Jacobi J. (ed). Pantheon, New York, pp. 50, 76

Poitevin B, Davenas E, Benveniste J. 1988. In vitro immunological degranulation of human basophils is modulated by lung histamine and apis mellifica. Br J Clin Pharmacol 25:439–444

Reilly DT, Taylor MA, Beattie NGM, et al. 1994. Is evidence of homeopathy reproducible? Lancet 344: 1601–1606

Reilly DT, Taylor MA, McSharry C, Aitchison T. 1986. Is homoeopathy a placebo response? Controlled trial of homoeopathic potency, with pollen in hayfever as model. Lancet ii:881–885

Resch G. 1987. Physical Chemistry of Highly Attenuated Remedies. Proceedings, 42nd Congress of the International Homeopathic League, Washington, pp. 300–304

Resch G, Gutmann V. 1987. Scientific Foundations of Homeopathy, English ed. Barthel & Barthel Publishing, Germany

Shepperd J. 1994. Chaos theory: implications for homeopathy. J Am Inst Homeopat 87:22–29

Shipley M, Berry H, Broster G, et al. 1983. Controlled trial of homeopathic treatment of osteoarthritis. Lancet i:97–98

Starr P. 1982. The Social Transformation of American Medicine. Basic Books, New York, pp. 30–59, 99–123

Steel K. 1981. Iatrogenic Illness on a General Medical Service at a University Hospital. N Engl J Med 304:638

Stephenson J. 1955. A review of investigations in the action of substances in dilutions greater than 1×10^{-24} (microdilutions). J Am Inst Homeopat 48:327–35

Swander H. 1994. Homeopathy: medical enigma attracts renewed attention. Am Acad Fam Pract Rep XXI(6):1–2

Ullman D. 1991. Discovering Homeopathy. North Atlantic Books, Berkeley, California

Ullman D. 1991. The international homeopathic renaissance. Berl J Homeopat 1(2):118–120

Warkentin D. 1991. MacRepertory, Version 3.41. Kent Homeopathic Associates, San Anselmo, California

Wharton R, Lewith G. 1986. Complementary medicine and the general practitioner. BMJ 292:1498–1500

6
Osteopathy

Glenn N. Wagner

*O*steopathy, or osteopathic medicine, celebrated its 100th birthday in 1992. This field is a distinctly American development. Although Andrew Taylor Still formulated this unique philosophy years earlier, 1892 is considered the birth date of osteopathic medicine because it marks the founding of the American School of Osteopathy in Kirksville, Missouri. Today, there are 15 osteopathic schools graduating an average of 1600 students per year, and approximately 32,000 DOs (doctors of osteopathy) providing care to 20 million Americans—roughly 10 percent of the population. Ten of these schools are affiliated with universities and publicly funded.

Definitions of Osteopathy

- That system of the healing arts which places the chief emphasis upon the structural integrity of the body mechanism as being the most important single factor in maintaining the well-being of the organism in health and disease (Magoun 1978).
- Perrin T. Wilson (1957) defined osteopathy as a comprehensive system of diagnosis and therapeutics based on utilizing the interrelationship between
(Continues)

---

anatomy and physiology for the study, prevention, and cure of disease (Wilson 1957).

- Leon Chaitow (1993), a British osteopath active in alternative medicine, defined osteopathy as a form of physical medicine that helps to restore the structural balance of the musculoskeletal system combining joint manipulation, physical therapy, and postural reeducation (Chaitow 1993).
- Alan Stoddard, another British osteopath and author of several frequently referenced texts on osteopathic principles and techniques, defined osteopathy as a system of healing in which chief emphasis is placed on the structural and mechanical problems of the body. The practice of osteopathy, while recognizing that human beings are complex entities influenced by a wide range of environmental and inherent factors, is concerned primarily with the mechanics of the body—how far the body is structurally normal or where it is abnormal, how that abnormality influences its health, and how to restore normal mechanics or when that it is not possible how best to
(Continues)

help the body adapt itself to its structural weakness (Stoddard 1959).

- A clinical art and science augmented by special methods and skills directed to the regulation and correction of musculo-skeletal function. . . . He notes that the reason for this biologic emphasis is not only that osteopathic medicine views the musculoskeletal system as a prime factor in functional derangement, but in addition that the body structure is recognized as an important source of physiologic derangement and as a major avenue for the application of therapy designed to assist natural defenses and to repair and restore physiologic adaptive functions (Northup 1969).

- A system of therapy founded by Andrew Taylor Still (1828–1917) and based on the theory that the body is capable of making its own remedies against disease and other toxic conditions when it is in normal structural relationship and has favorable environmental conditions and adequate nutrition. It utilizes generally accepted physical, medicinal, and surgical methods of diagnosis and therapy, while placing chief emphasis on the importance of normal body mechanics and manipulative methods of detecting and correcting faulty structure (Dorland 1974).

History

Andrew Taylor Still was born in Virginia in 1828. His father was a Methodist minister, physician, farmer, and millwright. During his youth, the family moved west to bring religion to the frontier. Despite the rigors of frontier life in Kansas, Andrew Taylor Still had a nearly continuous formal education until the age of 20. Then—with aspirations of becoming a physician, but hundreds of miles from the nearest medical school—Andrew "read medicine" for three years and served as an apprentice to his father. In 1854, he was listed on the roll of licensed physicians, and for the next 20 years maintained a traditional allopathic practice. (During this period, he also was elected to the Kansas State Legislature on the Abolitionist ticket, and served as a surgeon in the Union Army during the Civil War, holding the rank of Major at his discharge.)

In 1864, an epidemic of spinal meningitis claimed the lives of three of Andrew Taylor Still's children. This personal catastrophe caused him to re-examine medicine, particularly the subject of disease in humans and animals, based on detailed dissections and clinical observations. In 1874, Still broke with traditional medicine and announced his philosophy of osteopathy. Despite the fact that he initially applied his new philosophy and therapies in conjunction with accepted allopathic remedies, his theories generated considerable opposition from local colleagues.

Still became an itinerant physician and traveled throughout Kansas and Missouri before finally settling in Kirksville, Missouri, in 1887. He gradually reduced the use of drugs in his practice, and apparently rejected their use altogether by 1884. In 1892, in response to numerous requests, Still joined with William Smith, MD, MRCP (an Edinburgh graduate with 7 years of formal medical education) to establish the American School of Osteopathy in Kirksville, Missouri. The school was granted a charter by the state to grant the MD degree, but Still rejected this option in favor of a *DO* degree to distinguish its graduates from those of allopathic programs. Declared open to "negroes and women," the first class was comprised of 18 students, including three women (Suter 1988, Greenman 1989).

Still published four works: the Autobiography of Andrew T. Still (1897), Philosophy of Osteopathy (1899), Philosophy and Mechanical Principles of Osteopathy (1902), and Osteopathy Research and Practice (1910). He died in 1917, at the age of 89.

Considerable discussion has revolved around Andrew Taylor Still's rejection of drugs in medical therapy. His contemporaries, William Osler and Oliver Wendell Holmes, also denounced the widespread use of drugs—particularly the often toxic polypharmacy—in favor of other therapeutic modalities. (Suter 1988, Cushing 1925, Osler 1892). Considering the drugs used during this time, such as heavy metals, this attitude is not surprising.

Still is probably best recognized for his philosophy on the role of the musculoskeletal system in health and disease, and the importance of unobstructed vascular and neural pathways. He believed that health and disease were not dependent on sharply compartmentalized anatomic or self-limiting physiologic systems. The body functioned as a unit, and to understand health and disease, one had to consider the total body.

Still maintained that the unity of the body could not be understood without the musculoskeletal system, which comprises 60 percent of the body mass. Although joint strains and sprains resulting in pathologic limitations of normal joint motion manifest their more obvious effects in the local area of the lesion, joint dysfunction may mimic the symptomatology of disease in more remote body systems, and the possibility that local disorders in the musculoskeletal system affect the function of other body systems requires further study. In 1898, the American School of Osteopathy in Kirksville installed one of the earliest diagnostic x-ray machines and performed the first arteriography study (Peterson 1974, Northup 1975). Total medical care, including surgery, was part of osteopathic medicine from its inception (Still 1899).

Growth and Development

The succeeding years saw a continued spread of the osteopathic profession, legal recognition, and the development of educational meetings, publications, and research programs. Several of the early schools consolidated, and the first osteopathic hospitals were built. Formal standards for the accreditation of osteopathic colleges were adopted by the American Osteopathic Association in 1902, and enforced the following year by on-site inspections. The American College of Osteopathic Surgeons was formed in 1926, the American Osteopathic Hospital Association in 1934, and the Advisory Board for Osteopathic Specialists in 1939; by 1945, there were 11 specialty boards (History of the American College of Osteopathic Surgeons 1980).

Licensing legislation and the growth of osteo-

pathic hospitals made certain states more attractive to DOs. Concentrations of osteopathic physicians and institutions developed primarily in California, Michigan, Ohio, Pennsylvania, Missouri, Arizona, Florida, Texas, New Jersey, and New York (American Osteopathic Association History 1980).

A landmark court decision in Audrain County, Missouri, in 1950 established the right of DOs to practice in public hospitals as complete physicians and surgeons. This provided opportunities for DOs in places where there were no osteopathic hospitals; today, joint-staff hospitals are commonplace.

The longtime struggle for military recognition of DOs reached its climax in the 1950s. Osteopathic physicians had been drafted in the two World Wars, but were not permitted to serve as medical officers. Subsequent legislation made DOs eligible for military commissions but, because of opposition from allopathic physicians, was not implemented for 10 years. By 1967, DOs were accepted into the uniformed services on the same basis as MDs.

Full practice entitlement was obtained in all states by 1973, and today, there are DOs in every state. Osteopathic physicians also are scattered throughout the world, especially in Europe and Canada. The scope of practice for these osteopathic physicians differs from country to country; in many cases, it is limited to manipulative techniques and therapy similar to that of chiropractic.

Principles

Andrew Taylor Still offered three definitions of osteopathy: legal, historical, and technical (Still 1897). Legally speaking, osteopathy represents a system, method, or science of healing. The historical definition reflects Still's reasoning that "a natural flow of blood is health; and disease is the effect of local or general disturbance of blood, that to excite the nerves causes muscles to contract and compress venous blood flow to the heart; and the bones could be used to relieve pressure on nerves, veins and arteries."

The technical definition is more comprehensive: "Osteopathy is that science which consists of such exact, exhaustive, and verifiable knowledge of the structure and functions of the human mechanism, anatomic, physiologic, and psychologic, including the chemistry and physics of its known elements, as has made discoverable certain organic laws and remedial resources, within the body itself, by which nature under the scientific treatment peculiar to osteopathic practice, apart from all ordinary methods of extraneous, artificial, or medicinal stimulation, and in harmonious accord with its own mechanical principles, molecular activities, and metabolic processes, may recover from displacements, disorganizations, derangements, and consequent disease, and regain its normal equilibrium of form and function in health and strength."

Observation, natural law, normal function, and the total human mechanism remain hallmarks of osteopathic medicine focusing on the individual rather than the disease. Osteopathy, then, is a therapeutic system based on the belief that the body—in normal structural relationship and with adequate nutrition—is capable of mounting its own defenses against pathologic conditions. This is achieved through normalization of body mechanics and the neuromusculoskeletal system; structure governs function, with local and distant effects.

The Role of Manipulation

The use of manipulation as a therapeutic modality appeared first in ancient Egypt, and has been disappearing and reappearing ever since that time. In its broadest connotation, manipulation ranges from manual reduction of fractures, dislocations, subluxations, and other simple joint dysfunctions, to the application of manually applied external cardiac massage and postural drainage techniques commonly used in pulmonary diseases.

The role of manipulation in the history and development of osteopathic medicine has been important and controversial. The founders and advocates of osteopathic medicine did not build a system of medical practice around this single therapeutic modality during the past 100 years, but rather established a comprehensive system of healing utilizing manipulative diagnostics and therapy as well as other clinical modalities.

For example, Andrew Taylor Still never wrote a book on manipulative therapy, although he considered it to be a central portion of the osteopathic physician's therapeutic approach to illness and trauma. He viewed manipulation in the total context of the profession's basic philosophy. The Still thesis is based on five major concepts: (1) the unity of the body and the interrelationships of all its systems, (2) the healing power of nature and the ability of the body to mobilize its healing substances to preserve health and to protect against disease, (3) the somatic component of disease, based on the musculoskeletal system and its reciprocal communication with other systems, (4) the interdependence of structure and function; structure governs function, and function influences structure, (5) manipulative therapy in which biomechanical techniques are applied to restore and maintain normal structure-function relations in the musculoskeletal system not only for the normal functioning of the system itself but also through its neural-hormonal communication with other body systems. (Still 1902, Northup 1965).

Manipulative therapy is a potentially useful medium both for maintaining normal function and for correcting of dysfunction (Northup 1972, Stark 1975, Buzzell 1970). The principles and philosophy of osteopathic medicine apply not only to manipulative therapy but also to all aspects of health maintenance and disease prevention and treatment traditionally subsumed by allopathic medicine, such as surgery, obstetrics, pediatrics, emergency medicine, internal medicine, and geriatrics.

In fact, according to public statements made by the American Osteopathic Association, a patient's decision to see an osteopath, rather than an MD is based partially on the following (Northup 1965):

1. DOs are qualified and licensed to practice in all recognized branches of clinical medicine.
2. Their education is essentially the same as MDs, except that DOs receive additional training in diagnosis and treatment of the musculoskeletal system as osteopathic manipulative therapy (OMT).
3. DOs and MDs take the same state license examinations.
4. A larger percentage of DOs are in general practice and primary care because of their emphasis on treating the whole person.
5. A larger percentage of DOs practice in small communities and rural areas.

Osteopathic medicine is not necessarily an alternative medicine system, but rather as a healing system utilizing alternative medicine. Treatment modalities are chosen based on the patient's signs and symptoms, as well as a comprehensive patient history and examination in which the structure and function of the musculoskeletal system provides important clues to dysfunction. Manipulative treatment is a therapeutic means of correcting these dysfunctions that is used in conjunction with other clinical modalities.

Today, those precepts include (Martinke 1991):

1. The body is a unit.
2. Structure and function are reciprocally interrelated.
3. The body possesses self-regulatory mechanisms.
4. The body has the inherent capacity to defend and repair itself.
5. When environmental changes overcome the body's capacity for self maintenance, disease may ensue.
6. Movement of body fluids is essential to the maintenance of health.
7. The nerves play a crucial part in controlling the fluids of the body.
8. There are somatic components to disease that are not only manifestations of disease but also are factors that contribute to maintenance of the diseased state.

It is noteworthy that manipulative therapy is not mentioned in the eight current precepts of osteopathic philosophy. Osteopathic medicine generally is applicable to all disease states. The osteopathic physician does not address one organ system or structure at the expense of another, but rather evaluates the body as an integral unit. Somatic dysfunction, the so-called osteopathic lesion, is based on the diagnosis of local asymmetry, restriction of motion, and textural changes reflecting fixed postural tension (Martinke 1991). Literally, it means impaired or altered function of related components of the somatic (body framework) system: skeletal, arthrodial, and myofascial structures, and related vascular, lymphatic, and neural elements (Rumney 1976). The notion that manipulation is effective treatment is implicit in the term *somatic dysfunction* (Mitchell 1974).

These are classified as type I and type II lesions according to Fryette's physiologic motion principles (Fryette 1954). Type I are group curves involving more than one vertebra, in which rotation of affected vertebral segments is opposite to the side bending. Type II lesions demonstrate vertebral segments in which rotation and sidebending occur in the same direction, and are often traumatic in origin, resulting in a single dysfunction. The osteopathic spinal lesion demonstrates (1) spinal articular strain, (2) fixed postural tension, and (3) altered mechanics or somatic dysfunction with three pathways of stimuli—somatic to somatic, somatic to visceral, and visceral to somatic.

These dysfunctions follow the three laws of physiologic motion (Cathie 1969).

Laws of Physiologic Motion

- Motion into the concavity of the curve. In normal position, most weight-bearing goes through the anterior aspects of the vertebral bodies with the facets in neutral position. With sidebending, the vertebral bodies rotate to the opposite side.
- Simple motion or motion into the convexity of the curve. Sidebending cannot occur if the facets are locked, unless preceded and accompanied by rotation of the vertebral body to the same side. Locking of the facets implies a partial forward or backward bending motion.
- One motion occurs on top of another. Whenever a spinal joint has transversed any portion of the normal range of one or more of its physiologic movements, other physiologic movement is restricted, and the joint is forced to make a second movement. Trauma and somatic dysfunction occur with less stress than if the area were free to accommodate to the applied forces.

This is the concept of a facilitated segment which states that because of abnormal afferent or sensory inputs to a particular area of the spinal cord, that area is kept in a state of constant increased excitation, causing both skeletal and visceral organs innervated by the affected segment to be maintained in a state of overactivity (Korr 1975, Patterson 1976).

Theory of Correction

The theory of correction is to retrace the pathway of the osteopathic lesion. Predisposing factors include habitual and occupational posture, gravity, vertebral anomalies, transitional areas (occipito-atlantal, C7-T1, T12-L1, and L5-S1), muscle hyperirritability from stress, infection, reflex, physiologic locking of a joint, adaptation to stressors, and stable compensation for other structural deficits. Type I somatic dysfunctions may be due to muscle imbalance, short leg, trauma, visceral reflexes, occupation, or disease or infection (Martinke 1991).

Somatic dysfunction demonstrates alterations of the bony triangle composed of at least two vertebral segments, the separating disc, and the superior and inferior facets of both segments; soft tissue thickening of para-articular structures; muscle reaction; and vascular and neurologic interferences. Still's Law states that any position or condition of a spinal segment that interferes with its mechanical function may immediately or ultimately interfere with the nutrition of that segment and the sympathetic and somatic output of the cord (Cathie 1969). Head's Law states that where a painful stimulus is applied to a part of low sensitivity in close connection with a part of higher sensitivity, the stimulus is transferred to spinal centers through the part of higher sensitivity and vice versa (Cathie 1969). The basis for this observation is the sympathetic nervous system and its equilibration of sensitivities and the basis for referred pain.

Hilton's Law reflects the effects of regional innervation (Cathie 1969). Nerve trunks supplying muscles to any joint also supply the muscles that move the joint and the skin that covers the insertion of such muscles. This local adaptive process is the basis for osteopathic diagnosis.

Tension

Emotional tension, infection, physical training, and immobilization all contribute to irritation, pain, and muscle tension. Muscle tension results in internal tissue ischemia, retained metabolites, edema, and inflammation. Inflammation can result in a fibrous reaction and functional disability (Cailliet 1966). These adaptation concepts are fundamental principles in osteopathic structural analysis (Patriquin 1969, Selye 1950).

This cause-and-effect process is similar to that seen with the effects of aging on the musculoskeletal system; postural changes and attitude lead to joint strain, periarticular change, increased fascial tension, and connective tissue proliferation. Muscular contraction results in restricted motion, bone resorption, and alterations in the forces of gravity that disturb balance and reduce height.

Heilig's Summary of the Factors of Somatic Dysfunction

- Occasional palpable displacement of bony parts and loss of normal voluntary and/or involuntary movement.
- Presence of a synovial membrane with varying effects of trauma and strain.
- Effects of disturbance of the continuity of synovial and capsular elements.
- Involvement of tendinous insertions of long and short muscles proximal to the joints.
- Irritation of the rich supply of proprioceptive receptors for sense of position and pressure found in the articular cartilage.
- Possibility of microscopic entrapments of materials such as meniscoids or synovial material.
- Possibility of nerve trunk impingement caused by limiting membranes in the intervertebral area.
- Possibility of a rapid resetting of the γ-motor spindle reflex in the small muscles as a result of sudden stress.
- Possibility that the stimulus from the area of articulation enters into competition with central motor input, which may be responding to suprasegmental reflexes.

The stage of acute or chronic pathology, the amount of splinting involved, and the degree of pain all contribute to the decision concerning the type of manipulative technique used.

Categories of Lesions

Cathie defines primary lesions as being either structural, traumatic, or segmental reflexes, whereas secondary lesions primarily result from gravity with compensatory postural reflexes (Cathie 1969). Hoag classifies three categories of osteopathic lesions: primary, secondary, and compensatory. The primary osteopathic lesion is the result of an abnormal stimulus, frequently in the spinal area, which is strong enough or lengthy enough to produce an alteration of the body. The secondary osteopathic lesion is an area of spinal dysfunction resulting from visceral irritation or functional disturbance. The former activates an abnormal viscerosomatic reflex through the afferent fibers of the autonomic nervous system, then through the efferent portion of the reflex arc, to the vasculature of the paravertebral muscles, the fascia, ligaments, and articular structures. The compensatory osteopathic lesion is a similar area of musculoskeletal disturbance that follows the general pattern of primary or secondary lesions, exhibiting the same signs and symptoms. These lesions often are a result of postural abnormalities (Hoag 1969).

Treatment involves correcting the lesions in reverse order using relaxation techniques, stretching, and movement. Fisher classified syndromes likely to benefit from manipulation as articular or periarticular adhesions; subluxations or dislocations of joints, tendons, or intra-articular disks; adhesions of muscles, tendons, or fascia; and certain functional or hysterical conditions of the joints and of the spine (Fisher 1967).

Somatic dysfunctions or motion disturbances associated with the osteopathic lesion can be described according to the direction of increased freedom of motion, the position in lesion, and the direction of limitation of motion. There is usually an asymmetric pattern of motion in somatic dysfunction, with restriction in one direction and increased freedom of motion in the opposite direction. In most cases the position and direction of free motion are the same. The term *barrier* is used to describe the end point of permitted motion in the direction of limitation (Kappler 1981).

Treatment

Muscle Energy Techniques

Muscle energy techniques are a form of osteopathic manipulative treatment in which the patient actively directs muscles against a distinct counterforce (Martinke 1991, Greenman 1989). Muscle energy techniques are used to mobilize joints in which movement is restricted, to strengthen weak muscles, to stretch tight muscles and fascia, and to improve local circulation. These are classified as isotonic (concentric or eccentric) or isometric contractions.

Muscle energy techniques are carried out within a range of movement against increased tension or resistance. Localization of force is more important than the intensity of force. Monitoring forces, and confining them to the muscle group or the level of somatic dysfunction involved are important in achieving the desired results (Goodridge 1981).

Greenman describes four muscle contraction types: isometric, concentric isotonic, eccentric isotonic, and isolytic. The latter is a nonphysiologic contraction in which an external force is applied to a concentric isotonic contraction in the opposite direction. Success depends on control, balance, and localization (Greenman 1989).

These techniques use active muscle contraction to mobilize specific articulations and also engage the barriers to motion. Several principles should be followed:

1. The positioning of the somatic dysfunction into its physiologic motion barriers should be specific in all three planes (flexion-extension, side bending, and rotation).
2. The patient statically contracts muscles toward the freedoms of motion of the somatic dysfunction.
3. The patient relaxes muscle-contracting efforts.
4. The physician re-engages the joint into its new motion barriers.

These techniques are effective especially in patients with acute somatic dysfunction such as a whiplash injury, or injuries suffered in a fall.

Myofascial Techniques

Myofascial techniques are among the soft tissue techniques used to bring about relaxation of contracted muscles, increase circulation to an area of ischemia, increase venous and lymphatic drainage, and a stimulatory affect of the stretch reflex in hypotonic muscles (Murphy 1991). The physiologic principles include the extensibility of the connective tissues, the stretch reflex, heat, the muscle spindle reflex, the Golgi tendon organ reflex, reciprocal inhibition, and the crossed extensor reflex. There are active and passive techniques. Current interest in trigger points apply these same principles to achieve results in conditions such as fibromyalgia and myofascial pain syndrome (Travell & Simons 1983, Rachlin 1994, Cantu & Grodin 1992, Kraus 1984).

Counterstrain Techniques

Counterstrain techniques, the newest form of osteopathic manipulation, was devised by Lawrence Jones and is based on the belief that somatic dysfunction has a neuromuscular basis (DiGiovanna 1991, Jones 1981). The diagnosis is made by finding reflex tender points either anterior or posterior to the segmental lesion. The treatment technique is positional, and can be defined in two ways: relieving spinal or other joint pain by passively pulling the joint into its position of greatest comfort; and relieving pain by reduction and arrest of the continuing inappropriate proprioceptor activity by markedly shortening the muscle that contains the malfunctioning muscle spindle by applying mild strain to its antagonists (Jones 1981). The most important advantage of the counterstrain technique is that positioning can be carried out in almost every patient, and that the patient does not have to be cooperative to be treated. Thus, this technique is ideal for an acutely ill, inpatient population (Schwartz 1986).

Thrusting Techniques

Thrusting techniques are usually direct techniques in which the dysfunctional unit is placed into at least one of its barriers to motion, and a motion or impulse is applied through that barrier (DiGiovanna 1991, Greenman 1989, Magoun 1978, Nicholas 1974). There are three techniques: high velocity, low amplitude; low velocity, high amplitude; and the springing maneuver (generally considered a variant of the high velocity, low amplitude technique). These maneuvers are the techniques most commonly associated with osteopathic manipulative treatment.

Based on the patient's presentation, as well as a comprehensive history and physical examination including a structural diagnosis and a manipulative prescription, one or more of the principles and techniques described may be applied. These fall within six general principles and techniques (Greenman 1989).

1. Mobilization without impulse for soft tissue and articulatory tissues.
2. Muscle energy techniques.
3. High-velocity, low amplitude thrust technique (mobilization with impulse).
4. Functional or indirect technique.
5. Myofascial release technique.
6. Craniosacral or inherent force technique.

There are specialized techniques for each portion of the anatomy including the skull, vertebrae, pelvis, and extremities (DiGiovanna 1991, Greenman 1989, Magoun 1978, Nicholas 1974).

Applications

The application of osteopathic medicine is germane to the entire spectrum of human disease and trauma. It is a comprehensive system of healing, but is best known for its reliance on the diagnostic and therapeutic value of the musculoskeletal system and osteopathic manipulative therapy (OMT).

The basic concepts of osteopathic medicine are centered around holism, the unity of the body, ecology, health versus disease, homeostasis, and the mechanisms maintaining homeostasis (Hoag 1969, DiGiovanna 1991).

Osteopathic manipulative techniques are based on a comprehensive structural analysis of the patient which may involve palpatory, postural, and range of motion assessments, combined with radiographic (radiography, computerized tomography, magnetic resonance imaging, nuclear medicine) as well as clinical laboratory studies to define the scope of the problem and evaluate the signs and symptoms relative to the diagnosis or the differential diagnosis. Treatment focuses on correcting that problem by a variety of clinical modalities including medication, surgery, physical therapy, and OMT, as well as educating the patient in nutrition and other lifestyle factors. The patient is treated rather than the disease. This probably is the single greatest difference between osteopathy and allopathic medicine, which focuses on the disease process and its treatment.

Although applicable to all disease states, osteopathic manipulative treatment accordingly has special value in the treatment of whiplash injuries, scoliosis, the thoracic outlet syndrome, lumbar radiculopathies (herniated nucleus pulposus, spinal stenosis, sacroiliac joint syndrome, posterior facet joint syndrome, and the piriformis syndrome), spondylolisthesis and spondylolysis, coccygodynia, dysmenorrhea, as well as other disorders in pulmonary and cardiac patients (DiGiovanna & Schiowitz 1991).

Research and The Future

Osteopathic medicine is an evolutionary healing system that stresses the importance and use of the neuromusculoskeletal system in the diagnosis and therapy of a wide variety of maladies. Much of the research that has been published since its inception focuses on the techniques and scientific principles behind osteopathic manipulative therapy (Stark & Tilley 1975), although a wide range of studies are routinely reported in the osteopathic literature on all aspects of clinical medicine.

The A.T. Still Research Institute, which merged with the American Osteopathic Foundation in 1935, funds research for investigations specifically directed to osteopathic manipulative treatment, osteopathic principles, and osteopathic practices. The American Osteopathic Association (AOA) Research Grants Program began in 1937, and awards one-year research grants for biologic and clinically scientific projects, preferably directed toward answering questions traditionally or currently associated with the osteopathic medical profession. An emphasis on manipulative therapy is evident in their current programs. The AOA Clinical Investigator Development

Award (CIDA) began in 1990 to establish a training program to recruit and prepare osteopathic physicians for research and teaching careers in the medical sciences.

The AOA Annual Research Conference began meeting in 1955, as a forum for scientists and clinical investigators from osteopathic medical institutions. A number of special awards are presented at the research conference. These programs are directed at increasing the number of researchers within the osteopathic profession and continuing the evolutionary development of osteopathic medicine. Information on these programs can be obtained from the 1993 Osteopathic Research Handbook.

In recent years there has been a perceived convergence of osteopathic and allopathic medicine, which has increased the utilization of manipulative medicine as a treatment modality (Mennell 1992, Cyriax & Russell 1980, Cyriax 1982). Concern for the future of osteopathic medicine in this environment still exists despite the growing number of osteopathic schools and practicing osteopathic physicians. Emphasis has been placed on the role of osteopathic physicians as primary care physicians, and their importance in the delivery of health care is focused into managed care formats. Osteopathic community hospitals are being absorbed by larger health care facilities or organizations. Osteopathic physicians continue postgraduate training in allopathic programs, where there is potential loss of manipulative medicine skill, especially with the institution of practice parameters being patterned after allopathic principles of diagnosis and therapy. These issues are current concerns of the American Osteopathic Association and its members and receive a significant amount of discussion. A number of corrective measures aimed at the expansion of postgraduate osteopathic training programs have been proposed and are in variable states of institution; their success remains to be determined.

The continuing success of osteopathic medicine as it begins its second century of development will depend on its practitioners adhering to osteopathic principles, techniques, and the scientific basis for those principles and practices. Continuing research and education is fundamental to this effort (Northup 1987). According to the current President of the American Osteopathic Association, Dr. William G.

Anderson, traditional osteopathic medicine is an idea whose time has come.

References

American College of Osteopathic Surgeon. 1980. History of the American College of Osteopathic Surgeons: Membership Directory and By-Laws. Coral Gables, Florida. pp. 4–8

American Osteopathic Association. 1980. American Osteopathic Association History: Dates, Events and People. Yearbook and Directory of Osteopathic Physicians. Chicago. pp. 377–381

American Osteopathic Association. 1993. Osteopathic Research Handbook. Chicago

Buzzell KA. 1970. The cost of human posture and locomotion. In The Physiological Basis of Osteopathic Medicine. Postgraduate Institute of Osteopathic Medicine and Surgery, New York. pp. 63–72

Cailliet R. 1966. Cailliet Pain Series. FA Davis, Philadelphia

Cantu RI, Grodin AJ. 1992. Myofascial Manipulation: Theory and Clinical Application. Aspen Publishers, Gaithersburg, Maryland

Cathie AG. 1969. Textbook of Osteopathic Philosophy and Principles. Philadelphia College of Osteopathic Medicine Press. Philadelphia

Chaitow L. 1993. Osteopathy. In Alternative Medicine: The Definitive Guide. Burton Goldberg Group (eds). Future Medicine Publishing Inc. Puyallup, Washington. pp. 405–411

Cushing H. 1925. The Life of Sir William Osler. Oxford Press. Oxford

Cyriax J. 1982. Textbook of Orthopaedic Medicine: Volume I Diagnosis of Soft Tissue Lesions. 8th Ed. Bailliere Tindall. London

Cyriax J, Russell G. 1980. Textbook of Orthopaedic Medicine: Volume II Treatment by Manipulation, Massage and Injection. 10th Ed. Bailliere Tindall. London

DiGiovanna EL. 1991. Counterstrain. In DiGiovanna EL, Schiowitz S (eds). An Osteopathic Approach to Diagnosis and Treatment. JB Lippincott. Philadelphia. pp. 85–87

DiGiovanna EL. 1991. Thrusting techniques. In DiGiovanna EL, Schiowitz S (eds). An Osteopathic Approach to Diagnosis and Treatment. JB Lippincott. Philadelphia. pp. 87–88

Dorland's Illustrated Medical Dictionary. 1981. 26th Ed. WB Saunders. Philadelphia

Fisher. 1967. Symposium: manipulative treatment. Med J Aust 1278–1280

Fryette HH. 1954. Principles of Osteopathic Technique. Academy of Applied Osteopathy. Carmel, California

Goodridge JP. 1981. Muscle energy technique: definition, explanation, methods of procedure. J Am Osteopath Assn 81(4):249–254

Greenman PE. 1989. Principles of Manual Medicine. Williams & Wilkins. Baltimore

Heilig D. 1981. The thrust technique. J Am Osteopath Assn 81(4):244–248

Heilig D. 1975. Manipulation in the osteopathic management of the geriatric patient. In Stark EH, Tilley RM (eds). Clinical Review Series: Osteopathic Medicine. Publishing Sciences Group, Inc. Acton. pp. 89–100

Heilig D. 1969. Treatment of osteopathic lesions: illustrative points in technique. In Hoag JM, Cole WV, Bradford SG (eds). Osteopathic Medicine. McGraw-Hill. New York. pp. 197–203

Heilig D. 1969. Pathogenesis of structural disorders related to osteopathic lesions. In Hoag JM, Cole WV, Bradford SG (eds). Osteopathic Medicine. McGraw-Hill. New York. pp. 164–178

Hix EL. 1970. Viscerovisceral and somatovisceral reflex communication. In The Physiological Basis of Osteopathic Medicine. Postgraduate Institute of Osteopathic Medicine and Surgery. New York. pp. 85–100

Hix EL. 1970. The trophic function of visceral nerves. In The Physiological Basis of Osteopathic Medicine. Postgraduate Institute of Osteopathic Medicine and Surgery. pp. 101–113

Hoag JM. 1969. Concepts of osteopathic medicine. In Hoag JM, Cole WV, Bradford SG (eds). Osteopathic Medicine. McGraw-Hill. New York. pp. 13–19

Hoag JM. 1969. The osteopathic lesion: basic considerations. In Hoag JM, Cole WV, Bradford SG (eds). Osteopathic Medicine. McGraw-Hill. New York. pp. 100–107

Jones L. 1981. Strain and Counterstrain. American Academy of Osteopathy. Colorado Springs

Kappler RE. 1981. Direct action techniques. J Am Osteopath Assn 81(4):239–243

Korr IM. 1970. The sympathetic nervous system as mediator between the somatic and supportive processes. In The Physiological Basis of Osteopathic Medicine. Postgraduate Institute of Osteopathic Medicine and Surgery. New York. pp. 21–38

Korr IM. 1970. Vulnerability of the segmental nervous system to somatic insults. In The Physiological Basis of Osteopathic Medicine. Postgraduate Institute of Osteopathic Medicine and Surgery. New York. pp. 53–62

Korr IM. 1970. The segmental nervous system as mediator and organizer of disease processes. In The Physiological Basis of Osteopathic Medicine. Postgraduate Institute of Osteopathic Medicine and Surgery. New York. pp. 73–84

Korr IM. 1975. Proprioceptors and somatic dysfunction. J Am Osteopath Assn 74:638–650

Korr IM. 1975. The facilitated segment: a factor in injury to the body framework. In Stark EH, Tilley RM (eds). Clinical Review Series: Osteopathic Medicine. Publishing Sciences Group, Inc. Acton. p. 27–34

Korr IM. 1975. Proprioceptors and the behavior of lesioned segments. In Stark EH, Tilley RM (eds). Clinical Review Series: Osteopathic Medicine. Publishing Sciences Group, Inc. Acton. pp. 183–216

Korr IM. 1976. The spinal cord as organizer of disease processes: some preliminary perspectives. J Am Osteopath Assn 76:35–45

Kraus H. 1984. Treatment of myofascial pain. In Ruskin AP (ed). Current Therapy in Physiatry: Physical Medicine and Rehabilitation. WB Saunders. Philadelphia. pp. 103–113

Luciani RJ. 1975. The somatic-visceral autonomic reflex: one mechanism in acupuncture therapeutics. In Stark EH, Tilley RM (eds). Clinical Review Series: Osteopathic Medicine. Publishing Sciences Group, Inc. Acton. pp. 291–299

Magoun HI. 1978. Practical Osteopathic Procedures: the 'Birthright of Osteopathy.' Journal Printing Co. Kirksville, Missouri

Martinke DJ. 1991. The philosophy of osteopathic medicine. In DiGiovanna EL, Schiowitz S (eds). An Osteopathic Approach to Diagnosis and Treatment. JB Lippincott. Philadelphia. pp. 3–6

Mennell JM. 1992. The Musculoskeletal System: Differential Diagnosis from Symptoms and Physical Signs. Aspen Publishers. Gaithersburg, Maryland

Mitchell FL, Sr. 1958. Structural Pelvic Function. Yearbook American Academy of Osteopathy. pp. 71–89

Mitchell FL, Jr. 1979. Towards a definition of somatic dysfunction. Osteopath Ann 7:12–25

Mitchell FL, Jr. 1975. The influence of Chapman's reflexes and the immune reaction. In Stark EH, Tilley RM (eds). Clinical Review Series: Osteopathic Medicine. Publishing Sciences Group, Inc. Acton. pp. 179–182

Mitchell FL, Jr, Moran PS, Pruzzo NA. 1979. An evaluation and treatment manual of osteopathic muscle energy procedures. Valley Park

Murphy T. 1991. Myofascial Techniques. In DiGiovanna EL, Schiowitz S (eds). An Osteopathic Approach to Diagnosis and Treatment. JB Lippincott. Philadelphia. pp. 81–84

Nicholas NS. 1974. Atlas of Osteopathic Techniques. Philadelphia College of Osteopathic Medicine. Philadelphia

Northup GW. 1969. Orientation in Osteopathic Medicine. In Hoag JM, Cole WV, Bradford SG (eds). Osteopathic Medicine. McGraw-Hill. New York. p. 3

Northup GW. 1975. History of the development of osteopathic concepts, with notes on osteopathic terminology. J Am Osteopath Assn 75:405–409

Northup GW. 1965. Osteopathic medicine: a medical reformation. J Am Osteopath Assn 64:787–794

Northup GW. 1972. The role of manipulative therapy in the practice of medicine. J Am Osteopath Assn 71:537–542

Northup GW. 1987. Osteopathic Research: Growth and Development, American Osteopathic Association. Chicago

Osler W. 1892. The Principles and Practices of Medicine. D. Appleton Co. New York

Patriquin DA. 1969. Stress and adaptation. In Hoag JM, Cole WV, Bradford SG (eds). Osteopathic Medicine. McGraw-Hill. New York. pp. 214–227

Patterson MM. 1976. A model mechanism for spinal segmental facilitation. J Am Osteopath Assn 76:62–72

Peterson B. 1974. Radiology in Kirksville. J Am Osteopath Assn 74:167–172

Rachlin ES. 1994. Myofascial Pain and Fibromyalgia: Trigger Point Management. CV Mosby. St. Louis

Rumney I. 1976. The relevance of somatic dysfunction. In Yearbook of the American Academy of Osteopathy. Colorado Springs

Schwartz HR. 1986. The use of counterstrain in an acutely ill in-hospital population. J Am Osteopath Assn 86(7):433–442

Selye H. 1950. The General Adaptation Syndrome and Diseases of Adaptation. Yearbook of Pathology and Clinical Pathology. Chicago

Stark EH, Tilley RM. 1975. Clinical Review Series: Osteopathic Medicine. Publishing Sciences Group, Inc. Acton

Steiner C. 1994. Osteopathic manipulative treatment: What does it really do? J Am Osteopath Assn 94(1):85–87

Still AT. 1897. Autobiography of Andrew T. Still, the author. Kirksville, Missouri

Still AT. 1899. Philosophy of Osteopathy, the author. Kirksville, Missouri

Still AT. 1902. Philosophy and mechanical principles of osteopathy. Hudson-Kimberly Publishing. Kansas City, MO

Still AT. 1910. Osteopathy research and practice, the author. Kirksville, Missouri

Stoddard A. 1959. Manual of Osteopathic Technique. Hutchinson Medical Publishers. London

Stoddard A. 1969. Manual of Osteopathic Practice. Harper & Row Publishers. New York

Suter RE. 1988. Hippocratic thought: its relationship to and between Andrew Taylor Still and Sir William Osler. J Am Osteopath Assn 88(10):1243–1254

Travell JG, Simons DG. 1983. Myofascial Pain and Dysfunction: The Trigger Point Manual. Williams & Wilkins. Baltimore

Upledger JE. 1977. Integration of Acupuncture and Manipulation. Osteopathic Medicine. pp. 19–27, 103–111

Van Buskirk RL. 1990. Nociceptive reflexes and the somatic dysfunction: A model. J Am Osteopath Assn 90(9):792–808

Wilson PT. 1957. The definition of osteopathy. In Cathie AG (ed). Textbook of Osteopathic Philosophy and Principles. Philadelphia College of Osteopathic Medicine Press. Philadelphia. p. 94

Yale SD. 1991. Muscle Energy Techniques. In DiGiovanna EL, Schiowitz S (eds). An Osteopathic Approach to Diagnosis and Treatment. JB Lippincott. Philadelphia. p. 84

7
Chiropractic

Daniel Redwood

*C*hiropractic was forged in a crucible of controversy. Born in the American Midwest a century ago in reaction to the medical status quo, this manual healing art has matured to mainstream status while largely preserving its essential tenets. The modern chiropractic profession has scaled the walls of the health care establishment, with licensure, an increasingly strong scientific research base, widespread insurance coverage, and approximately 20 million patients per year in the United States, while maintaining strong roots in the alternative health community with a philosophy that emphasizes healing without drugs.

Chiropractic is the third largest independent health profession in the western world, following allopathic medicine and dentistry. Its practitioners are portal-of-entry providers, licensed both for diagnosis and treatment. Unlike dentistry, podiatry, and optometry, chiropractic practice is limited not by anatomic region but by procedure. The chiropractor's scope of practice excludes surgery and pharmaceutical therapy, and centers on the manual adjustment or manipulation of the spine.

The United States is home to 52,000 of the world's approximately 56,000 chiropractors (Peterson 1995). Chiropractors are licensed throughout the English-speaking world, and in an increasing number of other nations. Rigorous educational standards are supervised by government-recognized accrediting agencies, including the Council on Chiropractic Education (CCE) in the United States. After fulfilling science prerequisites in college, chiropractic students must complete a four-year program that includes coursework in anatomy, physiology, pathology, and diagnosis, as well as spinal adjusting, nutrition, physical therapy, and rehabilitation.

According to an American Chiropractic Association survey, nearly 90 percent of chiropractic patients present as neuromusculoskeletal cases—principally back pain, neck pain, and headaches—the conditions for which spinal manual therapy (SMT) is most effective (Plamondon 1995). Current research seeks to further define the role of SMT in the management of various musculoskeletal conditions, as well as to evaluate its effectiveness for visceral organ disorders such as dysmenorrhea, hypertension, infantile colic, asthma, and otitis media.

As chiropractic observes its centennial and enters the twenty-first century on the threshold of integration into mainstream health care, a thorough evaluation of the profession's role in health care delivery is underway. This calls for honest self-criticism within the chiropractic profession, and a spirit of genuine open-mindedness from the medical profession.

Historical Roots, Evolutionary Process

Precursors in Western Traditions

Spinal manipulation has been practiced for millennia in cultures throughout the world. Chiropractic's western progenitors include some prominent figures from the history of medicine. Hippocrates was an early practitioner of spinal manipulation (Withington 1959), using manipulation not only to reposition vertebrae, but also thereby to cure a wide variety of dysfunctions (Leach 1994). Galen, a Greek-born Roman physician whose approach to healing set the standard in western medicine for 1,500 years after his death, also used spinal manipulation and reported the successful resolution of a patient's hand weakness and numbness through manipulation of the seventh cervical vertebra (Lomax 1975, Copland-Griffiths 1991).

As Europe entered the Dark Ages, these healing traditions were preserved in the learning centers of the Middle East by the ascendant Arabic civilization. Later, this body of knowledge returned to Europe, and the works of Hippocrates and Galen helped form the foundations of Renaissance medicine. Ambroise Paré, sometimes called the "father of surgery," used manipulation to treat French vineyard workers in the sixteenth century (Paré 1968, Lomax 1975).

In the centuries that followed, manipulative techniques were passed down from generation to generation within families—often from mother to daughter. These "bonesetting" methods played an important role in the history of nonmedical healing in Great Britain, and similar methods are common in the folk medicine of many nations (Bennett 1981).

During the second half of the nineteenth century, the United States became a vibrant center of natural healing theory and practice. Osteopathy and chiropractic, two manipulation-based healing arts, trace their origins to that era. Both began in the American Midwest.

Beginnings of a New Profession

Daniel David Palmer (Figs. 7-1 and 7-2), a self-educated healer in the Mississippi River town of Davenport, Iowa, founded the chiropractic profession in 1895 on two fundamental premises: that the vertebral subluxation* (a spinal misalignment causing abnormal nerve transmission) is the cause of virtually all disease, and that the chiropractic adjustment (a

---

* This differs from the medical definition of subluxation, which according to Dorland's Illustrated Medical Dictionary is an incomplete or partial dislocation. Palmer's use of the term refers to a more subtle malposition with neural involvement.

manual manipulation of the subluxated vertebra) is its cure (Palmer 1910).

This "one cause-one cure" philosophy has played a central role in chiropractic history. While few, if any, contemporary chiropractors would endorse this simplistic formulation, it remains true that the raison d'être of the chiropractic profession is the detection and correction of spinal subluxations. Chiropractors may do much more, but it is their ability to do this one thing well that has allowed their art to survive for a century under a constant barrage of medical opposition.

The one cause-one cure adherents had two major political effects on the development of the profession. First, their faith in the truth of their message, combined with the positive results of chiropractic adjustments, created a strong and steadily growing activist constituency of chiropractic supporters. Civil disobedience was an integral part of the early development of the chiropractic profession. Hundreds, including the founder himself, were arrested for practicing medicine without a license (Fig. 7-3). Incarcerated in 1906, Palmer said, "I have never considered it beneath my dignity to do anything to relieve human suffering."

Palmer administered the first chiropractic adjustment to Harvey Lillard, a deaf janitor in the building where Palmer had an office. Lillard was bent over with acute back pain. Noting an apparent spinal misalignment in the patient's upper back, Palmer administered the adjustment, after which Lillard stood up straight, was free of back pain, and even was able to hear for the first time in many years. This singular event demonstrates the two chief symptomatic benefits ascribed to the chiropractic art of healing: relief of musculoskeletal pain and disability, which is now well accepted, and restoration of proper internal organ function (which remains unresolved).

At first, there was hope that Palmer had discovered a cure for deafness, but similar results were not forthcoming with other deaf patients. Since then, there have been rare reports of hearing restored through spinal manipulation, including one by a Canadian orthopedist (Bourdillion 1982). The story of Lillard's dramatic recovery has been used repeatedly to disparage chiropractic, with charges that such an event is impossible, because no spinal nerves supply the ear.

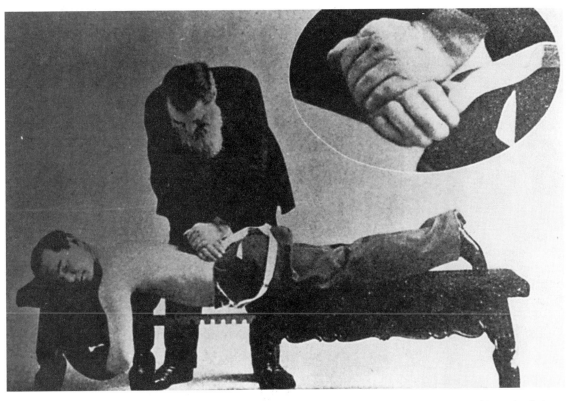

Figure 7-1. Daniel David Palmer, the founder of chiropractic, adjusting a patient, ca. 1906. (From the Palmer College of Chiropractic, with permission.)

Current knowledge of neurophysiology provides a theoretical basis for visceral organ responses to chiropractic adjustments. The underlying physiologic mechanism is the somato-autonomic reflex. Chiropractors and osteopaths assert that signals initiated by spinal manipulation are transmitted via autonomic pathways to internal organs.

In the case of Palmer's first adjustment, the relevant nerve pathway begins in the thoracic region, and courses up through the neck and into the cranium along sympathetic nerves that eventually lead to the blood vessels of the inner ear. Normal hearing depends on an adequate blood supply, which in turn depends on properly functioning sympathetic nerves.

Chiropractic and Allopathic Medicine in the United States

All nascent healing arts face serious challenges, most prominently to maintain the justifiable enthusiasm generated by positive therapeutic results, while distinguishing between the proven, the probable, and the speculative. Some of the harshest criticism of chiropractic has been in reaction to the tendency of some chiropractors to "globalize," making broad claims on the basis of limited anecdotal evidence (Gellert 1994).

Whatever the validity of these medical critiques (some of which mirror self-criticism within the chiropractic profession), the American medical establishment's view on chiropractic has never been that of a disinterested group solely seeking to serve the public good. This has caused generations of allopathic medical students to be taught that chiropractic is harmful or at best worthless.

That such a fiercely anti-chiropractic policy was pursued by the American Medical Association is no longer in dispute. In 1990 the United States Supreme Court affirmed a lower court ruling in which the AMA was found guilty of anti-trust violations for having engaged in a conspiracy to *contain and elimi-*

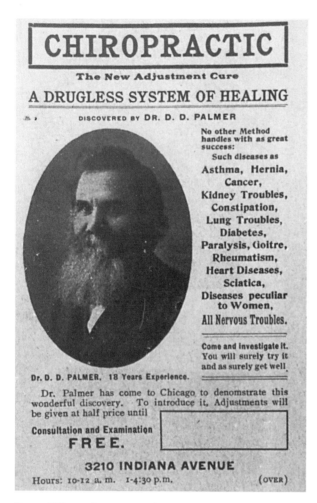

Figure 7-2. In this 1904 advertisement, Dr. Palmer touted chiropractic as a cure for virtually all human ailments. Such claims engendered great controversy. (From Palmer College of Chiropractic, with permission.)

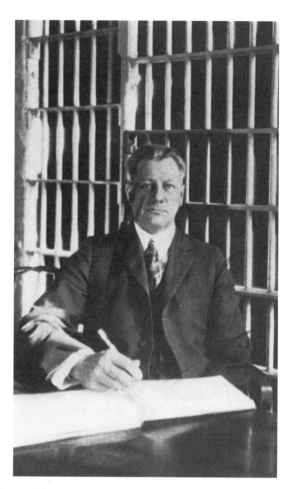

Figure 7-3. Hundreds of chiropractors served time in jail to secure the right to freely practice their healing art. Pictured here is Dr. D.S. Tracy, behind bars in Los Angeles, California. (From the Palmer College of Chiropractic, with permission.)

nate (the AMA's own words) the chiropractic profession (Wilk 1990). As a result, the AMA reversed its longstanding ban on interprofessional cooperation between medical doctors and chiropractors, agreed to publish the full findings of the court in the *Journal of the American Medical Association*, and paid a substantial sum, most of which is now being used for chiropractic research on visceral disorders.

These steps taken by organized medicine are a laudable milestone on the long road toward reconciliation between the chiropractic profession and the AMA.

Interprofessional Cooperation

While relations between the medical and chiropractic professions outside the United States also have been less than cordial, they have been sufficiently productive to permit closer collaboration between chiropractors and allopathic physicians. This has had particularly salutary effects on research. Many of the key clinical trials that first established chiropractic's scientific credibility were conducted in Europe and Canada in the past decade.

The tide is now turning in the United States as

well. Newly announced research projects funded by the federal government indicate an atmosphere of growing medical–chiropractic cooperation, and multidisciplinary organizations such as the American Back Society also reflect a newfound common ground. This spirit of reform may be penetrating to the grassroots level; a survey demonstrated that the majority of primary care physicians in the state of Washington refer at least some cases to chiropractors (Cherkin et al 1989). However, a later study by the same researcher showed that in hypothetical cases of patients with low back pain, only three percent of allopathic physicians surveyed would recommend spinal manipulation (Cherkin 1995).

AHCPR Guidelines: The Great Breakthrough

The 1994 Guidelines for Acute Lower Back Pain developed for the Agency for Health Care Policy and Research (AHCPR) of the U.S. Department of Health and Human Services by a blue-ribbon panel comprised of 21 medical physicians and 2 chiropractors, included a powerful endorsement of spinal manipulation (Bigos et al 1994).

The guidelines concluded that SMT hastens recovery from acute low back pain (LBP) and recommended it either in combination with or as a replacement for nonsteroidal, anti-inflammatory drugs (NSAIDs). The panel endorsed self-care methods including exercise, ergonomic seating, and low-heeled shoes. At the same time, the panel rejected numerous methods that for many years constituted the foundation of allopathic medicine's approach to acute LBP, such as bed rest, traction, and various other physical therapy and pharmaceutical modalities, and cautioned against lumbar surgery except in the most severe cases.

Perhaps most significantly, the guidelines state that spinal manipulation offers both symptomatic relief and functional improvement. Since none of the other recommended nonsurgical interventions offers both, one can infer that for acute LBP cases where none of the guidelines' diagnostic red flags (such as fractures, tumors, infections, or cauda equina syndrome) are present, SMT is the treatment of choice.

The release of the AHCPR guidelines was a truly seismic event. The medical press expressed amazement that the federal standards for the treatment of LBP—the nation's most prevalent musculoskeletal ailment and the most frequent cause of disability for persons under age 45—now assign a pivotal role to spinal manipulation, of which 94 percent is provided by chiropractors (Shekelle et al 1991).

Intellectual Foundations

The history of chiropractic, like all healing arts, is one in which empirical process preceded theoretical formulation. From the earliest days, practitioners have applied new treatment methods on an intuitive basis, noted those that were effective, and then theorized as to the underlying physiologic mechanisms. The resultant body of chiropractic theory, philosophy, and practice draws from principles shared by all natural healing arts, and also contributes uniquely to the cumulative sum and substance of health knowledge.

Common Domain Principles

Fundamental principles of natural healing are incorporated into the curricula at chiropractic training institutions.

The Natural Principles of Chiropractic

- Human beings possess an innate healing potential, an inner wisdom of the body.
- Maximally accessing this healing system is the goal of the healing arts.
- Addressing the cause of an illness usually should take precedence over suppressing its surface manifestations.
- Pharmaceutical suppression of symptoms can compromise the body's ability to heal itself.
- Natural, nonpharmaceutical measures (including chiropractic spinal adjustments) should be the approach of first resort, not last.
- A balanced, natural diet is crucial to good health.
- Regular exercise is essential to proper bodily function.

These principles, endorsed and elucidated by chiropractors for a full century, are recognizable today as the foundation of the emerging holistic health or wellness paradigm.

Core Chiropractic Principles

Other precepts, as well as those shared with such natural healing arts as homeopathy and naturopathy comprise the underpinning of chiropractic.

Precepts of Chiropractic

- Structure and function exist in intimate relation with one another.
- Structural distortions can cause functional abnormalities.
- The vertebral subluxation is a significant form of structural distortion and leads to a variety of functional abnormalities.
- The nervous system plays a prominent role in the restoration and maintenance of proper bodily function.
- Subluxation influences bodily function primarily through neurologic means.
- Chiropractic adjustment is a specific and definitive method for the correction of vertebral subluxation.

Although chiropractic is best known for relief of musculoskeletal pain, its basic axioms do not directly address pain relief. Instead, they focus on correction of the structural and functional imbalances that might cause pain. This paradox—that a profession renowned for the relief of musculoskeletal pain does not define its basic purpose in those terms—has been a persistent, and sometimes discordant, theme in chiropractic history.

Divergent Interpretations: Traditionalists and Modernists

A dichotomy exists between chiropractors who are labeled *straights* and *mixers*. Central to this controversy is the degree to which chiropractic practice should focus on symptom relief. Traditionalist, or straight chiropractors see their approach as being subluxation-based rather than symptom-driven; they confine their role to analyzing the spine for subluxations and then manually adjusting the subluxated vertebrae. A minority within the profession, traditionalists reject the use of symptom-oriented ancillary therapies such as heat, electrical stimulation, and dietary supplements. Some jurisdictions limit chiropractors to this circumscribed scope of practice.

While traditionalists seek to treat the cause (some even reject the term *treat* as excessively allopathic), broad-scope modernists seek to treat both the cause and the symptom. They contend that patient care is enhanced by such adjuncts as electrical physical therapy modalities, hands-on muscle therapies, and nutritional regimens including supplementation with vitamins, minerals, and herbs. Both groups agree that spinal adjusting is the paramount feature of chiropractic practice, and that advising patients on exercise and natural diet is appropriate within the chiropractor's scope.

Theoretical Constructs and Practical Applications

Bone-Out-of-Place

Early chiropractors, who followed Palmer's lead assumed that adjustments worked by moving misaligned vertebrae back into line, thereby relieving pressure caused by bony impingement on spinal nerves. As explained to patients, if you step on a garden hose, the water cannot get through; if you lift your foot off of the hose, the free flow of water is restored. Similarly, the chiropractic adjustment removes the pressure of bone on nerve, thus allowing free flow of nerve impulses.

Based on the information available in the nineteenth century, such concepts were plausible. Chiropractors were able to feel interruptions in the symmetry of the spinal column with their well-trained hands, and in many cases, could verify findings with radiographic images. When they adjusted the subluxated vertebra with manual pressure, patients often reported significant functional improvements and healing effects.

However, positive health changes have never been convincingly correlated with vertebral alignment. After an adjustment resulting in dramatic relief from headaches or sciatica, a radiographic study rarely shows any discernible change in spinal alignment. (Such comparative procedures are now considered inappropriate, because of the unnecessary radiation exposure.)

Motion Theory and Segmental Dysfunction

Alternative hypotheses are necessary to replace the outmoded bone-out-of-place concept. Chief among these is the theory of intervertebral motion and segmental dysfunction (SDF), the dominant chiropractic paradigm of our era. Though advocated by a minority of chiropractors for decades, this model first achieved attention profession-wide in the 1980s, and now enjoys broad acceptance in chiropractic college curricula throughout the world. This theory also allows a coherent explanation of chiropractic and the subluxation complex to be communicated in familiar terms to medical practitioners and researchers.

Motion theory contends that loss of proper spinal joint mobility, rather than positional misalignment, is the key factor in the subluxation complex. It posits that the subluxation always involves more than a single vertebra, and that subluxation mechanics involve SDF, an interruption in the normal dynamic relationship between two articulating joint surfaces (Schafer & Faye 1989). Anatomically, the vertebral motor unit, or motion segment, consists of an anterior segment of two vertebral bodies separated by an intervertebral disc, and a posterior segment, consisting of two adjacent articular facets, along with muscles, ligaments, blood vessels, and nerves interfacing with one another. Restriction of joint motion, a common feature of subluxation, is termed a *fixation*. Fixation-subluxations are the clinical entity most amenable to SMT.

> A Visual Model of Spinal Motion
>
> J. F. McAndrews, a former president of the Palmer College of Chiropractic and the current vice president for professional affairs of the American Chiropractic Association, was an early advocate of motion theory and practice. He offers a visual model of spinal motion principles:
>
> *(Continues)*

> View it as a mobile hanging from the ceiling, with many strings on which ornaments are suspended. As the mobile hangs there, it is in a state of dynamic equilibrium. Then, if you cut one of the strings, the whole mobile starts moving, because its balance has been upset. Eventually, it slows down and reaches a new state of dynamic equilibrium. But things have changed. It does not look the same. All those ornaments have shifted, in relation to the central axis and also in relation to each other.
>
> The body's musculoskeletal system works in much the same way. If its normal balance is disrupted, it must compensate. Structural patterns will be altered to a greater or lesser degree, depending on the nature and intensity of the forces that threw off the old pattern of balance (Fig. 7-4).

A triad of signs are classically accepted as evidence for the existence of SDF: point tenderness or altered pain threshold to pressure in the adjacent paraspinal musculature or over the spinous process; abnormal contraction or tension within the adjacent paraspinal musculature; and loss of normal motion in one or more planes (Leach 1994). Chiropractic education includes extensive training in the development of the psychomotor skills necessary to diagnose the subluxation complex/SDF and to perform the manipulative maneuvers best suited to its correction.

Subluxations characterized by ligamentous laxity are markedly more problematic than fixations and are frequently of traumatic etiology. Hypermobility is clinically diagnosed by eliciting a repeated click when a joint is moved through its normal range of motion. Hypermobile joints should not be forcibly manipulated, since this can increase the degree of hypermobility, but nearby articulations that have become fixated to compensate for the hypermobile joint should be manipulated, and muscles in the area should be strengthened and toned in order to minimize the stress on the hypermobile joint.

The motion segment is the initial focus of chiropractic therapeutic intervention, and is the site where the most direct and immediate effects of SMT

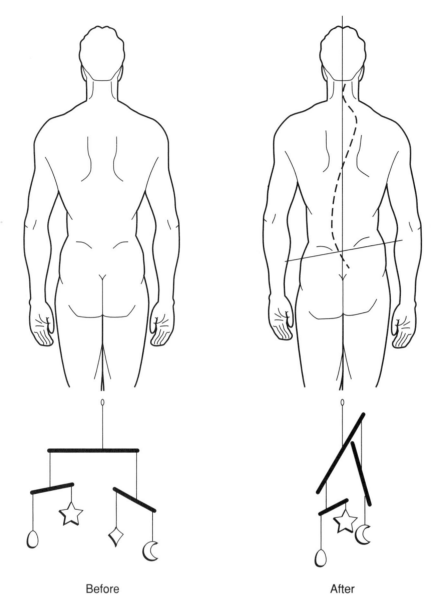

Figure 7-4. Visual model of spinal motion principles comparing mobile hanging from ceiling to body's musculoskeletal system before and after imbalance is introduced.

are likely to be noted. More far-reaching effects are possible through neural facilitation.

Facilitation

Segmental facilitation has been defined as a lowered threshold for firing in a spinal cord segment and is caused by afferent bombardment of the dorsal horn associated with spinal lesions (Korr 1976). Consequent effects can include local somatic pain or visceral organ dysfunction. Segmental facilitation is the dominant neurophysiologic hypothesis for how the vertebral subluxation complex or SDF influences autonomic function.

Some models for the specific mechanisms of facilitation postulate that inflammation is a key factor (Dvorak 1985, Gatterman & Goe 1990, Mense 1991). Inflammation alters the local milieu of the nerve, causing chemical, thermal, and mechanical changes and is likely to compromise its function. Such aberrant activity can disrupt nerve function and the homeostatic mechanisms essential to normal visceral organ function. Others have proposed neurologic models through which facilitation could occur even in the absence of inflammation (Korr 1975, Patterson & Steinmetz 1986).

A facilitated segment may result either in parasympathetic vagal dominance or excessive sympathetic output. "It appears that SDF is capable of initiating segmental facilitation and that certainly this is the most logical explanation for the use of [chiropractic] adjustment . . . for other than pain syndromes; certainly the segmental facilitation hypothesis is gaining greater acceptance and is based upon a large body of acceptable scientific research" (Leach 1994).

Rationale for the Chiropractic Adjustment

The central focus of chiropractic practice is the analytical process of determining when and where SMT is appropriate, and secondarily what type of adjustment is most appropriate in a given situation.

The chiropractor, after arriving at an overall diagnostic impression (not limited to the spine) and methodically ruling out pathologies that contraindicate SMT, proceeds to evaluate SDF in order to arrive at a specific chiropractic diagnosis (Fig. 7-5) (Leach 1994). This diagnostic process takes into account subluxations that are present, along with other clinical entities such as degeneration, disc involvement, or carpal tunnel syndrome. In certain cases, these entities require treatment additional to SMT, or affect the style of SMT, that is administered.

For example, the presence of advanced degenerative joint disease would rule out all forms of SMT that introduce substantial amounts of force into the arthritic joint. According to the Guidelines for Chiropractic Quality Assurance and Practice Parameters the high-velocity, low-amplitude thrust (HVLA) adjustment, the most common form of chiropractic SMT, is absolutely contraindicated in certain anatomic areas (Haldeman et al 1993).

Contraindications for HVLA

- Malignancies.
- Bone and joint infections.
- Acute myelopathy or acute cauda equina syndrome.
- Acute fractures and dislocations, or healed fractures and dislocations with signs of ligamentous rupture or instability.
- Acute rheumatoid, rheumatoidlike, or nonspecific arthropathies including ankylosing spondylitis characterized by episodes of acute inflammation, demineralization, and/or ligamentous laxity with anatomic subluxation or dislocation.
- Active juvenile avascular necrosis.
- Unstable os odontoideum.

These guidelines also rate, in descending order of severity, conditions that are relative to absolute contraindication, relative contraindication, and not a contraindication. Chiropractic diagnosis is geared toward evaluating where each case falls on this spectrum and then proceeding with appropriate medical referral, chiropractic treatment, or concurrent care.

Types of Manual Therapy Used by Chiropractors

HVLA, also known as osseous adjustment, is performed by manually moving a joint to the end-point of its normal range of motion, isolating it by local pressure on bony prominences, and then imparting a swift, specific, low-amplitude thrust. The thrust frequently is accompanied by a sound indicating joint cavitation, as the joint moves into the paraphysiologic space between normal range of motion and the limits of its anatomic integrity. Properly applied, the adjustment generally is a painless procedure.

Low-force chiropractic adjustments have also been developed for cases in which standard HVLA adjustment is contraindicated. Nonadjustive manual measures also employed by chiropractors (generally to supplement, not to replace SMT) include trigger point therapy, joint mobilization, and massage.

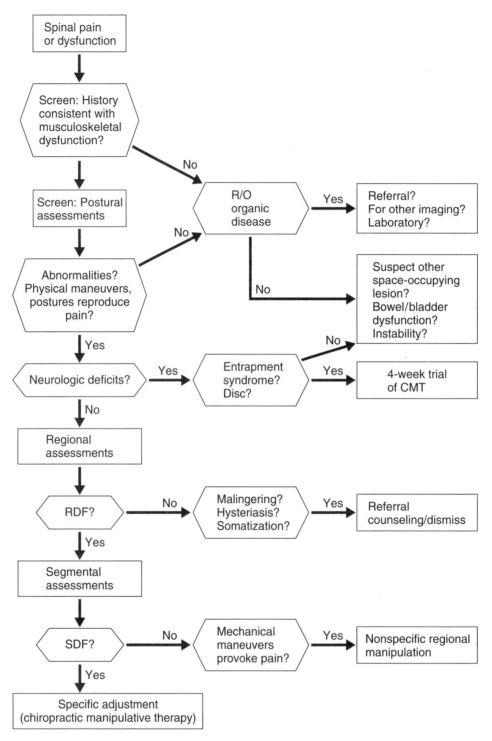

Figure 7-5. Proposed algorithm for the assessment of regional and segmental dysfunction. (Adapted from Leach RA. 1994. An algorithm for chiropractic management of spinal dysfunction. In The Chiropractic Theories: Principles and Clinical Applications. 3rd. Ed. Williams & Wilkins. Baltimore, with permission.)

Other Adjusting Methods

- High-velocity thrust with recoil.
- Low-velocity thrust.
- Flexion-distraction (originally an osteopathic technique for lumbar disc syndrome).
- Adjustment with mechanically assisted drop-piece tables.
- Adjustment with compression wave instruments.
- Various specific light-touch techniques.

Clinical Settings and Methodologies

Independence Born of Necessity

Chiropractic's long-time role as a dissenting wing of the Euro-American healing arts, has meant that its practitioners have functioned almost entirely in free-standing private practice. Chiropractic educational facilities have been private institutions, functioning almost entirely without public funding.

This status is gradually changing. Chiropractors serve on the staffs of some hospitals, and provincial universities in Quebec and Australia include chiropractic departments. Chiropractors serve in official capacities at the Olympic Games, and are playing an increasingly prominent role in the treatment of sports and workplace injuries. In 1993, J.R. Cassidy became the first chiropractor to be named research director of a university hospital orthopedics department, at the University of Saskatchewan in Canada. In 1994 John Triano became the first member of the profession to join the staff of the Texas Back Institute, in the dual role of staff chiropractic physician and clinical research scientist.

Such developments bode well for the future, but still remain more the exception than the rule. The most serious negative effect of chiropractic's peripheral status has been that the majority of patients who could benefit from chiropractic treatment have not received it. Referrals from allopathic physicians to chiropractors are more rare by far than referrals to other medical practitioners or to physical therapists.

The most positive salient aspect of operating outside the establishment for so many years is the encouragement of creative impulses and capacities. One of the greatest challenges currently facing the profession is developing uniform practice standards, while simultaneously maintaining the innovative atmosphere that has characterized the profession since its inception. The 1993 Guidelines for Chiropractic Quality Assurance and Practice Parameters, the "Mercy Document," is an initial effort.

Diagnostic Logic

First and foremost, chiropractors seek to evaluate individual symptoms in a broad context of health and body balance, not as isolated aberrations to be suppressed. This holistic viewpoint has much in common with both ancient and newly emerging models elsewhere in the healing arts.

Chiropractors recognize the need for a thorough evaluation of symptoms, and are trained to take histories and perform physical examinations. Chiropractors also are trained in state-of-the-art diagnostic techniques (Fig. 7-6). Examination procedures overlap significantly with those used by orthodox medical physicians, but chiropractors evaluate the information gleaned from these methods with a unique perspective that places great emphasis on the intricate structural and functional interplay between different parts of the body.

Chiropractic and Medical Approaches to Pain

Allopathic physicians engage in symptom suppression far more than chiropractors and also more frequently assume that the site of a pain is the site of its cause. Thus, knee pain is generally assumed to stem from a knee problem, or shoulder pain is assumed to stem from a shoulder problem. This pain-centered diagnostic logic frequently leads to increasingly sophisticated and invasive diagnostic and therapeutic procedures: If physical examination of the knee fails to clearly define the problem, imaging techniques are employed. If a radiograph fails to offer adequate clarification, the physician then uses MRI. In some cases, an arthrogram or a surgical procedure follows.

Like their allopathic colleagues, chiropractors use diagnostic tools, however, chiropractors are all too

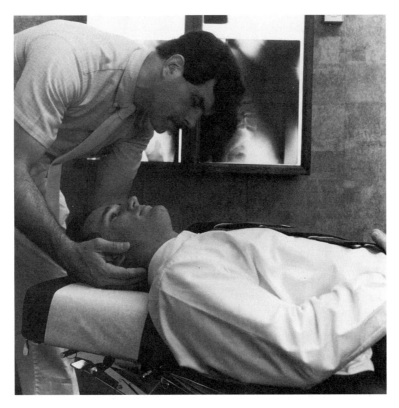

Figure 7-6. Contemporary chiropractors use state-of-the-art diagnostic and therapeutic methods.

familiar with cases in which this entire high-tech diagnostic scenario is played out, after which the knee problem is discovered to be compensation for a mechanical disorder in the low back. If the low back is mechanically dysfunctional and in need of spinal manipulation, this can place unusual stress on one or both knees.

The chiropractic approach to musculoskeletal pain involves evaluating the site of pain in a regional and whole-body context. Shoulder, elbow, and wrist problems can, of course, be caused by injuries or pathologies in the shoulder, elbow, and wrist, but can also have as their source segmental dysfunction in the cervical spine. In like manner, symptoms in the hip, knee, and ankle can originate in the lumbar spine. Not only pain, but other neurologically-mediated symptoms such as paresthesia can have a similar etiology. The ability to consider this chain of causation is central to chiropractic training.

Chiropractors from Palmer onward have intentionally refrained from assuming that the site of a symptom is the site of its cause. They assume instead that the source of the pain should be sought along the path of the nerves leading to and from the site of the symptoms. Pain in the knee might come from the knee itself, but tracing the nerve pathways between the knee and the spine reveals possible areas of causation in and around the hip, in the deep muscles of the buttocks or pelvis, in the sacroiliac joints, or in the lumbar spine.

Furthermore, if joint dysfunction does exist, it might have its primary source in the lumbar spine or it might represent a compensation for another subluxation elsewhere in the spine—perhaps in the lower or middle thoracics—or in a mechanical dysfunction of the muscles and joints of the feet. An integrative, whole-body approach to structure and function is of great value.

For patients whose presentation includes visceral organ symptoms, and if contraindications to SMT have been ruled out, chiropractic diagnostic logic includes evaluation of the spine with particular attention to those spinal levels providing autonomic nerve supply to the involved area, along with consideration of possible nutritional, environmental, and psychological factors.

Criteria for Referral to Allopathic Physicians

Chiropractic practice standards mandate timely referral to an allopathic physician for diagnosis and/or treatment for conditions beyond the chiropractor's domain, or when a reasonable trial of chiropractic care (current standards limit this to about one month in most cases) fails to bring satisfactory results (Haldeman et al 1993).

Chiropractors frequently seek second opinions in less dramatic cases, if chiropractic treatment fails to bring full resolution. Referrals from chiropractors to neurologists, neurosurgeons, orthopedic surgeons, internists, and other medical specialists are common. Referrals to complementary practitioners such as acupuncturists, homeopaths, and naturopaths also occur when appropriate.

Ethics of Referral

The medical profession has long had a clearly defined set of ethics for intraprofessional referral. A report is sent to the referring physician, and the patient remains the patient of the referring physician. When the medical establishment prohibited collegial relations with chiropractors, physicians receiving referrals from chiropractors frequently failed to extend such professional courtesies in return. At times this exerted a subliminal pressure on chiropractors not to refer. At a time when most chiropractic patients still elect not to inform their allopathic physicians that they are seeing a chiropractor, the need for breaking down all such barriers should be readily apparent (Eisenberg 1993).

Research

For years, chiropractors were attacked for offering only anecdotal evidence in support of their methods.

Spinal manipulation now has been shown by reputable researchers to be a superior healing method for low back pain. Over 30 randomized trials have compared SMT to other forms of treatment for LBP (Shekelle et al 1990, Anderson et al 1992). The majority have shown SMT to be superior to the other procedures, and none have shown it to be less effective than the comparison approaches or a control group. Each year brings the publication of new studies, in both medical and chiropractic journals, on the effectiveness of chiropractic care for an increasingly wide range of conditions.

Type M and Type O Disorders

A government commission of inquiry on chiropractic in New Zealand drew an instructive distinction between type M (musculoskeletal) and type O (internal organ) disorders. The initially skeptical commissioners concluded that chiropractic was safe and effective for type M, which in their definition included back pain and associated leg symptoms, neck pain and associated arm symptoms, and migraine headaches. Regarding type O disorders, the commission stated that while instances of therapeutic benefit from chiropractic treatment were undeniable, response for visceral organ problems was far less predictable than for type M disorders, and further research was necessary before any definitive conclusions could be reached (Chiropractic in New Zealand 1979).

A chiropractic research agenda has coalesced around the need to thoroughly document the effectiveness of SMT for both musculoskeletal and visceral disorders. Because approximately half of chiropractic patients present with low back pain, the initial research goal was to document chiropractic's effectiveness for that condition. The 1994 AHCPR guidelines indicate that this goal now has been largely achieved.

Early Chiropractic Research

B.J. Palmer, son of the founder of chiropractic, was among the premier early chiropractic researchers. He was one of the first in any health profession to use radiography as a diagnostic tool. He devised the neurocalometer (a thermographic instrument that detects paraspinal heat variances) and he developed a specialized method for adjusting the upper cervical spine.

Other researchers and developers noted for their seminal contributions to the field include Gillet, who formulated and refined motion theory (Montgomery et al 1985); Janse and Illi, whose anatomical dissections and cineroentgenographic studies of spinal and pelvic mechanics provided crucial documentation for that theory (Baker 1992); Gonstead, for his system of radiograph analysis; DeJarnette, for advances in postural analysis; and Goodheart, for his elaboration of manual muscle testing.

The University of Colorado Project

Beginning in the 1970s, Chung Ha Suh and colleagues at the Biomechanics Department of the University of Colorado undertook a series of studies which provided an extensive body of chiropractic-related basic science research. The project was funded with grants from the International Chiropractors Association, and added financial support from the American Chiropractic Association and the federal government of the United States.

The first American college professor, Suh, willing to defy the AMA boycott of chiropractic research, was a native of Korea, where he was not subjected to anti-chiropractic bias. In launching this research, he withstood intense pressure from powerful political forces within the American medical and academic establishments, which condemned chiropractic for lack of scientific underpinning, and did everything in their power to prevent chiropractors from obtaining the funding and university connections necessary for the development of a research base (Wilk v. AMA 1990).

The University of Colorado team pursued research in two major areas: development of a computer model of the cervical spine that allowed a deeper understanding of spinal joint mechanics and their relationship to the chiropractic adjustment (Suh 1974), and a range of studies on nerve compression and various aspects of neuron function (Triano et al 1982, Kelly et al 1975, Luttges et al 1976, MacGregor et al 1973, MacGregor et al 1975, Sharpless 1975, Simske et al 1994). Sharpless, for example, demonstrated that minuscule amounts of pressure on a nerve root (10 mmHg), resulted in up to a 50 percent decrease in electrical transmission through the nerve supplied by that root.

Chronic Lower Back Pain

The most influential original research in the 1980s and 1990s was done outside the United States. Three studies stand out as major landmarks: The University of Saskatchewan study on chronic LBP (Kirkaldy-Willis et al 1985); Meade's randomized clinical trial on LBP (Meade 1990); and Koes' study on persistent back and neck pain (Koes et al 1992). The study at the University of Saskatchewan involved approximately 300 subjects who had been totally disabled by back pain for an average of seven years, all of whom had gone through extensive, unsuccessful medical treatment. All were on government disability, and had been in pain for an average of 17 years before chiropractic treatment commenced.

After two to three weeks of daily chiropractic adjustments, between 79 and 93 percent of those patients without spinal stenosis had good to excellent results, reporting substantially decreased pain and increased mobility. After chiropractic treatment, over 70 percent were improved to the point of having no work restrictions. Moreover, follow-up after one year demonstrated that the improvements were long-lasting.

Even those with a narrowed spinal canal (classically considered a particularly difficult subset) showed a notable response. More than half improved substantially, and about one in five were free of pain and back on the job seven months after treatment. Extraordinarily enough, this research project was jointly administered at a university hospital by J.R. Cassidy, a chiropractor, and W.H. Kirkaldy-Willis, a world-renowned orthopedic surgeon.

The Cassidy-Kirkaldy-Willis study demonstrated the effectiveness of chiropractic for treatment of chronic, disabling LBP in cases where standard allopathic interventions had been exhausted (Kirkaldy-Willis 1985).

The Meade LBP study, a randomized clinical trial in 1990, compared chiropractic manipulation with standard hospital outpatient treatment for lower back pain in more than 700 patients. The medical treatment consisted of physical therapy and wearing a corset (Meade 1990).

Meade concluded that, "for patients with low-back

pain in whom manipulation is not contraindicated, chiropractic almost certainly confers worthwhile, long-term benefit in comparison to hospital outpatient management." The Meade study was the first randomized clinical trial to demonstrate both short-term and long-term benefits from chiropractic care, refuting the charge that chiropractic offers short-term relief, rather than lasting value (Meade, 1990).

A 1992 Dutch study compared the results of patients treated with physical therapy for persistent back and neck pain, against those given SMT, placebo treatment, and standard medical treatment by a general practitioner.

The results showed that both SMT and physical therapy were significantly more effective than a placebo treatment or treatment by a general practitioner. In addition, those receiving SMT showed more improvement than the physical therapy patients, and in fewer visits.

This was the first major research on SMT to expand its purview beyond lower back pain, to neck pain and pain in other areas of the back. It provided crucial support for the applicability of chiropractic treatment for these conditions (Koes 1992).

Headaches

Probably the most noteworthy chiropractic research to emerge from the United States by the mid-1990s is the ongoing work on headaches conducted at Northwestern College of Chiropractic in Minnesota in which chiropractic has been shown to be more effective than the tricyclic antidepressant amitriptyline for long-term relief of pain from muscle tension headaches (Boline 1991).

During the treatment phase of the trial, pain relief among those treated with medication was comparable to the SMT group. But the chiropractic patients maintained their levels of improvement after treatment was discontinued, while those taking medication returned to pretreatment status in an average of 4 weeks following its discontinuation. This implies that while medication suppressed the symptoms, chiropractic addressed the problem at a more causal level. The investigators are now pursuing comparative studies on migraine headaches.

Research on Type M Conditions

- An Australian study showed that patients treated by chiropractors lost four times fewer work days from LBP than those treated by medical doctors (Ebrall 1992).
- A cost-comparison study demonstrated that the compensation costs for lost work time were 10 times as high for those receiving standard, nonsurgical medical care than for those treated by chiropractors (Jarvis 1991).
- A study of worker's compensation cases indicated that patients receiving chiropractic care were temporarily disabled for half the length of time, were hospitalized at less than half the rate, and accrued bills less than half as high as patients receiving medical care for similar conditions (Wolk, 1987).
- A RAND Corporation study on the appropriateness of SMT for LBP declared spinal manipulation an appropriate treatment for some patients with that condition. The RAND protocol involved a multidisciplinary panel headed by an allopathic physician, which conducted an extensive review of the scientific literature, and a consensus process among the participants to determine areas of agreement (Shekelle et al 1991, 1992).
- An independent study commissioned by the Ontario provincial government found chiropractic to be safer and more effective than medical care for LBP. "On the evidence," the Manga Report stated, "particularly the most scientifically valid clinical studies, spinal manipulation applied by chiropractors is shown to be more effective than alternate treatments for low-back pain." Addressing the
(Continues)

pressing economic issues that precipitated the government's request for the report, they concluded, "there seems to be a comprehensive body of evidence, which can fairly be described as overwhelming, for the cost-effectiveness of chiropractic over medical management of patients with low-back pain." Manga and colleagues recommended a shift in policy to encourage and prefer chiropractic services for most patients with LBP, and called for placing chiropractors on the staffs of all hospitals (Manga 1993).

- A study found that patients seeing chiropractors for back pain were more satisfied with their care than patients of family practice physicians by a ratio of three to one. Interestingly, initial discussion of this study in medical journals generally assumed that the greater satisfaction rates among chiropractic patients were due to superior doctor-patient relationships, rather than the greater effectiveness of chiropractic treatment methods (Cherkin 1989).

- A clinical trial found that bed rest plus NSAIDs—long the standard method with which family practice physicians and general practitioners treated LBP—brought worse results than placebo treatment. This is particularly problematic in light of the fact that more people initially go to these primary care doctors for LBP than to any other type of practitioner. No study has shown chiropractic to be inferior to placebo (Gilbert 1985).

Research on Visceral Disorders

- Two trials evaluating the effects of chiropractic manipulation for primary dysmenorrhea have shown very encouraging results, including pain relief and changes in certain prostaglandin levels (Thomason et al 1979, Kokjohn et al 1992).

- A randomized, controlled clinical study demonstrated that diastolic and systolic blood pressure decreased significantly in response to chiropractic adjustments of the thoracic spine (T1–T5), while placebo and control groups showed no such change (Yates et al 1988).

- A study at the National College of Chiropractic showed a marked increase in the activity levels of certain immune system cells (PMNs and monocytes) after thoracic spine manipulation. These increases were significantly higher than in control groups, who were given either sham manipulation or soft-tissue manipulation (Brennan et al 1991).

- A study involving 73 Danish chiropractors in 50 clinics showed satisfactory results in 94 percent of cases of infantile colic. The results occurred within two weeks, and involved an average of three treatments (Klougart 1989).

- A series of studies by chiropractors working in concert with Italian medical doctors demonstrated promising effects of chiropractic treatment in cases of vertigo, tinnitus, headaches, and visual disorders (Mazzarelli 1982).

Beginnings of Type O Research

While the bulk of chiropractic research still focuses on musculoskeletal disorders, by the early 1990s, leading chiropractic clinicians and academics concluded that research on type O disorders must be expedited in order for the profession to survive and thrive.

Further exploration of chiropractic's effects on visceral disorders holds great promise, and is one of the most fertile areas for chiropractic research in the twenty-first century. Several studies underway indi-

Current Investigations

- A novel methodology, measurement of levels of a prostaglandin metabolite, will be used to evaluate the effects of chiropractic treatment on dysmenorrhea, which affects 50 percent of women of childbearing age. Prostaglandins have been implicated as agents responsible for uterine contraction and resulting pain during menstruation. Aside from utilizing this biochemical marker, changes in pain will be evaluated by a visual analog scale (VAS) and changes in menstrual distress by an independent questionnaire (MDQ). Patient groups will receive either SMT or a sham procedure. The study is designed to indicate not only whether SMT reduces pain in primary dysmenorrhea, but also whether it might correct the underlying cause altogether.

- Scientific evidence has not justified definite conclusions regarding the etiology or optimal treatment of infantile colic (IC). In this study active chiropractic treatment will be compared to a placebo chiropractic treatment, and also to the parental use of written systematic guidelines for responding to their baby's crying (Taubman's method), an approach that has already been suggested in a randomized clinical trial to be effective.

- A randomized clinical trial will evaluate the use of chiropractic adjustments and massage treatment for essential hypertension. The treatment period for this study is two months per patient, during which time each patient will be evaluated before and after each therapeutic intervention for both systolic and diastolic pressure. Follow-up measurements of blood pressure will be carried out to determine if lasting changes remain.

  (Continues)

- For several years, case data suggesting the efficacy of chiropractic care in the management of otitis media has been collected by both a chiropractor and collaborating pediatrician in Miami, Florida. This field study will feature the use of tympanometry as an objective measure of pressure within the ear before and after adjustments. A secondary study is also anticipated to provide either MRI or CAT scan data that has been digitalized to determine the diameter and/or inclination of the eustachian tubes before and after adjustments.

Chiropractic in the Health Care System of the Future

The greatest issue facing chiropractic in its first century was survival—whether it would remain a separate and distinct healing art, succumb to the substantial forces arrayed against it, or be subsumed into the great maw of allopathic medicine. This question has been resolved. Chiropractic has survived.

The key question for the next century, or at least the next generation, is, how can chiropractic best be integrated into the mainstream health care delivery system so that services are readily available to all who can benefit from their application? Furthermore, how can such integration be achieved without diluting chiropractic principles and practice to the point where chiropractic becomes a weak shadow of its former self?

An overwhelming majority of chiropractors (unlike osteopaths) do not wish to pursue the path toward becoming full-scope allopathic physicians. Moreover, they will not willingly opt for any system in which chiropractic services are available only on medical referral. Chiropractors will function gladly as contributing members of the health care team, but will not surrender their political independence, or the holistic, wisdom-of-the-body worldview that has always been the core of their profession. How can the desired integration be achieved?

cate the creativity being generated in this area (Johnson 1994).

Chiropractors, allopathic physicians, and the general public must agree upon a framework based on common goals. Fortunately, a common purpose does exist—all parties seek to create the most effective, efficient health care system possible for the greatest number of people. A framework for implementation also exists—at least in theory—based on the *level playing field* concept. This concept synthesizes the principles of democracy and hierarchy.

The democracy of science is one in which equal opportunity is enjoyed by all, and all hypotheses are innocent until proven guilty. Blind prejudice on the part of allopathic doctors, chiropractors, or anyone else, has no place in this environment. All methods, whether conventional or alternative, must prove themselves effective and cost-effective, and must demonstrate minimal iatrogenic effects. Approaches presently enjoying the imprimatur of the mainstream medical establishment are not exempt from this scrutiny.

Hierarchy also has a place on the level playing field, as long as it is based on demonstrable skills and proven methods. In those areas where conventional western medicine clearly has established its superior quality, such as trauma care, certain surgeries, and the treatment of life-threatening infections, this expertise should be honored. But when a complementary method such as chiropractic is proven superior, as in lower back pain, chiropractors must be accorded a similar role. This is a lateral conception of hierarchy rather than a vertical one, a relationship among equals; precedence is based on quality, which in turn is determined through adherence to mutually agreed upon standards.

There is an immediate and pressing need to broaden lines of communication between the chiropractic and medical professions, both on a one-to-one basis and in small and large groups, with the goal of offering a cooperative effort to all patients. Each side must learn to recognize its own strengths and weaknesses, as well as those of the other. No one has all the answers.

Although chiropractors have clear guidelines for referring to medical doctors, neither the medical profession as a whole nor its various specialty groups have developed formal guidelines for referring patients to chiropractors. In the post-AHCPR Guidelines era, such criteria are essential for informed decision-making. At a bare minimum, these guidelines should recommend referral to chiropractors of lower back pain patients who do not meet the AHCPR's tightly circumscribed criteria for surgical referral.

The future need not mirror the worst aspects of the past. It is incumbent upon all health care providers, and wholly consonant with our role that we heal not only sickness but old rifts among ourselves.

References

Anderson R, Meeker W, et al. 1992. Meta-analysis of randomized clinical trials on manipulation for low-back pain. J Manipulative Physiol Ther 15(3):181–194

Baker WJ. 1992. A clinical reformation in chiropractic: the research of Dr. Fred Illi. Chiro Hist 5:59–62

Bennett GM. 1981. The art of the bonesetter. Tamor Pierston, Isleworth

Bigos S, Bowyer O, Braen G, et al. 1994. Acute lower back problems in adults. Clinical Practice Guideline, Quick Reference Guide Number 14. Rockville, MD: U.S. Department of Health and Human Services, Public Health Service, Agency for Health Care Policy and Research, AHCPR Pub. No. 95-0643

Boline PD. 1991. Chiropractic treatment and pharmaceutical treatment for muscle contraction headaches: a randomized comparative clinical trial. Proceedings from the 1991 Conference on Spinal Manipulation. FCER. Arlington, Virginia

Bourdillion JF. 1982. Spinal Manipulation. 3rd Ed. Appleton Century-Crofts, East Norwalk, Connecticut

Brennan PC, Kokjohn K, Katlinger CJ, et al. 1992. Enhanced phagocytic cell respiratory burst induced by spinal manipulation: potential role of substance P. J Manipulative Physiol Ther 14:399–408

Cherkin D, Deyo RA, Wheeler K, Ciol MA. 1995. Physician views about treating low back pain. Spine 20:1–10

Cherkin D, MacCornack FA, Berg AO. 1989. Family physicians' views of chiropractors: hostile or hospitable? Am J Public Health 79:636–637

Cherkin D, MacCornack FA. 1989. Patient evaluation of low back pain care from family physicians and chiropractors. West J Med 150:351–355

Chiropractic in New Zealand: Report of the Commission of Inquiry. 1979. PD Hasselberg, Government Printer, Wellington, New Zealand

Copland-Griffiths M. 1991. Dynamic Chiropractic Today: The Complete and Authoritative Guide to this Major Therapy. Thorsons, Wellingborough

Curtis P, Bove G. 1992. Family physicians, chiropractors, and back pain. J Fam Pract 35:551–555

Ebrall PS. 1992. Mechanical low back pain: a comparison of medical and chiropractic management within the Victorian WorkCare scheme. Chiro J Aust 22(2):47–53

Eisenberg DM, Kessler RC, Foster C, et al. 1993. Unconventional medicine in the United States: prevalence, costs, and patterns of use. New Engl J Med 328:246–252

Gatterman MI, Goe DR. 1990. Muscle and myofascial pain syndromes. In: Gatterman MI (ed). Chiropractic Management of Spine Related Disorders. Williams & Wilkins, Baltimore, pp. 285–329

Gellert G. 1994. Global explanations and the credibility problem of alternative medicine. Advances 10(4):60–67

Gibbons R. 1992. The evolution of chiropractic: medical and social protest in America. In Haldeman S (ed). Modern Developments in the Principles and Practice of Chiropractic. Appleton Century-Crofts, East Norwalk, Connecticut

Gilbert JR. 1985. Clinical trial of common treatments for low back pain in family practice. BMJ 291:791–794

Haldeman S, Chapman-Smith D, Peterson DM. 1993. Guidelines for Chiropractic Quality Assurance and Practice Parameters: Proceedings of the Mercy Center Consensus Conference. Aspen Publications, Gaithersburg, Maryland

Jarvis KB, Phillips RB, et al. 1991. Cost per case comparison of back injury claims of chiropractic versus medical management for conditions with identical diagnostic codes. J Occup Med 33(8):847–852

Johnson M. 1994. The status of research at FCER: exploring the possibilities. J Am Chir Assn 31(12):43–48

Kelly PT, Luttges MW. 1975. Electrophoretic separation of nervous system proteins on exponential gradient polyacrylamide gels. J Neurochem 24:1077–1079

Kirkaldy-Willis W, Cassidy J. 1985. Spinal manipulation in the treatment of low back pain. Can Fam Physician 31:535–540

Klougart N, Nillson N, Jacobson J. 1989. Infantile colic treated by chiropractors: a prospective study of 316 cases. J Manipulative Physiol Ther 12:281–288

Koes BW, Bouter LM, et al. 1992. Randomised clinical trial of manipulative therapy and physiotherapy for persistent back and neck complaints: results of one year follow-up. BMJ 304:601–605

Kokjohn K, Schmid DM, Triano JJ, Brennan PC. 1992. The effect of spinal manipulation on pain and prostaglandin levels in women with primary dysmenorrhea. J Manipulative Physiol Ther 15:279–285

Korr IM. 1975. Proprioceptors and the behavior of lesioned segments. In: Stark EH (ed). Osteopathic Medicine. Publication Sciences Group, Acton, Massachusetts, pp 183–199

Korr IM. 1976. The spinal cord as organizer of disease processes: some preliminary perspectives. J Am Osteopath Assoc 76:89–99

Leach RA. 1994. The Chiropractic Theories: Principles and Clinical Applications. 3rd Ed. Williams & Wilkins, Baltimore

Lomax E. 1975. Manipulative therapy: a historical perspective from ancient times to the modern era. In Goldstein M (ed). The Research Status of Spinal Manipulative Therapy. Government Printing Office, Washington, DC, p. 11–17

Luttges MW, Kelly PT, Gerren RA. 1976. Degenerative changes in mouse sciatic nerves: electrophoretic and electrophysiological characterizations. Exp Neurol 50: 706–733

MacGregor RJ, Oliver RM. 1973. A general-purpose electronic model for arbitrary configurations of neurons. J Theor Biol 38:527–538

MacGregor RJ, Sharpless SK, Luttges MW. 1975. A pressure vessel model for nerve compression. J Neurol Sci 24:299–304

Manga P, Angus D, Papadopoulos C, Swan WR. 1993. A study to examine the effectiveness and cost-effectiveness of chiropractic management of low-back pain. Ministry of Health, Government of Ontario

Mazarelli J (ed). 1982. Chiropractic: Interprofessional Research. Edizioni Minerva Medica, Torino, Italy

Meade TW, Dyer S, et al. 1990. Low back pain of mechanical origin: randomized comparison of chiropractic and hospital outpatient treatment. BMJ 300:1431–1437

Mense S. 1991. Considerations concerning the neurobiological basis of muscle pain. Can J Physiol Pharmacol 69: 610–616

Montgomery DP, Nelson JM. 1985. Evolution of chiropractic theories of practice and spinal adjustment, 1900–1950. Chiro Hist 5:71–76

National Board of Chiropractic Examiners. 1993. Job Analysis of Chiropractic. NBCE, Greeley, Colorado

North American Spine Society (NASS) Ad Hoc Committee on Diagnostic and Therapeutic Procedures. 1991. Spine 16:10

Palmer BJ. 1951. Chiropractic Clinical Controlled Research. Palmer School of Chiropractic, Davenport, Iowa

Palmer DD. 1910. Text-book of the Science, Art and Philosophy of Chiropractic. Portland Printing House, Portland

Paré A. 1968. The Collected Works of Ambroise Paré (translated by Thomas Johnson). Milford House, New York

Patterson MM, Steinmetz JE. 1986. Long-lasting alterations of spinal reflexes: a potential basis for somatic dysfunction. Manual Med 2:38–42

Peterson DM. 1995. Dynamic Chiropractic. Motion Palpation Institute, Huntington Beach, California, 13(2)3

Plamondon RL. 1995. Summary of 1994 ACA annual statistical study. J Am Chir Assn 32(1):57–63

Schafer RC, Faye LJ. 1989. Motion Palpation and Chiropractic Technic. Motion Palpation Institute, Huntington Beach, California

Sharpless S. 1975. Susceptibility of spinal roots to compression block. In Goldstein M (ed): The Research Status of Spinal Manipulation. Government Printing Office, Washington

Shekelle PG, Adams AH, et al. 1991. The appropriateness of spinal manipulation for low-back pain: project overview and literature review (R-4025/1-CCR/FCER). RAND, Santa Monica

Shekelle PG, Adams AH, Chassin MR, et al. 1992. Spinal manipulation for low-back pain. Ann Intern Med 117(7):590–598

Simske SJ, Schmeister TA, et al. 1994. An experimental model for combined neural, muscular, and skeletal degeneration. JNMS 2:116–123

Suh CH. 1974. The fundamentals of computer aided x-ray analysis of the spine. J Biomech 7:161–169

Thomasen PR, Fisher BL, Carpenter PA, Fike GL. 1979. Effectiveness of spinal manipulative therapy in treatment of primary dysmenorrhea: a pilot study. J Manipulative Physiol Ther 2:140–145

Triano JJ, Luttges MW. 1982. Nerve irritation: a possible model of sciatic neuritis. Spine 7:129–136

Wilk v. AMA, 895 F2D 352 Cert den, 112.2 Ed 2D 524 (1990)

Withington ET (trans). 1959. Hippocrates: vol. III. Harvard University Press, Cambridge

Wolk S. 1987. Chiropractic medical care: a cost analysis of disability and treatment for back-related worker's compensation cases. Foundation for Chiropractic Education and Research, Arlington, Virginia

Yates RG, Lamping DL, Abram NL, Wright C. 1988. Effects of chiropractic treatment on blood pressure and anxiety: a randomized, controlled trial. J Manipulative Physiol Ther 11:484–488

8
Western Herbalism

Lisa Meserole

*P*lants have been used by human beings for food, medicine, clothing, tools, and in religious rites since before recorded history, more than 60,000 years ago (Solecki & Shanidar, 1975). No continent, island, climate, or geography that is home to human culture lacks a formal tradition of incorporating local flora into daily and ceremonial life as a means of enhancing health and welfare. Prehistoric plant life prepared the earth to be a viable and hospitable habitat for homo sapiens, and plant ecology continues to help maintain the oceans, continents, and atmosphere today.

> "It is the power of the truth that endures."
>
> —Imhotep (Egyptian physician, later exalted as the god of medicine, Papyrus, 2400 BC)
>
> "Through contention all things are made manifest."
>
> —Herakleitos the Dark.

Definition

Herbalism is the study and practice of using plant material for food, medicine, and health promotion. This includes not only treatment of disease, but also enhancement of the quality of life, physically and spiritually. Although a fundamental principle of herbalism is to promote preventive self-care and guided, simple self-treatment among the general population, an herbalist, or herbal practitioner, is someone who has undertaken specific study and supervised practical training to achieve competence in treating patients.

An herb can be an angiosperm, that is, a flowering plant, shrub, or tree, or a moss, lichen, fern, algae, seaweed, or fungus. The herbalist may use the entire plant, or specifically the flowers, fruits, leaves, twigs, bark, roots, rhizomes, seeds, or exudates (such as tapped and purified maple syrup), or a combination of parts. Botany defines an herb as a nonwoody, low-growing plant, but herbalists use the entire plant kingdom. In many herbal traditions, nonplants are used as healing agents, including animal parts (organs, bone, tissue), insects, animal and insect secretions, worm castings, shells, rocks, metals, minerals, and gemstones. These examples are recorded in ancient and contemporary materia medicae, formal manuscripts of healing agents and their indication and uses. Egyptian, Chinese, Tibetan, European, and American, and other worldwide material medicae are important references for herbal practitioners. This discussion will address only plant herbal agents.

Herbalism is a misleading term, for it implies that a single hidden root gives rise to the diverse ways in which all human cultures across the millenia have used plants for food, medicine, and ritual. The use of herbs by the peoples of the Americas, Europe, Africa, the Middle and Far East, the Pacific Islands, and other regions is specific to each society and paradigm. For example, contemporary Western scientists have been restricted until recently by the Western mechanistic premises of biology and physics (see Chapter 1).

Although there is no single, worldwide system of herbalism, all herbal traditions share certain themes.

Common Themes of Herbalism

- Optimization of health and wellness. Most traditions include specific systems of food, spice, and herb taboos and recommended inclusions; adherence to protects practitioners and users from undesirable consequences. A pregnant woman in Mexico avoids eggs because they could push her into a state of excess cold that could weaken her (see Chapter 15). During winter flu season, extra ginger and hot peppers are added to curries in Indian cuisine to protect against infection. Similarly, shitake mushrooms (powerful immunomodulators) are used in winter soups in traditional Japanese cooking.
- Emphasis on the whole person. This includes body, mind, soul; past, present, and future; and community.
- Emphasis on the individual. In Chinese herbal medicine, 10 patients with high blood pressure might receive 10 different herbal formulas. Furthermore, the same patient might take different hypertension formulas at age 45, and at age 65, and each formula might be adjusted repeatedly according to pulse, tongue, and other readings.
- Emphasis on the community. The illness or recovery of a member might influence the community itself, beyond emotional group empathy.

(Continues)

- Attention to finding and treating the root cause of a problem, not just the manifestations and symptoms. Although, like most healers and medicine suppliers, if the cause remains unidentified or untreatable, symptomatic treatment is offered.
- Application of the principle of duality between both the healing and the life threatening forces of nature. The fundamental assumption of this principle is that natural law is greater than the will of individual or community, and healing demands that the healer, the patient, and the community align with natural forces.
- Belief in the reality of the unmeasurable and abstract. Although dual, the abstract and physical worlds are inseparable. An herbalist who also is a true healer devotes himself or herself to maintaining balance and communication between the visible and invisible. This might be accomplished through communing with ancestors, spiritual forces, nature, or plants, and adjusting activities to natural cycles (for example, in Tibetan medicine, blending a formula during a specific season, moon phase, or auspicious date).
- Premise of recycling. Nature is inherently circular and repetitive; generally sequential, but not predominantly linear; and predictable, but seldom certain. This leads to the frequent traditional practice of offering an object or prayer, in return for healing plants and for addressing requests for healing to both the physical and spiritual worlds.
- Openness to exchange of knowledge. Most traditions incorporate new medicinal plants and new herbal uses and preparations that have been learned about through trade or travel.

(Continues)

- Regulation of the herbalist's practice through local accountability to his or her community. Success and prestige arise primarily from professional reputation that grows via word of mouth; not from image, business acumen, or material wealth.
- Humility generated from the healer's recognition of his or her own limits and skills. Since reputation depends generally on treatment efficacy and community standing, an herbalist would be reluctant to take on a case without reasonable confidence that he or she would succeed. Complex or incurable cases would be referred to another, or the patient would be advised that no treatment was available, other than minimization of suffering.

Classifications of Herbalists

Each cultural or medical system has different types of herbal practitioners, all consistent with its paradigm. However most paradigms identify professional herbalists, lay herbalists, plant gatherers, and medicine makers. (Professional or lay herbalists often collect their own plants and prepare their own medicines.)

Professional Herbalist

A professional herbalist undertakes formalized training or a long apprenticeship in plant and medical studies, or alternatively in plant and spiritual or healing studies. This knowledge includes extensive familiarity—often a relationship—with specific plants, which involves their identification, habitat, harvesting criteria, preparation, storage, therapeutic indications, contraindications, and dosing. A professional herbalist is not necessarily the primary healer (Iwu 1993). A professional herbalist might fol-

low a family tradition, or might be selected at a young age as being endowed with potential mastery of using plants as healing aids. In Europe and the United States, this group includes officially trained medical herbalists, clinical herbalists, licensed naturopathic doctors specializing in botanical medicine, licensed acupuncturists with training in Chinese herbal medicine, licensed Aryuvedic doctors, Native American herbalists and shamans, Latin American curanderos and other lineage or culturally recognized professional herbalists. The shaman from Madagascar who—although never acknowledged or compensated for his contribution—revealed the usefulness of Caranthas roseus, the greater periwinkle developed in the west as vinblastine and vincristine against certain cancers, exemplifies the spirit and expertise of a professional healer and herbalist.

Many herbalists consider the patient's direct involvement in his or her own healing, and the summoning of the patient's intellectual, emotional, physical, and spiritual attention to the process as critical. Partly for this reason, and because of traditional herbalism's emphasis on "right relationship," social context and self-responsibility, many herbal practitioners deliberately prescribe elaborate rather than convenient herbal therapies. For example, on a returning home visit to Ghana a merchant developed an infected leg ulcer. Instead of being supplied an herbal medicine by the herbalist, he was directed to the nearby, live plant source (a local tree bark). He collected and prepared the antimicrobial and vulnery poultice and applied it daily until his wound healed. Although self-collection and medicine preparation is impractical in the United States, self-involvement in the healing process is possible in many ways, and parallels the complex lifestyle changes now routinely recommended to patients with chronic ailments such as cardiovascular disease.

Lay Herbalist

A lay herbalist has a broad knowledge of plants useful for health problems, but does not have extensive training in medical and spiritual diagnosis and management. He or she may be an herb vendor with a sensitivity to the needs and desires of the marketplace, whose livelihood has been passed down as a family business. Evaluation of medicinal plant quality, strength, uses, and dose are included in the lay herbalist's domain. The Irish herbalist who uses specific herbal treatments for certain skin or stomach symptoms is an example.

Plant Gatherer, Grower, and Medicine Maker

Plant gatherers, growers, and medicine makers might consider themselves to be herbalists; actually, they are to the practicing herbalist what the contemporary pharmacist is to the clinical physician. In Chinese medicine, there is one specialist who produces and collects plants, one who processes and stores plants, and a clinical herbalist/doctor who prescribes the medicines. In some systems, preparing and handling medicines is considered a spiritual privilege and responsibility. Therefore, certain herbal medicines are prepared only by the herbalist or healer or a designated assistant.

Herbs and Medicinal Plants

Physicians in the United States studied and relied on plant drugs as primary medicines through the 1930s. Until that time, medical schools taught basic plant taxonomy and pharmacognosy, and medicinal plant therapeutics. The term *drug* derives from an ancient word for *root* and the roots and rhizomes of many medicinal plants continue to provide alkaloids, steroidal saponins, and many active constituents that are clinically useful today. The United States Pharmacopeia listed 636 herbal entries in 1870; only 58 were listed in the 1990 edition (Boyle 1991). Although some plants were dropped because they were found to be weak or unsafe, the majority of clinically useful plants were replaced with pharmaceuticals, which generated profits from patented drugs and helped support the industrialization of medicine.

Characteristics and Composition

In many traditional systems, the characteristics of a medicinal plant is emphasized without attention to its composition because techniques and equipment for plant analysis are new. Preanalytical, chemical knowledge of medicinal and food plants derived from direct perception through the five senses; from the herbalist's attentive, empirical observation of

plants' effects on animals and humans; and in some traditions, from sacred teachings and sixth sense intuition. Plants' healing uses and properties are paradigm-specific. In Chinese and Tibetan medicine, the "five tastes" are sweet, sour, salty, pungent, and bitter. Each flavor is associated with certain qualities and corresponding physiologic actions. For example, cinnamon (*Cinnamomum cassia*) bark is warm, sweet, and pungent, and is used to warm the channels and disperse cold. It is prescribed for certain infections, correlating with recent pharmacologic and clinical research which demonstrated that aqueous decoctions strongly inhibit *Staphylococcus aureus* and *Salmonella typhi* (Bensky 1986).

Knowledge of the chemical composition of food and medicinal plants is growing worldwide, as access to analytical technology improves. Perhaps the only disadvantage to identifying, categorizing, and researching molecular constituents from plants is the risk of equating the plant's therapeutic efficacy to its composition; analysis is reductionist in paradigm, and data cannot exist beyond the limits of the technology (and available funding to apply it) or the paradigm from which it arises.

Food, medicinal, and healing plants contain digestible fiber (carbohydrates and hemicellulose) and indigestible fiber (cellulose and lignins), nutritives (calories, vitamins, minerals, trace elements, amino acids, essential fatty acids, and water), and both inert and active constituents.

Adhering to a western paradigm, plant constituents can be classified according to their morphology, source plant taxonomy, therapeutic (pharmacologic) applications, or chemical constituents (Tyler, et al 1985). A classical organization of the active chemical constituents includes the following:

1. Carbohydrates: sugars, starches, aldehydes, gums, and pectins Glycosides: cardiac glycosides in digitalis purpurea leaf, anthraquinone glycosides in aloe sp latex, and rhubarb, (Rheum officinale) root and rhizome, flavinol glycosides (rutin and hesperidin used to reduce capillary bleeding), and other glycoside types.
2. Tannins: present in coffee and tea.
3. Lipids: fixed oils and waxes.
4. Volatile oils: essential oils such as peppermint and eucalyptus.

5. Resins.
6. Steroids: including the steroidal saponins from Mexican yam (*Diocorea* sp), the original source of early oral contraceptives.
7. Alkaloids: atropine from Atropa belladona, quinine from chinchona, morphine from Papaver somniferum.
8. Peptide hormones.
9. Enzymes: bromelain from pineapple.

Activities

Activities and correspondent indications for the use of plants are, again, paradigm-specific. In the

---

Influences on Plant Activities and Their Therapeutic Properties

- Specific plant species, variety, and sometimes individual plant itself.
- Habitat including latitude, longitude, exposure, humidity, rainfall, sun, shade, wind, temperature and daily and seasonal variation, soil, soil microorganisms, insects, birds, animals, companion plants, pests, plant diseases, and interaction with humans (damage, cultivation, harvesting, and pollution).
- Composition and constituents (presence of active and inert ingredients).
- How and when plant is collected, stored, processed, how herb is dispensed, and dosed.
- Presence of adulterants, pests, or disease.
- The prescriber—many traditional systems in Africa and Asia ascribe the ability to potentiate the plant's healing properties only to initiated healers or shamans.
- The patient's health status, disease, age, and receptivity to healing.
- The symbolic or cultural significance of the plant.
- The placebo effect.

United States alone, there are varying opinions regarding a particular plant's full spectrum of physiologic action. This is due to the complex nature of plants and their uses.

This list might threaten the confidence of the researcher, herbalist, or patient that the desired effect will be produced. However, every factor listed is present in the human food supply, which has supported human life since prehistory. A true scientist might agree that there is no way to control all variables, although identifying, controlling, or tracking those most suspected of producing specific outcomes is the tedious and honorable responsibility of all healers and researchers. Plant actions are recorded in the pharamacopeias through the first half of this century in archaic terminology. Many terms are similarly used to describe the actions of contemporary pharmaceuticals.

A sample of some classic plant actions—often but not always associated with identifiable nutritives or active constituents—are as follows:

Plant Actions

- Respiratory system: stimulating expectorant (*Marrubrium vulgaris,* hoarhound), relaxing expectorant (*Prunus serotina,* black cherry bark), antitussive (*Prunus serotina*), immunomodulator for upper respiratory tract infection (*Echinacea purpurea* and other species).
- Gastrointestinal system: emetic (Ipecehuana), anti-emetic (*Zingiber officinal,* ginger), laxative (*Plantago ovata,* psyllium seed), spasmolytic (*Papaver somniferum,* opium poppy).
- Nervous system: sedative (*Valerian officinalis*), stimulant (*Piper myristicum,* kava kava), cardiotonic (*Crataegus oxycantha* or monogyna, hawthorne), antidepressant (*Hypericum perforatum,* Saint John's wort).

These examples illustrate a few of the many actions ascribed to classical western paradigm herbs.

Often, contemporary research elucidates the constituents, mechanisms of action, and clinical responses that justify traditional uses. Occasionally, some plants are found to be inactive, ineffective, or to contain potential toxins, which allow for their discontinuance or for requiring special methods of preparation and dosing. Like most prescription medications today, some strong herbs must be dosed carefully to render them safe and effective. However, to provide a realistic perspective, casava root—one of the leading sources of calories and carbohydrates for people worldwide—contains cyanide-like compounds that produce permanent neurotoxicity, paralysis, and death if improperly prepared; traditional preparation involves cooking, which renders the toxins inert.

Other complications to the direct association of active constituents to in vivo and clinical medicinal actions are that many times the active compounds remain unidentified, or the physiological response to the medicinal part of the whole plant is distinct from the actions of the individual active constituents (as in the cases of Valerian and Echinacea). In addition, sometimes ingredients that appear inert are later found to be active when a more accurate mechanism of action or bioassay associated with the plant's effects is discovered. This occurred in the National Cancer Institute's screening program, when inactive plants were rescreened decades later with advanced methodologies and found to contain biologically active compounds.

From a nonreductionist paradigm, plant composition alone offers an incomplete explanation of the full scope of the properties and actions of food and healing plants. Traditional herbalists, turn of the century vitalists, naturopathic doctors, and many contemporary medical doctors and practitioners share a belief in a "life force" that is yet to be fully understood. Many herbalists hold that healing energy is inherent to plants; it is primarily this energy, rather than nutritive or chemical constituents, which promotes healing. Shamans, traditional healers, and alchemists used their skills, knowledge, and power to instill certain plants with special healing properties in this view.

Herbal Therapeutics

Different cultural paradigms use plants for healing in a manner founded on each paradigm's premises. Herbal practitioners in the United States, may rely primarily on the plant's pharmacologic actions (in some cases enhanced by specific processing and extractive solvents and techniques, or formulating plant medicines into standardized extract products to concentrate and guarantee unit doses of active constituents); individual plant pharmacokinetics (best preserved by using single, whole plants or their extracts); synergistic formulating (blending a number of medicinal plants together to achieve specific therapeutic effects unachievable by using a single herb alone); nutritive value (as when Urtica repens, or nettles, are recommended as a tea rich in absorbable iron); energetics; or a combination of these.

CASE EXAMPLE

A thirty-five-year-old patient in the United States consults with a Western naturopathic doctor or medical herbalist about experiencing mild anxiety. The patient's family history and personal and psychological health history are "unremarkable."

A health screening and physical examination within the last 6 months identified no health problems. The patient is evaluated for a "constitutional" physiological profile, a personal and social profile, and a lifestyle (stress, diet, exercise, recreation, and spiritual values) profile. Treatment for her simple, circumstantial, stress-induced anxiety is to increase exercise and gardening (time outdoors), make some minor adjustments to her diet and lifestyle, and soak her feet each evening in a lavender (*Lavandula officionalus*) foot bath (mildly relaxing) for 10 days. Use Passiflora incarnata tincture, specifically dosed, twice daily for 2 weeks; then consult with the practitioner on her progress and symptoms. Passiflora incarnata is listed in Martindale's Extra Pharmacopeia (Martindale 1994), and in the Pharmacopeia's of Egypt, France, Germany, Switzerland, and Brazil, although it is not listed in the US Pharmacopeia.

(Continues)

It acts as a mild sedative and antispasmodic. Among its constituents are a volatile oil (sedating on inhalation but of unknown composition), cyanogenic flavinoids 5-7-dihydroxyflavone ("chrysin," a monflavinoid shown to act as a partial agonist, displacing three H flunitrazepam from central benzodiazipine receptors from mice), and passiflorine (a harmane alkaloid).

Food and medicinal plants have multiple actions, due at least in part to their multiple constituents. This is in relative contrast to many pharmaceuticals, which typically have a single or few specific therapeutic actions. However, pharmaceutical side effects demonstrate how uncommon a true single action is physiologically—whether because of minor but concurrent nontherapeutic pharmacologic actions or because a single action provokes the desired therapeutic physiologic response along with unintended, nontherapeutic responses.

The multiple actions of plants—although a challenge to the isolation of single active constituents or primary single pharmacologic or physiologic actions—are only a problem if plants are classified as highly potent, synthetic pharmaceuticals. However, since the vast majority of medicinal plants are much less potent than pharmaceuticals, and since humans have evolved on plant based diets (each individual plant or animal food, a complex chemical soup of unknown formula), it seems appropriate to assume that humans are probably better adapted to plants as food and medicine than to strong pharmaceutical drugs that have 50 years or less of use in the population worldwide.

Herbal medicines can be delivered in many forms. Some plants are best used fresh, but are seldom marketed fresh since they are highly perishable. Dried, whole, or chopped herbs can be prepared as infusions (steeped as tea) or decoctions (simmered over low heat). Flowers, leaves, and powdered herbs are infused (chamomile or peppermint), while fruits, seeds, barks, and roots require decocting (rose hips, cinnamon bark, licorice root). Many fresh and dried herbs can be tinctured as preserved medicines in al-

cohol; some plants are suited to acetracts (vinegar extracts), while others are active and well preserved as syrups, glycerites (in vegetable glycerine), or miels (in honey). Powdered or freeze-dried herbs are available in bulk, tablets, troches, pastes, or capsules. Fluid and solid extracts—strong concentrates (four to six times the crude herb strength)—and fresh plant juices preserved in approximately 25 percent alcohol (as in the fresh plant echinacea succus) are other forms.

Nonoral delivery forms include herbal pessaries, suppositories, creams, ointments, gels, linaments, oils, distilled waters, washes, enemas, baths, poultices, compresses, moxa, snuffs, steams, and inhaled smokes and aromatics (volatile oils). The predominant plant delivery forms vary among different herbal traditions. Tinctures are widely used in Britain and the United States; tablets of standardized extracts of certain herbs (like Ginko biloba) are popular in Germany and the United States; decoctions are common in Tibetan, Chinese, and African traditions; therapeutic oils are used topically and internally in Ayurvedic treatments; teas, smokes, and compresses are used in the Native American tradition.

There is another point to be made regarding herbal therapeutics as distinct from contemporary over the counter and prescription pharmaceuticals. Herbal therapies have never been utilized nor do they show high efficacy when they are used as pharmaceutical substitutes. Crude or processed plant foods and medicines tend to work best preventatively or therapeutically as slow-acting, gradual, healing agents. They must be taken consistently, in the correct form and dose. (There are some medicinal plants that work rapidly.) Additionally, the herbal practitioner's familiarity with each medicinal plant or herbal formula usually is much greater than the medical doctor's familiarity with each individual pharmaceutical, and this permits the herbalist to precisely select a particular plant or formula for each patient. Three different patients each with a chief complaint of headache would each receive a different herbal prescription. The approach an herbalist uses to arrive at which herbs to prescribe is distinct from how a conventional western physician prescribes a pharmaceutical.

Herbs in Preventive Health and Patient Self Care

"What is more respectable than to take care of oneself within one's own means?"

—A H Banneran, World Health Organization

This discussion would be incomplete if it were not reemphasized that herbs are essentially "people's medicine." Traditional systems of herbalism generally make little distinction between food and medicinal plants and local accessibility to food, spice, and therapeutic herbs was a given in nonindustrialized societies.

Before this century, people everywhere had closer personal contact with food and medicinal plants. The modern era has brought many advantages to human health and sanitation, but one potential disadvantage of economic and occupational specialization is the loss of this contact with the source of plant medicines. The marketplace has become multileveled so that the consumer usually has no direct or personal relationship with the herb producer. Sometimes, because of costs of production, taxes, and marketing, the packaged herbal product costs 20 times the price of the crude herb. There are undeniable advantages to certain prepackaged or concentrated herbal products, but two disadvantages are accountability and economic access. If fresh or bulk crude herbs are abandoned in the marketplace for less perishable and higher return products, the patient has access to only highly processed products, and the cash-poor patient loses access altogether. This is particularly ironic in the case of medicinal plants; most traditional systems considered healing plants a gift of nature or God, and access to them a basic human right.

A partial solution to ensure access to high quality herbs is to support the renewed national interest in home gardens and urban "pea patches," thus embracing herbalism's unwritten dictum of self responsibility and direct individual contact in the cycles of nature. Many culinary herbs such as thyme, oregano, and rosemary contain antioxidants, antimicrobial volatile oils, and are digestive stimulants and antiseptics. Although specific herbs may vary depending on climate and region, such kitchen gardens could serve as preventive and therapeutic medicines for minor ailments.

In contemporary America, the context for using medicinal plants for preventive and therapeutic purposes already has been lost—except for subcultures in which it has been preserved, such as among the Amish and Native Americans. A restoration of the personal and symbolic relationship to food and medicinal plants could be linked with contemporary scientific knowledge of herbal applications. Appropriate self care could be encouraged with public education, access to consultation with professional herbalists and physicians, and access to fresh herbs and high quality, processed herbal medicines when needed. This improved patient involvement in the self care of the body and its signals might then improve the utilization of professional medical care.

Research in Food and Medicinal Plants

Although there is a relatively extensive contemporary literature on medicinal and healing plants, most of it exists outside of the United States and often in languages other than English. In addition, there is very little consistency in standard research designs and protocols among various countries.

There is a great need for more research on food, spice, and medicinal plants, especially for their potential use in syndromes and diseases poorly treated by conventional western medicine. The challenge is to conduct the research in the holistic spirit. This requires creative funding of research unlikely to provide high profit returns to a single source. Fortunately, research on crude or extracted traditional plant remedies is relatively inexpensive, compared to the astronomical costs of new drug development by pharmaceutical companies. Many medicinal plants eliminated from the United States Pharmacopeia over the years were dropped because they lacked contemporary research documentation of efficacy, not because they were proven to be ineffective (although there were some plants that proved less useful clinically than newly developed drugs).

Retaining a holistic context in medicinal plant research also involves addressing differences in paradigm. Involving traditional herbalists as research design consultants would protect against inadvertently eliminating a critical element of the paradigm in which the herb is used. In the past, plant collection for research has sometimes proved an environmental threat (habitats, species, or traditional knowledge were lost or threatened). The holistic approach to contemporary plant collection and research must be conducted in a way so as to conserve the traditional knowledge and ecology of the source plant, in order to avoid transgression of intellectual property rights, destruction of the plant habitat, or an imbalance of economic or intellectual returns to the source habitat and community.

There is a need for simple, well-documented analysis and outcomes research of crude and whole plant medicines, to determine their greatest potential applications and benefit to human health. British sailors were cured of scurvy with limes, originally presumed to be therapeutic against the disease solely because of their vitamin C content. However, limes and citrus proved more effective against scurvy than vitamin C supplementation; this was largely explained by the presence of bioflavonoids, later isolated and discovered to be prevalent in citrus pulp. The desirability of performing bioassays and clinical efficacy studies on whole herbs and herbal formulas, as well as on identified active constituents within the plants, is clear.

Increasing contemporary research on medicinal plants is critical, but the importance of documenting and incorporating the empirical knowledge of healing plants cannot be overemphasized. One of the greatest disadvantages of modern research is its highly selected—often single sex age group, ethnicity, or locality—human cohort; its relatively brief treatment and monitoring intervals; and its failure to fully document subclinical or seemingly irrelevant symptoms of the participating individuals. Sample populations are relatively tiny compared to the worldwide population. If, however, information gleaned from research is linked with empirical knowledge (usually derived from hundreds of years of human use across many generations and ethnic groups), along with contemporary clinical reporting from patients and practitioners on tolerance and efficacy, then herbal therapeutics and preventative protocols can reach the threshold of the 21st century

positioned to enhance the health of future generations.

Challenges for Contemporary Herbalism

The greatest opportunity for human benefit from food, spice, and healing plants will be afforded only if at least some elements of the traditional contexts and paradigms in which herbs have been used are preserved. The special relationship of humankind to the plant world is one of these traditions.

Challenges for the future include the preservation of germ plasm; the conservation of biodiversity and plant habitat; training professional and other herbalists, exchanging information with traditional healers; providing physicians and other health care professionals with a familiarity with plant medicines; educating the public in the appropriate use of herbs for self care; ensuring the funding of medicinal plant research that focuses on public health, clinical therapeutics, and wellness—not just drug development; and preserving public access to inexpensive, tonic, and therapeutic herbs through economic, environmental, market, legislative, and health policy.

In a recent study, the most trusted professional chosen by a sample of the American public was the pharmacist. This survey reveals the value and need of many people to have a personal, face-to-face relationship with the one who prepares and provides them with medicine. Traditionally, this was the role of the herbalist and healer, as well as the turn-of-the-century medical doctor. Today, many pharmacists are becoming interested in learning about herbal medicines, and students in herbal training and naturopathic medical schools are becoming more interested in natural products chemistry. This appears to be a timely example of nature's principle of reciprocity.

The re-emergence of herbalism in the west might have been predicted by traditional herbalists and healers centuries ago, who believed in the recycling patterns of nature. All

(Continues)

herbal traditions rely predominantly on an ecological relationship between the natural environment, the community, the herbal practitioner, and the individual. Self-sufficiency and personal responsibility are emphasized amidst the irrevocable interdependence of human society with nature. The role of "herbalism" in contemporary Western society is not to serve as a substitute for the pharmaceutical advances of the last decades, but to serve as an ancient paradigm that was less mechanistic and more holistic and humane in scope and that, if responsibly reclaimed and integrated, could greatly benefit future health care worldwide. This is illustrated in the following quote by Paiakan, a contemporary Kayapo Indian leader.

"I am trying to save the knowledge that the forest and this planet are alive, to give it back to you who have lost the understanding" (Odum 1971).

References

Bensky D, Gamble A. 1986. Chinese Herbal Medicine Materia Medica. Eastland Press, Seattle, pp. 34–35

Boyle W. 1991. Official Herbs in the United States Pharmacopoeias 1820–1990. Buckeye Naturopathic Press, East Palestine

DeFeudis FV. 1991. Ginkgo biloba Extract (Egb 761): Parmacological Activities and Clinical Applications. Elsevier, Paris

Donden Y. 1986. Health Through Balance: an Introduction to Tibetan Medicine. Snow Lion Publications, Ithaca

Farnsworth NR, Bunyapraphatsara N. 1992. Thai Medicinal Plants Recommended for Primary Health Care Systems. Medicinal Plant Information Center, Bangkok

Hoffmann DL. 1987. The Herb User's Guide: The Basic Skills of Medical Herbalism. Thorsons Publishing Group, Wellingborough

Iwu MM. 1993. Handbook of African Medicinal Plants, CRC Press, Boca Raton, pp. 343–349

Junius MM. 1993. The Practical Handbook of Plant Alchemy. Healing Arts Press, Rochester

Odum H. Environment, Power and Society. John Wiley & Sons, New York, p. 8

Scudder JM. 1874. Specific Diagnosis: A Study of Disease with special reference to the administration of remedies. Wilstach, Baldwin and Co, Cincinnati

Solecki RS, Shanidar IV. 1975. A neanderthal flower burial in northern Iraq. Science 190:880–889

Stetter C. 1993. The Secret Medicine of the Pharaohs—Ancient Egyptian Healing, Edition Q, Chicago

Suzuki D, Knudtson P. 1992. Wisdom of the Elders: Sacred Native Stories of Nature. Bantam Books, New York

Tyler VE, Brady LR, Robbers JE. 1988. Pharmacognosy. Lea and Febiger, Philadelphia

Wood M. 1986. Seven Herbs: Plants as Teachers. North Atlantic Books, Berkeley

Wren RC, revised by Williamso EM, Evans FJ. 1988. Potter's New Cyclopaedia of Botanical Drugs and Preparations. CW Daniel Company Limited, Saffron Walden, pp. 294–298

9
Healing Touch

Victoria E. Slater

Victoria E. Slater

Energetic Healing

Healing touch (HT) is one of a long line of healing traditions based on the belief in a universal healing energy. As one of these energetic healing strategies, HT includes new techniques, as well as modern variations of indigenous practices found around the world. Energetic strategies are credited with relieving physical and emotional distress. Some approaches use a practitioner's hands to sense and interact with a person's energy flow; others, such as meditation and biofeedback, use the person's mind (Slater 1995a, Slater 1995b).

Hand-Mediated Healing Modalities

- Healing touch
- Therapeutic touch
- Polarity
- Reiki
- Jin shin jyutsu
- External qigong
- Touch for health
- Reflexology
- Acupressure and shiatsu massage

History

The earliest reference to universal energy was in India, 5000 BC. Since then, many cultures have developed rich philosophies and healing traditions around this concept (Brennan 1993, Bruyere 1989). Some terms used to describe the phenomenon are *prana* in India; *ch'i, qi,* and *ki* in China, Thailand, and Japan; and *mana* in Hawaii. In 500 BC, Pythagoras called it *vital energy.* Mesmer who developed hypnosis in the 1800s, named it *animal magnetism* (Brennan 1993). Some believe it is the essence of the Christian holy spirit (Baginski & Sharamon 1988, Gordon 1978). In the Western scientific world, physicists' descriptions of quantum and electromagnetic fields closely resemble descriptions of *prana, ch'i, mana,* and magnetic fluid.

Residents of industrialized nations have few terms and almost no culturally sanctioned healing approaches that use this energy that is recognized by many cultures around the world and has spawned healing traditions for at least 7000 years, among them Hindu pranic healing, Eastern qigong, Hawaiian kahuna, and Native American medicine. Perhaps westerners are not aware of the energetic practices because we often are enclosed in air conditioned and heated buildings, distracted by television, radio, and even books. Few of us just sit and sense our environment and ourselves.

Although many energetic approaches are practiced throughout the world, there is only one energy. Dora Kunz, a noted healer, says "healing energy is

121

a beneficent power available to all living beings. . . . [Since] this healing power or energy is available to everyone, it is essentially the same, no matter how it may be described" (Kunz 1991). Because many systems use the same healing energy couched in different philosophies and names, this author coined the phrase "hand-mediated energetic healing" (HMEH) to refer to all healing methods in which a practitioner's hands are the medium of transfer or exchange of something that subjectively feels like energy (Slater 1995a).

Hand-Mediated Energetic Healing Practices

The two most prominent HMEH approaches used in nursing are Healing Touch (HT) and Therapeutic Touch (TT). HT refers to approaches taught in the American Holistic Nurses' Association's (AHNA) Certificate Program in Healing Touch for Health Care Professionals, and TT refers to the Krieger-Kunz Method of Therapeutic Touch.

Actually, the word 'touch' is a misnomer in HT and TT. Research results demonstrate that one need not physically touch a recipient to achieve the desired effects during and following a hand-mediated energetic healing session (Quinn 1984). Techniques usually are performed inches and sometimes feet from the recipient's body. Outcomes are attributed to energy for two reasons: it is the closest image to what practitioners and recipients describe feeling during a session, and it is a tacit recognition that, because actual physical touch is not necessary, the results attributed to HMEH cannot be due to physiologic responses to physical touch.

With the western penchant for innovation, new techniques have been created or adapted from ancient practices. Most of these practices fit one of four models: intuitive trial and error; a combination of many approaches; a relatively traditional approach; or the selective use of many techniques. Two techniques developed by intuitive trial and error were created for use with animals (Fox 1990, Tellington-Jones 1992).

Polarity, an example of blending techniques, is a result of Dr. Randolph Stone's 60-year study and practice of osteopathy, naturopathy, chiropractic medicine, acupuncture, herbology, reflexology, and

other Eastern massage techniques, and Arabic healing arts (Gordon 1978). A close look at a session indicates the practices from which polarity originated, although it is a widely practiced energetic healing approach with a tradition of its own.

The most classic modern energetic healing approach is the Krieger-Kunz Method of Therapeutic Touch (Krieger 1979, 1987, 1993). This is a type of pranic healing, a modern interpretation of several ancient healing practices, traditionally known as the "laying on of hands." Unlike polarity, it is not a blending of widely different traditions but a transplantation of similar ones. Other practices that were transplanted to western society are reflexology, Reiki, and acupressure.

HT, simply defined as an energy based therapeutic approach to healing (Mentgen & Bulbrook 1994), is midway between polarity and TT in its philosophy and approach to healing. Like polarity, it is an amalgam of many techniques; however, HT relies more on the practitioner's ability to interpret the recipient's energy flow and select appropriate techniques than on rules and protocols. Like TT, it is built upon ancient energy practices, but HT includes recent ones and is not cast in a dominant tradition.

Hand-mediated energetic approaches differ in the time allotted for treatment. TT sessions should last no longer than 25 minutes (Krieger 1993). Reiki, a Tibetan/Japanese technique, the Japanese practice of Jin shin jyutsu, and polarity average one hour. HT treatments might last five minutes or as long as necessary, depending on the problem, the technique chosen, the practitioner's skill, and the recipient's responses.

HT and TT are best known among nurses and are considered nursing techniques, although practiced widely by non-nurses, and even non-health care professionals. TT was the first to be introduced to nurses; it is a grassroots phenomenon which started with a few nurses and has expanded into thousands practicing a variety of approaches. Nurses generally are cautious, adhering to the status quo of health care delivery; even if they disagree with the system, they stay within its boundaries. Not so with HMEH. Nurses have defended it against often hostile attacks. Many are so convinced of its effectiveness that they leave traditional health care settings to establish private energetic healing practices. Those choosing to remain in institutional settings use HMEH in these hospitals, home health care practices, and nursing homes. The Presbyterian Hospital in Denver, Colorado, has a Department of Energy that oversees energetic healing within the institution. Many hospitals include HT or TT as part of standard nursing protocols. HMEH is taught in nursing schools and has a growing research base.

Why do nurses become aware of this energy and seek to interact with it before most physicians? This might have something to do with education and spheres of practice. Nursing students traditionally are introduced to their craft by giving bed baths to each other and then to patients; medical students first dissect cadavers that have been soaking in formaldehyde for 3 years. Thus, nursing students first encounter people who are suffused with the energy of life. Later, in practice, most nurses regularly share intimate space, time, and feelings with patients; physicians often are necessarily more separated. Nurses might have difficulty becoming aware of peoples' energy flows because they are constantly surrounded by them, much as fish are always surrounded by water. Physicians may sometimes have the opposite problem; it is difficult for them to appreciate something they may seldom have the opportunity to experience.

HMEH has been described by its detractors as a placebo, a hoax, voodoo, and witchcraft. However, a glance at the speed with which its popularity has grown among a traditionally conservative group suggests that there might be more to it. Only research will determine in which category HMEH belongs—placebo, fad, hoax, or valuable healing approach.

Intellectual Tradition

Even though HMEH traditions have been practiced for centuries, allopathic medicine and nursing largely considered them quackery until TT was introduced. Why did TT make such a difference? Dolores Krieger, a professor of nursing at New York University, and Dora Kunz, her teacher of healing, developed TT as a sequential approach slightly resembling the nursing process. In the early 1970s, Krieger courageously offered a TT elective to nursing students and began teaching TT workshops nationwide.

Krieger describes the first step, centering, as the ground state from which Therapeutic Touch proceeds (Krieger 1993). To center, one becomes still within oneself. Kunz describes it as a conscious effort to free oneself from one's anxieties and inner disturbances, and to be at peace within oneself (Kunz 1991). Centering resembles the concentration necessary to hear the heart beat—one must "become" his or her ears, or hands, not just use them. People who meditate, pray, or practice biofeedback are familiar with a centered state of consciousness.

Once centered, the practitioner uses hands to assess the recipient's energy field and provide treatment. The practitioner slowly moves her or his hands in the space above the recipient's body, as if smoothing out a piece of fabric or gently moving soap bubbles around. The hands may be positioned on or above the skin, to direct energy to a specific location and hold that position for a short time. The two actions are alternated as often as desired until the practitioner decides TT is finished, for the moment. Evaluation and reassessment is a continuous process. Several of Krieger's graduate students were convinced TT had value and began researching TT for theses and dissertations, the results of which are described in this chapter.

Krieger's approach flourished partly because of her timing. At the time Krieger began teaching TT, quantum physics was being presented in ways that nonphysicists could understand (Capra 1984, Zukav 1979, Bohm 1980). Capra's book, *The Tao of Physics* compared quantum physics with Eastern mysticism; Zukav's *The Dancing Wu Li Masters: An Overview of the New Physics* proved easy to read, and Bohm's *Wholeness and the Implicate Order,* clearly presented the quantum theory of undivided wholeness. The images of the quantum realm presented by Capra, Zukav, Bohm, and other writers matched the subjective experiences that practitioners were having during TT and other HMEH treatments. HMEH providers avidly read these books and began speaking in terms of frequencies, waves, energy, vibrations, and balanced or congested fields.

Janet Mentgen, a nurse in Colorado, developed HT. Mentgen had been practicing HMEH for many years when introduced to Therapeutic Touch and added it to her large healing repertoire. During several years of teaching HMEH, she refined a five-course sequence of hand-mediated and personal healing. In 1990, her Healing Touch for Health Care Professionals became the first certificate program offered by the AHNA.

HT techniques are developed intuitively and pulled from various approaches, such as those of Dolores Krieger, Barbara Brennan (Brennan 1988, 1993), Brugh Joy (Joy 1979), and Native American medicine. Specific techniques are used, for example, to relieve back and other pain; to clear anesthesia, drugs, and tobacco smoke from a person's system; to ease dying; to counteract depression; and to energize or to relax. Adjuvant hypnotherapy is taught to interested advanced practitioners. HT practitioners blend existing techniques, thus creating new ones. Mentgen uses new techniques a minimum of 100 times with volunteer clients before she adopts them.

The HT curriculum places a strong emphasis on "healer, heal thyself." People involved in a healing practice must strive to heal their own emotional issues, to avoid bringing these issues into another's healing session. Each HT workshop teaches and reinforces the use of multiple personal healing strategies including hearing others' stories of dramatic changes in their lives. One person's success often inspires others to do their own healing work.

People who seek certification as Healing Touch practitioners from the AHNA are required to sample the energetic healing waters and experience different modalities. Extensive reading is expected, including books about techniques, healing traditions, self-healing, and possible theoretical explanations. Persistent students can complete all training and individual preparation necessary for certification in 2 to 3 years. Certified practitioners may apply to become instructors. The AHNA is aware of criticism leveled against practitioners of an approach that seems as simple as hand-mediated energetic healing, yet achieves extraordinary success. Every effort is taken to insure that the education and evaluation of prospective HT practitioners is comprehensive.

HMEH practices differ strikingly from allopathic medicine in approach and philosophy. Allopathic medicine is concerned with cure; HMEH, with healing. To cure implies that a physician fixes a problem in the patient, which that person cannot fix for him or herself. Only one actor is recognized. Healing requires either one or two actors. The person being healed is primary; the assistant, such as a HMEH practitioner, is useful. Energetic healers unanimously assert that each person is his or her own healer (Carlson & Shield 1989). Quinn, a TT practitioner, compares a healer to a midwife who is able only to assist a woman to deliver her own baby. A midwife does not force, but facilitates; does not push, but receives; does not insist, but accepts (Quinn 1989). All hand-mediated energetic approaches are based on this view. The recipient is the healer; the provider is a midwife privileged to assist. The mechanism for healing is something that feels like energy.

Theoretical Basis

Because a recipient need not be touched during a treatment, HMEH cannot be explained directly by physiologic and psychologic effects of physical touch such as those described by psychoneuroimmunology. HMEH techniques and responses suggest a twofold explanation based on electromagnetic and quantum physics and transpersonal psychology.

Electromagnetic and Quantum Physics

Newtonian physics applies to structures larger than molecules, such as bones, joints, buildings, and airplanes. It does not adequately describe subatomic phenomena as do electromagnetic and quantum theories.

Physicists Davies and Gribbin portray matter as a culturally-constructed concept, or a myth (Davies 1992). If all matter in the human body were collapsed together, the resulting volume would be less than a grain of sand; the rest is electromagnetic interactions within the quantum realm. The person you see walking down a street or the book from which you are reading these words are images constructed of light. Your certainty that the person you touch is solid contrasts strikingly with the quantum fact that this simply is not so. Your touch is an electromagnetic and quantum interaction.

Humans may be considered electrical devices that produce magnetism, heat, and phosphorescence (Wolf 1982). An electromagnet, which usually has an iron core encircled by electrical coils, produces a radiating field that periodically decreases in density.

Similarly, human beings have an inner circulating core containing iron (hemoglobin). When one is alive, electricity surges through the body and produces an electromagnetic field that surrounds the iron. The body also has heat (body temperature). This EM field may be what HMEH healers describe as the various energetic bodies of a human (Brennan 1988), depicted in Figure 9-1 (Mentgen & Bulbrook 1994).

Phosphorescence may be the aura. Phosphorescence is the glow produced by some materials when in the presence of electricity, such as a television or florescent lights. Both rely on electricity surging through phosphorescent-producing material. Because electrical devices produce phosphorescence, and humans have electrical properties, the human body might be phosphorescent. Perhaps that glow is not easily recognized because—like the water to the fish—it is ever-present. It also may be that our phosphorescence is beyond the range of visible light.

Light is radiant electromagnetic energy. Its frequency is measured in cycles per second (cps), ranging from 10 cps in power and telephone lines to 10^{24+} cps in gamma rays. Visible light is a tiny section of the whole with frequencies between 10^{14} and 10^{15} cps. We see that range of light because it is the only part of the electromagnetic spectrum that propagates in water, as shown in Figure 9-2 (Jackson 1975). During the evolution of life on earth, biological organisms developed eyes that were only able to see the electromagnetic frequencies to which they were exposed. It is not inconceivable that some people develop the ability to see beyond the range of what we label "visible light," to see the "invisible" light that exists around people, known as "auras." Perhaps the halos depicted in paintings of saints are the artists' depictions of phosphorescence.

Within quantum theory, there are eight strikingly different subtheories that all mathematically predict the same experimental results, so that any one can be used to describe a phenomenon (Herbert 1985). Physicists continually search for a grand theory that will subsume the different quantum theories.

Holography and Undivided Wholeness

Among the popular quantum theories that offer a tentative explanation for HMEH is undivided wholeness, similar to a hologram (Gerber 1988, Talbot 1991). Holographic images are familiar to many because of Hollywood and Disneyland. A hologram is a collection of interfering wave patterns created by splitting a laser light beam in two, as shown in Figure 9-3. One of the beams illuminates an object being photographed, such as an apple, and reflects off the apple onto a photographic plate. When the other beam—which has increased in size from pencil-thin to a flashlight-like beacon—hits the same photographic plate, the two beams interfere. When a laser

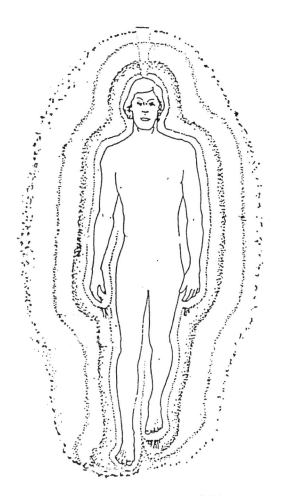

Figure 9-1. Model of the human energy field. (From Mentgen J, Bulbrook MJ. 1994. Healing Touch: Level I Notebook. Healing Touch, Lakewood, Colorado, p. 3, with permission.)

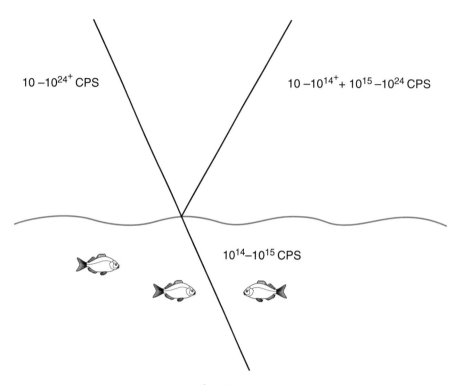

$10 - 10^{24^{+}}$ CPS

$10 - 10^{14^{+}} + 10^{15} - 10^{24}$ CPS

$10^{14} - 10^{15}$ CPS

Figure 9-2. Range of visible light penetrating water.

beam strikes this interference pattern, a three-dimensional image of the object previously photographed is revealed.

Interference wave patterns resemble the waves that ripple out when several pebbles are thrown into a pond at the same time. Each sends out rippling waves. When these waves meet, they interfere with each other and create what are called interference patterns. In holography, the information about the photographed object is stored in those nondescript interference wave patterns.

The patterns created by interfering light waves can be described by mathematical equations called Fourier transforms. The human brain translates the information collected by the eyes, ears, nose, taste buds, and skin into Fourier transforms. Somehow, the mind interprets the equations and the person experiences sight, sound, smell, taste, and touch. It is as if one's experiences are recorded as holograms and then interpreted as experiences (Talbot 1991). What we perceive as real may be more our mind's interpretation of holographic interference patterns

projected by other humans, trees, animals, rocks, and stars.

The oddity of holograms is that information is not localized on any one part of the photographic plate or device on which interference patterns are recorded. If you chop a holographic image into many pieces and expose them to the proper laser light, each piece will contain the entire holographic image. Even the tiniest corner of a hologram contains the entire picture because it contains all of the information needed to reproduce the image (Fig. 9-4). The picture produced by one minced piece will be blurry, but whole. As one adds pieces, the image will become clearer.

If humans are like holograms, each piece, cell, and atom contains all the information needed to project the whole. The image produced by one cell would be blurry, but complete.

The holographic phenomenon closely resembles a healer's experiences. During HMEH sessions, the healer often senses energetic movement within a recipient that simulates the interference patterns de-

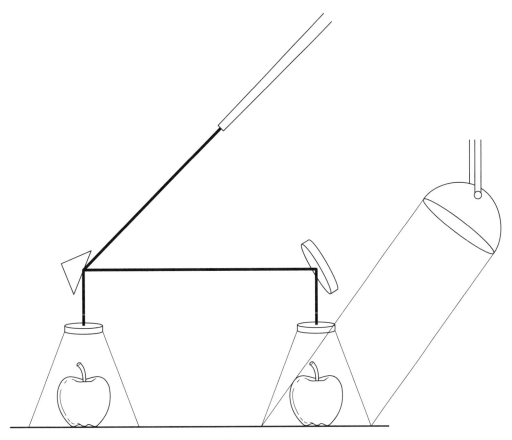

Figure 9-3. Holographic imaging process.

scribed by holography. Much of the information and memories that surface have a wholeness and freshness about them that suggest a type of holographic storage. However, holography does not fully explain, to this author, the human condition. Even though the skin, eyes, ears, nose, and taste buds may receive and process information as Fourier transforms and humans somehow store that material, such computer-like processing does not explain fully the sensation of being touched or of being human.

Holographic theory describes the universe, and the human being, in terms of information interference patterns. Other theories describe the universe and humans as collections of quantum and electromagnetic interactions. Perhaps both or neither are true. The human state may be processed as holographic information; the experience of being a three-dimensional human might be due to quantum

and electromagnetic interactions. Both perspectives, seemingly separate, apply to HMEH experiences.

Other quantum theories useful to students of energetic healing are potentiality/actuality, consciousness-created reality, and many worlds or parallel universes. Physicist Werner Heisenberg proposed that the quantum world consists of two phenomena—potentialities and actualities (Herbert 1985). To understand the differences, one must recall the dual nature of light. Light can act either like a wave and spread across a room, or like a particle, triggering a light-sensitive device.

The matter of the universe acts like particles; the force acts like waves. For example, a wave moving across the surface of the ocean is pure energy; successive water droplets along the wave path just react to and interact with the energy's force. Each water droplet seems insignificant, but their actions com-

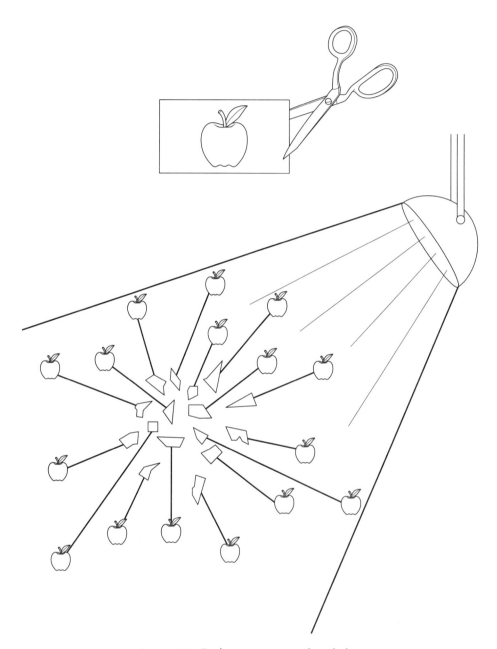

Figure 9-4. Each piece contains the whole.

bine with the energy to create the movements of the ocean. In the quantum realm, transient particles interact, creating and destroying particles and emitting electromagnetic waves. According to Heisenberg, the unseen quantum wave-like force represents possibilities and probabilities. A particle is the manifestation of one of these possibilities. Until that happens, no material reality exists. If one considers that each human body contains the volume of less than a grain of sand, we consist of very little matter and a great deal of potential. This is true psychologically and philosophically, as well as physically.

A persistent question among quantum physicists is what causes a wave to "collapse" into a particle, or an unseen potentiality to become a discernable actuality. One theory is called observation-created reality (Herbert 1985). Something must observe a wave, and by doing so, selects it to collapse. Something must observe the array of potential (wave) in order for an actual phenomenon (particle) to manifest. Anything, even an experimental device, can be the observer.

However, some physicists argue that only a conscious observer, such as a human being, can select a potentiality to become actuality. The theory of consciousness-created reality demands a reflecting consciousness, not just an aware one. Consciousness-created reality implies that consciousness is fundamental, not a property that simply emerges from biological processes. Religious traditions such as Christianity, Judaism, and Islam have name this consciousness God or Allah. Eastern religions identify a Oneness. However, the proponents of consciousness-created reality go beyond the actions of a divine consciousness and suggest that "only an apparatus endowed with consciousness (even as you and I) is privileged to create reality" (Herbert 1985). The nature of this consciousness will be considered shortly.

In the many worlds theory, or parallel universes, each observation of a wave creates more than just the reality you experience. It creates all possible realities. If you choose to eat cereal for breakfast in one reality, you choose eggs in another, and skip the meal altogether in a third. Each possible choice is manifested, but you are aware of only one.

Flipping coins is a simple example of parallel universes. When one flips a coin, both heads and tails are selected, just manifested and experienced in different universes, as shown in Figure 9-5. Each successive flip creates more universes. In just a short time, multiple universes of experience exist. Many are very similar (all heads), but some are drastically different (tails). An individual's particular experiences are consciously selected from among all possibilities (Wolf 1988). The ones not selected reside in parallel universes of which we are not readily aware. Because many possibilities overlap, few people experience drastic life changes—but the possibility exists.

One often hears that giving or receiving HMEH treatments has changed people's lives. Kunz observed that practitioners who open themselves to these energies . . . have found that the practice has begun to change them as well, in subtle but meaningful ways (Kunz 1991). HT practitioners claim that the accumulation of subtle, but meaningful, differences through repeated sessions has been crucial to their emotional and physical healing. Perhaps, the parallel universe theory helps explain such statements. If HMEH involves altering one's electromagnetic frequencies ever so slightly and doing so is the same as selecting a different one of the parallel universes or many worlds, then HMEH assists a recipient to select a universe with a different present and different possible futures.

Physicist Fred Alan Wolf applies quantum theory to his experiences with indigenous shamanic healing. He concludes that "shamans see the universe as made from vibrations, shamans choose what is physically meaningful and see all events as universally connected, shamans enter into parallel worlds, and shamans perceive reality in a state of altered consciousness" (Wolf 1991). In a few brief statements, he effectively blends four physical theories—electromagnetism, holography, many worlds, and consciousness-created reality—with healers' acts of centering.

Quantum physics seems to offer tentative explanations for HT experiences, but remains speculative until an experimental test can be devised. This author suggests that HMEH involves the interaction of two holographic, three-dimensional, solid-appearing quantum and electromagnetic humans who are able to select actualities from potentialities, which may be the equivalent of selecting different universes. The healer has learned to regulate internal electromagnetic frequencies, enabling the recipient to passively alter his or her own electromagnetic state. Holography implies that the slightest holographic/quantum/electromagnetic change in even one cell reflects throughout the entire body and vice versa. If the result of such a change is perceived as beneficial, it may be called therapeutic or healing. Perhaps the important question is not which quantum theory best helps describe HMEH, for they all can, but what is the nature and role of a consciousness that is able to alter one's quantum/electromagnetic/holographic state and select potentialities or universes.

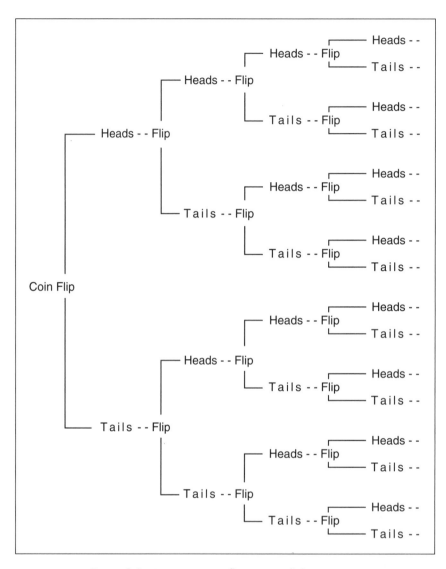

Figure 9-5. Repetitive coin flips in parallel universes.

Transpersonal Psychology

In Freudian and behavioral psychologies, one's consciousness is separate from and subordinate to physical processes. The physical world (as explained by Newtonian physics, chemistry, and physiology) is the primary reality; your conscious experiences emerge from the physical processes of your living body. The physical is independent of and superior to one's consciousness. In the extreme view, consciousness dies with the body's demise.

Such a view is incompatible with HMEH experiences, in which one's consciousness is fundamental to and in unity with the physical. More congruous is the relatively new transpersonal psychology. In the transpersonal psychologies, consciousness is primary; it precedes and even might orchestrate physical experiences. Variously described as one's eternal soul, spirit, or self, it pervades all realities and is the primary source or creative principle of existence (Mack 1993). As such, it is not viewed as a separate phenomenon from the physical. The two are intertwined like two dancers twirling to the music of a waltz, with consciousness leading. Mystics are most often associated with hearing the music of the consciousness, but the experience is not limited to those we might call mystics. All greater-than-self experiences are transpersonal.

GREATER-THAN-SELF EXPERIENCES

The emerging transpersonal psychology . . . is concerned specifically with . . . becoming, individual and species-wide meta-needs, ultimate values, unitive consciousness, peak experiences, B-values, ecstasy, mystical experience, awe, being, self-actualization, essence, bliss, wonder, ultimate meaning, transcendence of the self, spirit, oneness, cosmic awareness, individual and species-wide synergy, maximal interpersonal encounter, sacralization of everyday life, transcendental phenomena, cosmic self-humor and playfulness, maximal sensory awareness, responsiveness and expression, and related concepts, experiences, and activities (Sutich 1975).

Transpersonal psychologies include Eastern and Western mystical traditions such as Buddhism, Sufism, and Christianity; psychological and spiritual development; parapsychology; altered states of consciousness; metaphysics, energetic healing, placebos, and the role of mythology in viewing the world (Tart 1975). This list is not exhaustive—any area of study involving a view of eternal consciousness is considered a transpersonal psychology.

The Institute of Noetic Sciences was founded in 1973 to explore and research consciousness. It is sponsoring current studies of spontaneous remission and evidence of consciousness after death. Mind-body interactions are of primary interest, as are various self- and assisted-healing approaches such as HMEH (McNeill & Guion 1991).

Transpersonal psychologists seem to use the words *spirit* and *consciousness* interchangeably, and the dictionary's definitions imply they are similar. Spirit is defined as the intelligent or immaterial part of man as distinguished from the body; consciousness is the state of mental activity including emotion and thought (New Lexicon 1989). Transpersonal experiences have been described as spiritual (Tart 1992), and the investigation of spiritual and religious experience (Mishlove 1993). Perhaps both spirit and consciousness are what Kunz calls the *timeless self* . . . a principle of being which provides continuity during life, and persists after death (Kunz 1991).

Assagioli, a student of Jung's, concluded that human consciousness consists of several dimensions, including one's daily reality and several levels of higher consciousness (Assagioli 1993). His dimensions of the psyche resemble both Kunz's timeless self, as well as the consciousness that is the creative principle of existence and pervades all realities. Assagioli believed that one's primary psychological task is to synthesize one's different psychological dimensions. His system of strategies is called psychosynthesis.

Hand-mediated energetic healing is applied transpersonal psychology and quantum/electromagnetic physics. A HMEH practitioner learns to alter her or his state of consciousness to enter the dimension of the timeless self and to alter her or his quantum/EM core. The process by which a HMEH practitioner alters the EM state acts like biofeedback. Rather than relying on instruments for feedback, however, the practitioner learns to be sensitive to subtle changes within her or himself.

ALTERING CONSCIOUSNESS

When Elmer Green of the Menninger Foundation tested people who were called or called themselves healers, he found they altered their electrical states at will. In some of the healers we have studied, we found voltage surges . . . of maybe 80 volts. The whole body will change voltage by 80 volts and it will last for a second or two and then come back down again. That is not possible, except for the fact that it happens. But the healers are not surprised by it because they say, "Oh, well, I generated this charge and I sent it" (Walsh 1992).

The healers' actions of generating an electrical surge resemble Green's descriptions of biofeedback (Green 1977). Both match this author's experiences as she gradually has learned to sense the more delicate nuances within her own electromagnetic state.

Settings

A Healing Touch Session

During a HT session, the practitioner first assesses the recipient's energetic state. Developing sensitivity to subtle differences in the energy in and around the recipient requires practice, but almost everyone can learn. Those who practice develop the ability to distinguish nuances within what initially appears to be slight differences, and some will learn to see differences as well as feel them (Brennan 1993, Bruyere 1989, Kunz 1991). For most people, all it takes is a will to try and approximately 30 minutes of relaxed practice to detect activity in the space around a person.

In HT and related approaches, the practitioner generally uses her or his hands to feel for differences in the space around a person. Such variations often are described as heaviness, congestion, holes, leaks, vibrations, stagnation, temperature variations, and other differences in the space around the physical body. Ideally, the field surrounding a person should feel like a symmetrical, and like a barely perceptible, but steady breeze.

The energy also resembles the controlled power of a river. The strength of the current carries your canoe downstream. Its power is palpable when you choose to concentrate on it; otherwise it seems just part of the environment. When the river banks narrow or the water encounters rocks, trees, or other obstructions, the current loses its steady flow. Water speeds up, backs up, swirls, spits, and crashes. Ripples or tiny white caps form, indicating turbulence. Debris may collect in hollows, behind rocks, and in trees, further disturbing the current's flow.

An approaching obstruction is readily apparent to the experienced canoeist but novices will not know what to look for. Until they learn to interpret white caps and flow patterns properly, people often hit a submerged rock and are left at the mercy of the rock

and the river. Sometimes it is hard to get off the rock without help.

An individual's energy flows like a river. If there are no obstructions, it is smooth, gliding, and barely perceptible. People whose energy flows smoothly usually report being at peace with themselves and others. However, if debris—such as pain, rage, depression, broken bones, cancer, bleeding, or any physical or emotional problem—is in the way, the energy stream reflects the interference.

A HT practitioner learns to sense changes in the stream of energy, perhaps detecting something that feels like turbulence, eddies, holes, and white caps. The person being assessed might talk about his or her sadness, rage, depression, physical pain, cancer, poor marriage, or any obstruction. A goal of HT is to smooth the flow, to mobilize it if stuck, and to leave the recipient with an energy flow that feels smooth, powerful, and unobstructed. When a practitioner senses that the recipient's energy has become as smooth as possible, the recipient often will talk about how relaxed he or she feels, and how much the pain and depression have lessened.

As the HT practitioner alters his or her own quantum/EM state, he or she offers the recipient an opportunity to do the same, just more passively. To the degree that the recipient is passive, a HT treatment is a temporary measure; it helps pull people "off the rocks." Until people learn to interpret their own currents, they might keep getting stuck. Each time a person receives a treatment, obstructions get smaller because the energy flow does not revert to the pretreatment state.

Ultimately, however, healing is each individual's personal responsibility. Through strategies such as meditation and centering, one can access dimensions of consciousness other than the daily reality. When a person begins to actively study and work with the energetic state through counseling, meditation, visualization, guided imagery, biofeedback, and other similar methods, one's personal obstructions disintegrate rapidly. HT, alone, can relieve a wide variety of physical and emotional pains; it can heal when combined with personal emotional explorations.

This might make healing and HT sound too simple, and too good to be true. However, thousands of people have experienced HT and discovered for themselves the power of the energy flow; how to interact with it for their own physical, emotional, and spiritual healing; and how to offer the same capabilities to others.

Applications

HMEH is used in every conceivable location and with virtually all medical and nursing diagnoses. Nurses use it in hospitals, nursing homes, home health care, hospice, and, most visibly, in their private practices. It is used in newborn nurseries, neonatal intensive care units, labor rooms, recovery rooms, medical-surgical and pediatric units, and in psychiatric settings. It has been taught to Lamaze classes. It has been used to help reduce edema, temperatures, hives, pain, anxiety, premenstrual syndrome, fatigue, depression, diarrhea, headache, as well as during chemotherapy and following radiation therapy. It has been used to relieve unpleasant HIV positive symptoms. One nurse works on players' injuries in the locker room of a football team. Another set up a practice in the back room of a bar, treating injured alcoholics and people who will not seek standard health care (Krieger 1993).

All HMEH practitioners have their own stories. Some tell of healings so rapid, so difficult to believe. This author has seen small tumors disappear, severe constipation and sunburn quickly resolve, systolic blood pressure drop from over 200 to approximately 150 within 5 minutes, Fifths' disease run its course in 3 days, panic attacks disappear in 5 minutes, severe fractures heal remarkably fast, steady paroxysmal ventricle contractions (PVCs) and migraines disappear.

Anecdotal reports are wonderful topics of conversation, but do not demonstrate to anyone other than the practitioner and recipient that HMEH is more than wishful thinking. Research is required to provide substantial support or to disprove the effects attributed to HMEH.

Research and Evaluation

Most published research on hand-mediated energetic healing modalities is on TT. Because it is believed that all HMEH techniques are similar, research on TT is applied to all approaches. Such an assumption is efficient, but not necessarily correct. In time, the effects of each modality must be studied; for this discussion, research in HMEH will be considered applicable to all similar approaches.

TT has been shown to statistically significantly reduce state anxiety in patients on a cardiovascular unit ($p < .001$) (Heidi 1981, Quinn 1984), and in oncology patients receiving chemotherapy ($p < .05$) (Guerrero 1985). In one of the two studies on cardiovascular patients, patients were touched during the TT and mock TT (MTT) treatments; in the other, they were not touched at all, and the results of both studies were essentially the same.

TT has relieved tension headache pain ($p < .0001$) (Keller & Bzdek 1986) and was followed by significant changes in neonate behavior (Fedoruk 1985). Behaviors of hospitalized psychiatric patients treated with TT were compared both to their own pretreatment and post-treatment behaviors and to nontreated patients. Those who received TT were judged more amenable to talking, calmer, more self-disclosing, and more cooperative than usual, and more so than patients who did not receive TT (Kline & Durham 1992, Potter Hughes 1994).

Studies on the physiologic effects of TT have mixed results. TT was tested against postoperative narcotics and found to be statistically less effective (Meehan 1985). Responses to measures such as pulse, galvanic skin response, peripheral skin temperature, muscle tone, electromyography, and skin conductance have been inconsistent. About half of the studies using such measures have had statistically significant results (Kramer 1990, Post 1990, Quinn 1988). Interestingly, the studies in which results have been statistically insignificant used healthy volunteers as subjects; those in which results were significant used actual patients in real life situations of illness and hospitalization. Randolph suggested that the choice of ill versus well subjects may influence the significance of results in TT studies; she attempted to alter healthy 'fight or flight' responses in healthy volunteers who were exposed to a stressful situation and was unable to do so (Randolph 1984). This indicates that TT is a safe modality that relieves unhealthy stress levels but does not affect appropriate ones (Quinn 1988).

Three studies have tested blood and immune responses to HMEH. One found significant changes in hemoglobin count, which rose following TT (Krieger 1979); another revealed similar results after Reiki (Wetzel 1989). In a small pilot test, researchers found a lower level of suppressor T cells following TT (Quinn 1993). Such an effect is the equivalent of enhancing the immune system, because the self-suppression of immune activity is retarded.

In the most dramatic study, 44 healthy male volunteers received identical full-thickness dermal punch biopsies for which rate of wound healing was measured. Half received TT to the wound. On the 16th day after the biopsy, 12 of the 23 subjects who received TT had completely healed wounds. None of the wounds in the control group had healed (Wirth 1992).

In 1989, Quinn analyzed published TT research to discover methodological problems. She found a time discrepancy between TT research and TT practice. In research, five minutes are allotted for treatments; in actual practice, TT treatments range from 9 to 32 minutes. A more serious concern was that TT practitioners were used to give MTT treatments. Study participants receiving MTT described it as peaceful, safe, and indescribable (Quinn 1989b). She discovered that experienced TT practitioners assisting with studies were unable to avoid centering and sending energy, even when trying. When practitioners began moving their hands as prescribed in TT, they immediately entered a centered state of consciousness. The mock treatments were not truly mock. Nevertheless, many studies had statistically significant results suggesting that even five minutes of the prescribed hand motions of TT, alone, might be effective, and that concentrating on a TT treatment increases the effects.

As a result, Quinn made several suggestions for future research (Quinn 1989): first, TT treatments during research should be longer and more closely follow standard practice. Second, providers of mock or control treatments should have no experience with TT. Finally, investigators should give no treatments of any kind. She was concerned that an investigator cannot be researcher (ideally objective) and provider (believing in the treatment) concurrently.

No results are yet available from ongoing HT research. Sharon Scandrett-Hibdon, past-president of the AHNA, told this author that a holistic study can-

not be done in parts. HMEH treatment involves the presence of the provider; the provider's state of consciousness, here-and-now or altered; hand movements; and recipients' and providers' responses. Therefore, HMEH studies should combine quantitative and qualitative approaches. Information about treatment effects alone is insufficient; one also must consider the effects of the presence of a centered or uncentered provider and discover the personal experience of both provider and recipient.

Because holistic studies should not be done in parts, and because the researcher should not give treatments, the logistics of conducting quality research will limit the number of individual studies. Working nurses do not have the time, support, or funding to invest in complex studies. A research consortium within the AHNA is in the planning stages and a pilot study for multisite data collection is currently underway in nine cities nationwide. AHNA members intend to select research topics, coordinators, and designs annually, and to participate in data collection. The AHNA research consortium will help relieve the burden of studying a complex, often misunderstood practice, and allow all who are interested to participate.

Extraordinary claims require extraordinary results. It remains to be seen if future research can provide extraordinary results to support the extraordinary claims of HMEH practitioners and recipients.

Summary

HMEH looks odd. One wonders how any effect at all can come from waving your hands over another person. One also must wonder whether or not the person doing the waving is a charlatan. HMEH's appearance, alone, creates detractors. The lack of an easily understood explanation increases them.

Physiologic and psychoneuroimmunologic responses do not easily explain HMEH, because the recipient often is not physically touched. Quantum and electromagnetic theories seem to offer the best explanations for HMEH, but they are hard to understand and usually are not taught to students of the health care sciences. While anecdotal reports abound of salutary effects, relatively few research studies of HMEH have been published. The results of these studies appear mixed at first, until one takes a closer look. For people experiencing real distress, HMEH *has* been shown to offer effective relief.

Although HMEH looks strange, and its explanations are obscure, the number of providers and recipients who unwaveringly claim that the techniques are therapeutic is increasing rapidly. Many are certain that giving or receiving HMEH treatments has changed their lives for the better.

> Dora Kunz wrote that in the holistic view, the universe is a living, dynamic, and orderly realm suffused with consciousness. She thinks of the individual consciousness of each person, the self, as the point or principle of integration within a human being. It is around such a point that mental and emotional configurations center, and thereby become meaningful to us and useful in our experience. The self, she writes, (which should not be confused with the ego or egotism) is the thread which not only connects us to reality, but also gives ultimate shape, meaning and value to our experience.
>
> A scientific framework for a holistic view that involves consciousness giving shape to reality may require a blending of quantum theories and transpersonal psychology. Kunz suggests that even a conservative assessment must conclude that this new holistic view of reality ranges from a fruitful working principle to a promissory note for the future (Kunz 1991).

The best and fairest advice for anyone intrigued by one intervention, HMEH, that closely resembles a blending of transpersonal psychology and quantum physics: "You don't need to believe that this system will work in order to profoundly experience it. You don't need to believe in the ocean to get wet; however, you do have to jump in" (Gordon 1978).

References

Amdahl K. 1991. There Are No Electrons. Clearwater, Arvada

Assagioli R. 1993. Psychosynthesis. A Collection of Basic Writings. Penguin. New York

Baginski BJ, Sharamon S. 1981. Reiki. Universal Life Energy. Life Rhythm. Mendocino, California

Bohm D. 1980. Wholeness and the Implicate Order. Ark, London

Brennan BA. 1988. Hands of Light. A Guide to Healing Through the Human Energy Field. A New Paradigm for the Human Being in Health, Relationship, and Disease. Bantam. New York

Brennan B. 1993. Light Emerging. The Journey of Personal Healing. Bantam. New York

Bruyere R. 1989. Wheels of Light. A Study of the Chakras. Bon. Sierra Madre

Capra F. 1984. The Tao of Physics. An Exploration of the Parallels Between Modern Physics and Eastern Mysticism. 2nd Ed. Bantam. Toronto

Carlson R, Shield B. (eds). 1989. Healers on Healing. JP Tarcher, Los Angeles

Davies P, Gribbin J. 1992. The Matter Myth. Dramatic Discoveries that Challenge our Understanding of Physical Reality. Touchstone. New York

Fedoruk RB. 1985. Transfer of the relaxation response: therapeutic touch B as a method for reduction of stress in premature neonates. Dissertation Abstracts International 46:978B

Fox MW. 1990. The Healing Touch. New Market. New York

Gerber R. 1988. Vibrational Medicine. Bear, Santa Fe, New Mexico

Gordon R. 1978. Your Healing Hands. The Polarity Experience. Wingbow. Oakland

Green E, Green A. 1977. Beyond Biofeedback. Knoll.

Guerrero MS. 1985. The effects of therapeutic touch on state-trait anxiety level of oncology patients. Masters Abstracts Int 42:24(3)

Heidi P. 1981. Effect of therapeutic touch on anxiety level of hospitalized patients. Nurs Res 30:32–37

Herbert N. 1985. Quantum Reality. Beyond the New Physics. Doubleday. New York

Jackson JD. 1975. Classical Electrodynamics 2nd Ed. John Wiley & Sons. New York

Joy WB. 1979. Joy's Way. A Map for the Transformational Journey. An Introduction to the Potentials for Healing with Body Energies. JP Tarcher, Inc. Los Angeles

Keller SK, Bzdek VM. 1986. Effects of therapeutic touch on tension headache pain. Nurs Res 35:101–108

Kline T, Durham LL. 1992. Responses of persons with schizophrenia to therapeutic touch. Paper presented at the meeting of the Society for Education and Research in Psychiatric-Mental Health Nursing, Chevy Chase, Maryland, November 5

Kramer NA. 1990. Comparison of therapeutic touch and casual touch on stress reduction of hospitalized children. Pediatr Nurs 16:483–485

Krieger D. 1976. Therapeutic touch. Nurs Times April 15: pp. 572–573

Krieger D. 1979. The Therapeutic Touch. How to Use Your Hands to Help or to Heal. Prentice Hall. New York

Krieger D. 1987. Living the Therapeutic Touch. Healing as a Lifestyle. Dodd, Mead & Co. New York

Krieger D. 1993. Accepting Your Power to Heal. The Personal Practice of Therapeutic Touch. Bear. Santa Fe, New Mexico

Krieger D, Peper E, Ancoli A. Therapeutic touch: searching for evidence of physiological change. Am J Nurs 79: 660–662

Kunz DVG. 1991. The Personal Aura. Quest. Wheaton

Mack JE. 1993. Foreword. p. xi. In Walsh R, Vaughan F (eds). Paths Beyond Ego. The Transpersonal Vision. JP Tarcher. Los Angeles

McNeill B, Guion C (eds). 1991. Noetic Sciences Collection 1980–1990. Ten Years of Consciousness Research. Institute of Noetic Sciences. Sausalito, California

Meehan MTC. 1985. The effect of therapeutic touch on the experience of acute pain in postoperative patients. Dissertation Abstracts Int 46:795B

Mentgen J, Bulbrook MJ. 1994. Healing Touch: Level I Notebook. Healing Touch, Lakewood. Colorado, p. 3

Mishlove J. 1993. The Roots of Consciousness. The Classic Encyclopedia of Consciousness Studies Revised and Expanded. Council Oak. Tulsa, Oklahoma

Montagu A. 1971. Touching. The Human Significance of the Skin. Harper & Row. New York

The New Lexicon Webster's Dictionary of the English Language. 1989. Lexicon. New York

Post NW. 1990. The effects of therapeutic touch on muscle tone. Masters Abstracts Int 28:587

Potter Hughes P. 1994. The experience of therapeutic touch as a treatment modality with adolescent psychiatric patients. Unpublished master's thesis

Quinn JF. 1984. Therapeutic touch as energy exchange: testing the theory. Adv Nurs Sci 6:42–49

Quinn JF. 1988. Building a body of knowledge: research on therapeutic touch 1974–1986. J Holistic Nurs 6: 37–45

Quinn JF. 1989a. Healing: the emergence of right relationship. In Carlson R, Shield B (eds). Healers on Healing. JP Tarcher. Los Angeles

Quinn JF. 1989b. Future directions for therapeutic touch research. J Holistic Nurs 7:19–25

Quinn JF. 1989c. Therapeutic touch as energy exchange: replication and extension. Nurs Sci Q 2(2):79–87

Quinn JF, Strelkauskas AJ. 1993. Psychoimmunologic effects of therapeutic touch on practitioners and recently bereaved recipients: a pilot study. Adv Nurs Sci 15(4): 13–36

Randolph GL. 1984. Therapeutic and physical touch: physiological response to stressful stimuli. Nurs Res 33(1):33–36

Slater VE. 1995a. Toward an Understanding of Energetic Healing. Part 1: Energetic Structures. 13(3):209–224

Slater VE. 1995b. Toward an Understanding of Energetic Healing. Part 2: Energetic Processes. 13(3):225–238

Sutich A. 1975. Introduction to the original edition. In Tart CT (ed). Transpersonal Psychologies: Perspectives on the Mind from Seven Great Spiritual Traditions. Harper San Francisco, San Francisco, p. 1

Talbot M. 1991. The Holographic Universe. Harper-Collins. New York

Tart CT. (ed). 1975. Transpersonal Psychologies: Perspectives on the Mind from Seven Great Spiritual Traditions. Harper-San Francisco, San Francisco

Tellington-Jones L. 1992. The Tellington TTouch. A Breakthrough Technique to Train and Care for Your Favorite Animal. Penguin. New York

Walsh P. 1992. Bioenergy. A Healing Art. New World Media Alliance,

Wetzel WS. 1989. Reiki healing: a physiologic perspective. J Holistic Nurs 7:47–54

Wirth DP. 1992. The effect of non-contact therapeutic touch on the healing rate of full thickness dermal wounds. Subtle Energies 1(1)1–20

Wolf FA. 1982. The Body Quantum. MacMillan. New York

Wolf FA. 1988. Parallel Universes. The Search for Other Worlds. Touchstone. New York

Wolf FA. 1991. The Eagle's Quest. A Physicist Finds Scientific Truth at the Heart of the Shamanic World. Touchstone. New York

Zukav G. 1979. The Dancing Wu Li Masters. An Overview of the New Physics. Quill. New York

10
Aromatherapy

Caroline J. Stevensen

Aromatherapy is the therapeutic use of essential oils extracted from plants. The term *aromathérapie* was coined by the French chemist René-Maurice Gattefossé in 1928. (His book of the same name was published in 1937.) Gattefossé is considered by many to be the father of the modern day scientific use of essential oils.

The food and perfume industries are the largest users of essential oils. Some confusion about the therapeutic potential of aromatherapy may be due to this link with the cosmetic industry. The dictionary definition of aromatherapy is a method of treating bodily ailments using essential plant oils (Chambers 1988). Aroma is defined in chemical terms as belonging to the closed chain class of organic compounds or benzene derivatives. Therapy is defined as a treatment used to combat a disease or abnormal condition. Essential oils are described as oils forming the odiferous part of plants, and as ethereal, suggesting not only a chemical constituent, but also a heavenly, spirit-like or airy quality. Based on these definitions, aromatherapy is a treatment using a range of organic compounds of which the odor or fragrance play an important part.

Jean Valnet, the French physician well known for his invaluable work on aromatherapy, speaks of aromatherapy as the medicinal use of aromatic essences derived from plants (Valnet 1990). Kusmirek, an aromatherapist based in England, describes aromatherapy as an industry combining perfumery, science, psychoaromatherapy, and aromacology, saying that the use of essential oils seeks to influence or change body, mind, or spirit (Kusmirek 1992).

Tisserand, an English aromatherapist, refers to essential oils from plants as the blood of a person. "They are not the whole plant, but are whole organic substances in themselves. Like blood they will die if not properly preserved. The essential oil is like the most ethereal and subtle part of the plant, and its therapeutic action takes place on a higher more subtle level than that of the whole organic plant . . . having in general a more pronounced effect on the mind and emotions than does herbal medicine" (Tisserand 1988).

Statements such as these are not based in scientific fact and no trials have been performed to support their validity. It is unfounded, anecdotal comments like this that have helped keep aromatherapy from being considered a serious science. Valnet states that forgotten and ignored for many years, aromatic essences are coming back into their own, for many researchers and for a large section of public opinion, as the stars of medicine. Many patients are now unwilling to be treated except by natural therapies, foremost amongst which plants and their essences have a rightful place (Valnet 1990). It is evident that both the scientific and the more subtle qualities of aromatherapy are important to those working with aromatherapy oils.

Essential oils are extracted from different parts of plants such as the roots, bark, stalks, flowers, or leaves. These extracts are mostly distilled, although other methods might be used. Essential oils might be applied to the body via massage with a vegetable oil, inhaled, used as a compress, mixed into an ointment, or inserted internally via the rectum, vagina, or mouth. The latter method is used chiefly by the medical profession in France.

Aromatherapy appears to be one of the fastest growing complementary therapies in the United Kingdom. Aromatherapy was brought to the United Kingdom from France by Madame Marguerite Maury, born in Austria. She was the first layperson to study and utilize the effects of essential oils absorbed through the skin. Her research was based on that of Gattefossé and her own clinical work with her husband, a French homoeopathic doctor. She promoted the modern day use of massage with essential oils, the *aromatherapy massage,* and began teaching aromatherapy to beauticians. This training has gradually filtered from the cosmetic into the therapeutic domain and is increasingly being used by nurses, physiotherapists, and other health care professionals.

Modern day aromatherapy is one of the fastest growing complementary therapies. This growth includes not only training and practice of aromatherapy, but also production of essential oils. In the United Kingdom, it is hard to pick up a magazine or watch a program on alternative medicine that does not mention aromatherapy. Trained aromatherapists in the United Kingdom currently number approximately 5,000 without the existence of a central register. In a recent survey, over 21,000 people members responded to a questionnaire on alternative medicine. Of the respondents, 7 percent had used aromatherapy, compared to 25 percent for osteopathy, 14 percent for chiropractic, 12 percent for homeopathy, and 9 percent for acupuncture.

Aromatherapy gradually is becoming more accepted in the orthodox medical field as a treatment to enhance both physical and psychological aspects of patient care. Skeptics might reject the therapy because of a lack of clinical trials—a criticism levelled at other branches of complementary medical treatments—as well as concern regarding the safety and quality of essential oils. These issues will be resolved as more research is performed and aromatherapy will have its full and appropriate place in modern health care.

History

Maurice-René Gattefossé was a French chemist and scholar who described aromatherapy as a particular branch of science and therapeutics in 1928. He be-

came interested in the study of essential oils following an accident in his laboratory. Gattefossé burnt his hand badly following a chemical explosion. He applied lavender essential oil that was close by. The burn healed with remarkable speed, and without infection or scarring. Amazed at this result, Gattefossé began to investigate the properties of essential oils. He was the first person to analyze and record the individual chemical components in each oil, classifying the oils according to their properties (such as antitoxic, antiseptic, tonifying, stimulating, calming) (Franchomme 1990).

Gattefossé carried out experiments in military hospitals during World War I. He claimed to achieve remarkable results using essential oils preventing gangrene, curing burns, and obtaining cicatrization far more quickly than usual. However, after the war, his methods came under professional scrutiny, and were largely left behind (Maury 1964).

Essential oils from aromatic plants were used before 1928. Over what length of time distilled essential oils have been used is uncertain. Popular opinion claims that the Arabs discovered the distilling of plants in the middle ages, and Avicenna has been given credit for this achievement in the tenth century AD (Arcier 1990). However, an Italian research party led by Dr. Paolo Povesti, the director of the International Biocosmetic Research center in Milan, found a perfectly preserved terra-cotta distillation apparatus or still in the museum of Taxila, at the foot of the Himalayas. It was used for beauty products, and dated back 5,000 years to the Indus Valley civilization (Williams 1989).

Aromatic substances, which may or may not include essential oils as prepared today, were used in the ancient civilizations of Egypt, China, Greek, Rome, and Arab countries, in middle ages, during the scientific revolution, and up to the present day. The importance of this is captured in the comment of Marguerite Maury: Perfumes and aromatics have their own history and long past. The latter is so bound up in the story of mankind that it is impossible to separate the two (Maury 1964).

In Egyptian times, Nefertum was the God of perfumes, incense, and fragrant oils. He was the son of Ptah, the creator God, and Sekmet, the Goddess of fiery protection, healing, and alchemical distillation. In a hymn to Nefertum, he is described as the "Lord of oils and ungents, the soul of life. Nefertum smells the soul of the lotus and plants, purifies the body. In Egyptian life, fragrance was a means of communication between the gods and humanity, offering health to the living and assisting the dead in the next life (Steele 1992). There was some overlap between the use of aromatic products for spiritual well-being, health, and beauty. King Ramses III reportedly burned two million blocks of incense during the 30 years of his reign (Stoddart 1991). The medicinal properties of aromatic oils were understood by the later Egyptian periods, and a wide range of essential oils were used, including frankincense, myrrh, cedarwood, henna, and juniper. The essence of cedarwood was prepared by heating in clay vessels covered by a layer of woollen fibers. These fibers were then squeezed, allowing the essence to be extracted (Valnet 1990). When the tomb of Tutenkhamun was discovered in 1922, vases were found in the tomb, which, upon analysis, contained ointments of frankincense in a base of animal fat. The scent was apparently faint but still in evidence (Tisserand 1988).

The ancient Chinese are well known for their use of herbal medicine, acupuncture, and moxibustion (the burning of mugwort to balance the body's energy), but there seems to be little detail regarding the use of aromatic oils. The Hebrews gained their knowledge of aromatic oils from prisoners held by the Egyptians.

The ancient Greeks used the aromatic essences both for medicine and for perfumes. Hippocrates expounded the virtues of a daily bath and a scented massage to maintain health and well-being. Aristotle argued that pleasant smells contribute to the well-being of humanity. The Roman poet Lucretius described the particles of pleasant smells as being smooth and round, whilst the particles of unpleasant smells were barbed and prickly.

Biblical evidence of the use of aromatic substances is present in both the old and new testaments. God commanded Moses to make a holy anointing oil of myrrh, cinnamon, calamus, cassia, and olive oil (Exodus 30, 22–25); frankincense and myrrh were brought to the birth of Jesus Christ (Matthew 2, 11).

The middle ages saw a rise in the use of oils both as perfumes and medicines. Catherine de Medici, married to King Henry II, made fashionable the use of aromatic substances for ailments and perfumery.

Her perfumer Cosimo Ruggieri not only assisted her with her health and beauty, but was able to prepare much less pleasant substances to help dispose of her enemies. Aromatic oils also were used to block out the smell of poor hygiene, and ward off various plagues; pomanders and the fragrant tops on walking sticks were commonly used for this purpose. In 1589, a German pharmacopeia listed 80 essential oils for treating different conditions, and lavender essence was first prepared in France at this time (Arcier 1990).

Away from Europe, the Native American shamans were no strangers to the use of herbs and aromatics. The perfumeros, or healers, bathed their patients in scents and, by the skillful use of perfume, could transform the auric field—the energetic or emotional envelope that surrounds a person. The blowing of tobacco smoke over a person, combined with a perfume, also was seen as having curative powers. The use of fragrance enabled transformations in religious, magical, and healing rituals. An ancient connection exists between fumigating and perfuming in this culture (Steele 1992).

The scientific revolution and the manufacturing of synthetic substances that commenced in the 19th century saw the retreat of essential oils until the work by Gattefossé and his followers during this century. The perfume industry developed separately from the therapeutic field, with the introduction of such names as Coco Chanel, who launched the famous Chanel No. 5 in 1921. It was she who said that the most mysterious, most human thing, is smell. With the subsequent commercial development of the cosmetic industry, the gap between the cosmetic and the therapeutic use of essential oils became evident. Chanel and her scientific advisers, successfully used synthetic products to make modern perfumes. This process separated cosmetics completely from the therapeutic use of essential oils, except perhaps for good feelings experienced by people wearing and experiencing the perfumes.

Marguerite Maury's research into the cutaneous application of essential oils commenced the teaching of aromatherapy in the 1950s, as it is used today. Maury was influenced by the work of Valnet, who was an army doctor during the second world war. He recognized that essential oils could have been used to alleviate some of the infection experienced by the soldiers, instead of the massive amounts of penicillin that were prescribed. He obtained consistent results using essential oils with his wartime patients in Tonkin (Valnet 1990). Madame Maury identified two uses of aromatherapy in France: first as part of allopathy in its use by doctors, and second as a beauty treatment in the form of massage. She also acknowledged the more subtle aspect of aromatherapy and mentioned its link to vibratory medicine.

Development

Madame Maury influenced the beginnings of the practice of aromatherapy in the United Kingdom. Micheline Arcier, a well known aromatherapist in London, met Madame Maury at a beauty conference in 1959. Arcier and three other masseuses asked Maury to run a course for them. Madame Maury had clinics in London, Paris, and Switzerland, and Madame Arcier worked with her in London. Madame Arcier then began working with the oils and teaching small numbers of masseuses in the 1960s and 1970s. She also met Valnet, who worked and consulted from her London clinic.

Aromatherapy was still little known at this time. In fact, this method only earned widespread popularity in the 1980s. It is interesting to note the recent growth of aromatherapy, and yet, how few people have been responsible for its development over the last few decades.

Since the 1980s, numerous schools of massage and aromatherapy have opened. There are nearly 5000 aromatherapists trained in the United Kingdom, although not all practice full-time. The number of people receiving aromatherapy is less than those receiving osteopathy, and there are only 2000 registered osteopaths. Training in aromatherapy has continued in schools for lay massage practitioners, but has grown to be included in nursing colleges and universities of higher education where the courses may be undertaken as part of a diploma or degree program.

The skills of therapeutic massage, usually the Swedish style, were taught to masseuses as well as physiotherapists as part of their professional training. Massage was part of the curriculum at nursing schools at the turn of this century, but was excluded as their training became more scientific and technically orientated. It is now recognized as a valuable skill in terms of pain management and stress relief, and is slowly being reintroduced into their training.

Fifty books were published on the topic of aromatherapy in the United Kingdom in the 7 years before 1995, indicating the rise in its popularity. Unfortunately, these books do not add new research-based information about essential oils. They often are published for commercial benefit, rather than to further the science of aromatherapy. Most books are aimed at both lay and professional audiences, indicating the lack of sophistication in this field. Many books offer recipes of essential oils, losing sight of the fundamental principles involved. The exceptional work by Franchomme and Pénoël gives detailed chemical analysis of each oil and conditions, indications, and contraindications for each oil (Franchomme & Pénoël 1990). Two new books by Vickers and Tisserand and Balacs address this problem by providing more scientific information, including the available research on essential oils, their chemical constituents, and the clinical practice of aromatherapy (Vickers 1996, Tisserand & Balacs 1995). To this author's knowledge, there have been no books on aromatherapy published and virtually no research performed in North America, except for a study on the inhalation of essential oils for the treatment of respiratory conditions (Boyd 1946).

Theoretical Basis

Essential oils are volatile, fragrant, organic constituents that are obtained from plants either by distillation, which is most common, or by cold pressing, which is used for the extraction of citrus oils. Oils may be extracted from leaves (eucalyptus, peppermint), flowers (lavender, rose), blossoms (orange blossom or neroli), fruits (lemon, mandarin), grasses (lemongrass), wood (camphor, sandalwood), barks (cinnamon), gum (frankincense), bulbs (garlic, onion), roots (calamus) or dried flower buds (clove). Varying amounts of essential oil can be extracted from a particular plant; 220 pounds of rose petals will yield less than two ounces of the essential oil, while other plants such as lavender, lemon, or eucalyptus give a much greater proportion. This accounts

Table 10-1. Chemical Components of Essential Oils and their Therapeutic Actions

Chemical Component	Therapeutic Action
Aldehydes	Anti-infectious, litholitic, calming
Ketones	Mucolitic, litholitic, cicatrising, calming
Esters	Antispasmodic, calming
Sesquiterpenes	Antihistamines, anti-allergic
Coumarins, lactones	Balancing, calming
C15 and C20 alcohols	Estrogen-like action
Acids, aromatic aldehydes	Anti-infectious, immunostimulants
Phenols, C10 alcohols	Anti-infectious, immunostimulants
Oxides	Expectorant, antiparasitic
Phenyl methyl ethers	Anti-infectious, antispasmodic
C10 terpenes	Antiseptic, cortisone-like action

(From Franchomme P, Pénoël D. 1990. L'aromatherapie Exactement. Roger Jallois. Limoges, with permission.)

for the variation in price amongst essential oils. Essential oils come from sources worldwide—lavender from France, eucalyptus from Australia, and sandalwood from India.

Essential oils are commonly a mixture of over 100 organic compounds, which may include esters, alcohols, aldehydes, terpenes, ketones, coumarins, lactones, phenols, oxides, acids, and ethers. A list of the major chemical components and their attributed therapeutic effects may be found in Table 10-1. Within the oils, there might be more of some active constituents than others, which give the oil its particular therapeutic value. For example, oils containing large amounts of esters (50 to 70 percent), such as neroli *Citrus aurantium aurantium* are thought to be calming, while other oils such as tea tree *Melaleuca alternifolia terpineol* − 4 are regarded as antibacterial, antiviral, and immune system-boosters due to the large amounts of alcohol (45–50%) in their composition (Franchomme & Pénoël 1990). Critics of aromatherapy may say that the idea of an active ingredient goes against the desire for a whole natural substance. There is a question of the naturalness of any oil removed from a plant; immediately after the flower is cut, chemical changes occur. Other chemicals may appear in the oil which were not originally in the plant (Dodd 1991).

Aromatherapy is used for a wide range of physical, mental, and emotional conditions, including burns, severe bacterial infections, insomnia, depression, hypertension, and arrhythmias. Some of the findings that support these claims will be discussed in the research section of this chapter.

The process of liquid gas chromatography is used to identify the quantity of each chemical constituent within the oil (Franchomme & Pénoël 1990). As with grapes grown for wine, the quality of the yield varies according to the climate and other growing conditions of the plant. Lavender oil is popularly thought to be harmless, but according to its chemical type, or chemotype, it might not be suitable for use as a therapeutic oil. True lavender, *Lavandula angustifolia*, grown at approximately 1000 meters in the French alps, has a high degree of purity and therapeutic constituents, while Stoechas lavender, *Lavandula stoechas*, grown at sea level by the Mediterranean, contains high quantities of ketones, and so may be neurotoxic and abortive and is contraindicated in pregnant women, babies and children (Franchomme & Pénoël 1990).

Potential side effects of essential oils include the neurotoxic and abortive qualities already mentioned, as well as dermal toxicity, photosensitivity, allergic reactions, problems with internal usage, and liver sensitivity (Franchomme & Pénoël 1990). Unless oils are labelled with the full botanical data in Latin, it is impossible to tell whether or not they are dangerous or contraindicated. Lack of legislation over labelling and quality control of essential oils in the United Kingdom has contributed to the unease in some health care settings about their use. The fact that essential oils can be purchased at retail stores also gives the general public a false idea as to the relative safety of these oils.

The quality of essential oils also can be affected by their producers, who might add chemicals to extend the oil's capabilities, or pesticides to act as contaminants. Gas chromatography will identify the chemical make up of any oil, but it is not a complete assurance of quality. A certain degree of adulteration is common in the essential oil world, and often is impossible for the consumer to detect. Reputable oil suppliers who perform their own quality control are currently the only safeguard.

There are few principles for the treatment of aromatherapy. Many aromatherapists discuss the concept of synergy at some length, that the whole natural essence is more active than its principle constituent. Those constituents that form a smaller percentage of the whole are found to be more active than the principle constituent (Valnet 1990). As early as 1919, Heurre is quoted as saying it is not enough to place side-by-side the principle chemical elements which analysis shows to be present in a particular vegetable essence, in order to obtain a product which, therapeutically speaking, is as active as that of the natural essence (Valnet 1990).

The basis of the action of aromatherapy is thought to be the same as that of modern pharmacology, using smaller doses. The chemical constituents are absorbed into the body, affecting particular physiologic processes. Aromatherapy oils are taken into the body via the oral, dermal, rectal, or vaginal routes, or simply by olfaction.

The cutaneous administration of essential oils mixed in a vegetable carrier oil in the form of an aromatherapy massage is a frequent method of administration. Benefits can be gained not only from the oils through the skin, but also from inhalation of the vapor, and from physical therapy in the form of massage. Once the oil reaches the upper dermis, it enters the capillary circulation where the oil can be transported throughout the body (Hotchkiss 1994). A massage oil made with lavender penetrated the skin after 10 minutes (Jäger 1992). Blood samples taken at intervals after massage, when analyzed by gas chromatography, showed that two major constituents of lavender oil, linalool and linalyl ace-

tate—reached maximal concentrations 20 minutes after the massage, although traces had been evident at five minutes. Levels returned to baseline after 90 minutes, indicating elimination of lavender from the bloodstream (Jäger 1992). Other studies support the passage of aromatic compounds through the skin of humans (Collins 1984, Bronough 1990).

Oral administration of essential oils carries more potential risks of poisoning or irritation to the gastric mucosa, if administered by unqualified hands. It might be useful for qualified medical practitioners to get larger doses of essential oils into the body for the treatment of serious infections. A more detailed knowledge of essential oil toxicology is required for administration via this route than is possessed currently by the average aromatherapist.

A significantly lower dose is administered to the body via the skin than when given orally (Tisserand & Balacs 1995). Rectal administration of oils in the form of suppositories may be useful for local problems, and to avoid the portal system of the body, thus allowing higher systemic concentrations of the oils to be absorbed (Tisserand & Balacs 1995). Vaginal administration in the form of pessaries or douches also are used for local problems.

Simple inhalation of the oils is a method used for respiratory conditions, insomnia, and mood elevation and enhancement, or simply for making an environment more pleasant. It is not surprising that essential oils are absorbed via inhalation, considering that conventional medications such as those for asthma are administered in this way. Steam inhalers can be used for respiratory infections, and a variety of electrical and fan-assisted apparatus may be used to scent a room. Locomotor activity in mice increased after the inhalation of rosemary oil (Kovar 1987). A rise in serum levels of 1, 8-cineole, a major constituent of rosemary, corresponded with the rise in locomotor activity. Aromatic compounds of sandalwood, rose, neroli, and lavender all were present in the blood of mice after inhalation (Buchbauer 1993). Studies also have demonstrated the absorption of aromatic compounds by humans (Falk 1990, Falk-Filipsson 1993). Overexposure to oils absorbed via this method can result in headaches, fatigue, or allergic reactions such as streaming eyes and skin problems.

The influence of touch in the form of massage is a major aspect of aromatherapy treatment when the oils are administered cutaneously. One study was able to show additional psychological benefit, including reduction in anxiety, to cardiac patients who had aromatherapy massage with the essential oil of neroli (*citrus aurantium ssp. aurantium*) compared to those who had massage with a plain vegetable oil (Stevensen 1994). Other studies have shown positive psychological benefits from massage, including positive subjective response (Madison 1973); the perceived state of relaxation (Longworth 1982); reported pleasurable feelings (Bauer & Dracup 1987); and an improvement in the perceived level of anxiety (Dunn 1992). Physiological results from massage generally have shown no significant difference in heart rate or arterial blood pressure (Dunn 1992, Kaufmann 1964, Reed & Held 1988, Longworth 1982, Bauer & Dracup 1987) or respiratory rate (Dunn 1992, Kaufmann 1964, Reed & Held 1988, Longworth 1982, Bauer & Dracup 1987, Madison 1973). The importance of massage for both relaxation and release of physical and psychological stress should not be underestimated and can be seen only as a positive aid to the administration of essential oils, when administered appropriately.

It is suggested that aromatherapy would not have gained its rapid increase in popularity if the oils were not fragrant, thus affecting mood and emotions. Several references already have been made to the inextricable link between the development of human biology, the sense of smell, and the importance of aromas. Sigmund Freud developed the idea of "organic repression" of the sense of smell. He attributed this to upright gait, which elevates the nose from the ground where it had enjoyed pleasurable sensations previously (Freud 1929). This repression may not be complete, but many people have a diminished sense of smell, a sense more vital to the survival of animals than humans. It may be this need to satisfy pleasurable sensations via the sense of smell that is attracting so many people to aromatherapy.

The human response to aromas is associated with olfaction naturally. The neurons of the olfactory system, which are the chemical senses of the body, rest in the section of the midbrain known as the limbic system. The structures of the limbic system extend from the midbrain through the hypothalamus into the basal forebrain, which is concerned not only with visceral functions, but also with emotional expression. The cortical and medial nuclei of the amygdala, a body situated within this system, receive information from the olfactory system. The basolateral nuclei are involved with the expression of emotion (Shepherd 1983). Aromatherapy's effect on emotion and psychological state therefore is not surprising (Stevensen 1994, Hardy 1992). The emotional and psychological benefit of aromatherapy is important in many clinical situations, including chronic, life-threatening conditions such as cancer, heart disease, and AIDS.

Settings

Aromatherapy is used in a variety of settings throughout Europe and the United Kingdom. These include clinics run by private aromatherapists, clinics attached to general medical practices, and orthodox health care settings used by aromatherapists, or other health care professionals who have been trained in aromatherapy. With regard to the practice of aromatherapy, individual member countries of the European Union each have their own regulations.

Under English Common Law, a person is innocent until proven guilty. As there is no law currently stating a minimum level of training and practice in aromatherapy in the United Kingdom, practitioners can perform without attaining a minimum standard of competence. The British Department of Employment has granted funding for a working party to define national occupational standards for aromatherapy, reflexology, homeopathy, and hypnotherapy. A core curriculum for these complementary therapies also is being proposed. Meanwhile, aromatherapists are working towards Statutory Registration in line with what currently exists for osteopaths since 1993. The Aromatherapy Organisations Council, the governing body for aromatherapy, currently represents 80 percent of the profession, 13 professional associations, and 80 schools and colleges with set minimum standards.

In other European countries, legislation on the practice of complementary therapies including aromatherapy is different as European law differs from

English law. Under the Napoleonic Law developed from the Treaty of Rome, a person is guilty until proven innocent. The practice of complementary therapies in Switzerland, Germany, and France is illegal unless medically qualified, although nonmedical practitioners are tolerated to a certain extent. No therapist in Europe can advertise treatment of any kind or make medical claims except helping stress. Treatment is taken to mean a treatment of any physical or mental disorder by medical or physical means. Because of the legal difficulties of calling oneself a therapist in either Switzerland or Germany, practitioners of aromatherapy have coined the term aromatology and call themselves aromatologists (Ashby 1993).

Aromatherapists who work in practices with general medical practitioners generally do so on a session-by-session basis. The physician often maintains clinical responsibility for the patient referred to the aromatherapist. Aromatherapy in orthodox health care settings is being provided by lay aromatherapists and, increasingly, by trained nurses or other health care professionals such as physiotherapists with aromatherapy training. According to the United Kingdom Central Council (UKCC) Code of Professional Conduct, each nurse is accountable for her own actions, including standards of training to ensure competence in practice (UKCC 1992). The use of aromatherapy within nursing practice falls into this category. Professional bodies such as the Royal College of Nursing (RCN) will provide insurance for nurses using aromatherapy within their nursing practice. Chartered physiotherapists in the country have to take out separate insurance for the use of aromatherapy.

Growth in the use of and interest in aromatherapy have developed so rapidly in recent years that professional legislation has struggled to keep up. Aromatherapy and massage is being taught to professional audiences in Southeast Asia, Australia, and North America, while being reintroduced as a modern concept with cutaneous application for the use of health care professionals other than doctors in some European countries.

Settings in the United Kingdom where aromatherapy has been adopted are included in Table 10-2. The reasons for the use of aromatherapy in these settings are diverse and may include the reasons

Table 10-2. Conventional Medical Settings Where Aromatherapy Is Used in the United Kingdom

Intensive care units	Palliative care settings
Coronary care units	Hospices
Renal units	Pediatric units
Neurologic units	Midwifery units
HIV/AIDS units	Learning disability settings
Geriatric units	Burns units
Cancer units	

mentioned in Table 10-3. These tables are not conclusive, but research performed to support the use of aromatherapy in some of these settings is discussed later.

The United Kingdom is being used as a model for many other countries with regard to legislation regarding the practice of aromatherapy. In the European Union, debate in 1994 focused on the regulation of herbal medicines, including essential oils, in preparation for the single European market. Historically, English practitioners have been able to dispense herbal medicines using special rights afforded them by Henry VIII. In the 1994 debate, there was no undue pressure being placed on the United Kingdom to implement the directive and, in line with a discretionary caveat allowing each European member country to amend a directive, Germany chose to exempt herbal medicines from licensing. The British House of Commons tabled a motion on October 27, 1994 (Motion 1672) to discuss this matter. The British government decided that herbal medicines should continue to be exempt form licensing requirements and not subject to the new regulations

Table 10-3. Reasons to Administer Aromatherapy in Conventional Medical Settings

Relaxation
Stress and anxiety relief
Pain and discomfort relief
Insomnia and restlessness
Infections and wound healing
Burns
Enhancing self-image
Stimulating immune function
Treatment for constipation

required by the European directive. Notice was made of the valuable contribution of herbal medicines over the centuries and concern was raised at the large cost of providing the research data necessary to meet the licensing requirements, as well as the cost of licensing each product.

Research

As with many other complementary therapies, the research basis for aromatherapy is incomplete. Problems already have been noted regarding the attributes given to some essential oils that have their basis in herbal medicine rather than aromatherapy research. In fact, much of the research performed on the use of essential oils or their individual constituents has been performed in animal models and isolated tissue cultures. Few trials have been conducted in human subjects under clinical conditions. Kusmirek identifies the problem with the rapid development of aromatherapy: popular use has outstripped research (Kusmirek 1992). Members of the medical profession and those wishing to use aromatherapy in the conventional health care settings have found that this lack of research in essential oils precludes acceptance of aromatherapy in the clinical environment. Little is known about possible interactions with conventional medications or treatments, but it is presumed that because the dosages of essential oils absorbed in the body generally are small, and because there has been no reported incidence of difficulties, that essential oils administered in physiologic doses are safe given the contraindications mentioned earlier. Further research is required. This section presents a brief review of aromatherapy research data, with particular emphasis on the action of the essential oils. A more detailed description may be found in Vickers (1996).

Antimicrobial Activity

The effect of essential oils on a wide variety of pathogens is well known. Their chemical constituents of alcohols and aldehydes, terpenes and phenyl methyl ethers help to explain this action. The antimicrobial aspects of essential oils have been the most widely investigated. Janssen performed a useful review of the literature in this field from the 1970s to the early 1980s. He concluded that many essential oils do have antimicrobial effects, but found this difficult to qualify due to the variation in test methods and the insufficient description of essential oils and microorganisms in some studies. From the different chemotypes or chemical subgroups of *Thymus vulgaris* (common thyme), the strongest antifungal chemotype had eight times the effect of the weakest (Janssen 1987).

Another investigation reported antibacterial activity of a number of oils, including *Artemisia dracunculus* (tarragon), *Salvia officinalis L* (sage), *Salvia sclarea* (clary sage), and *Thymus vulgaris L* (thyme) (Zani 1991). Other studies support the antimicrobial actions of essential oils (Baylier 1979, Panizzi 1993). There also is evidence that the constituents of essential oils have antimicrobial properties. The alcohols geraniol, eugenol, menthol, and citral all showed high antibacterial activity in one investigation (Moleyar 1992).

Animal Models

Buchbauer performed perhaps the most extensive research on essential oils in animal models. After 1 hour of inhaling an essential oil or fragrance compound, mice became sedated by sandalwood, rose, neroli, and lavender. Some of the constituent compounds found to have a sedative effect on inhalation were anethole, bornyl salicylate, coumarin, 2-phenylethyl acetate, benaldehyde, citronella, and geranyl acetate. Compounds which stimulated after inhalation include geraniol, isoborneol, isoeugenol, nerol, methylsalicylate, alpha-pinene and thymol. Lavender oil was found to be a more effective sedative than either of its major constituents (linalool and linalyl acetate) in isolation (Buchbauer 1993). Again, this supports aromatherapists claims of synergy within essential oils (Tisserand 1988, Price 1995).

Tissue Cultures

Peppermint, commonly known for its benefit in digestive disorders, has been found to inhibit gastrointestinal smooth muscle in tissue models (Taylor 1983), and affects the flow of calcium across the cell wall of the gastrointestinal smooth muscle (Taylor 1985). High doses of peppermint might have been found to induce spasm. This idea would support findings that high doses in essential oils may produce opposite effects.

Pharmacologic Preparations in Animals

The effects of essential oils with pharmacologic preparations in animals has been studied. The concern from the medical profession and aromatherapists alike regarding the lack of information about interaction between aromatherapy oils and conventional drug preparations in humans already has been mentioned. Jori investigated the effects of essential oils on drug metabolism, using pentobarbital, a sedative drug, to induce sleep in rats. 1, 8-cineole, an oxide, was found to significantly interfere with pentobarbital. Both the sleeping times and the brain levels of the drug were reduced by about 50 percent after subcutaneous injection and aerosol inhalation. These effects were persistent even when the 1, 8-cineole was administered 36 hours before the Pentobarbital (Jorich 1969). Similar results were reported elsewhere (Wade 1986).

Psychological Effects

In Torri's 1988 study, inhalation of various essential oils was found to lead to a change in brain wave activity. The oils were measured for an increase (+) or decrease (−) of brain wave activity. The results of the oils were as follows: basil (+ +), bergamot (− − −), rosewood (+/−), chamomile (− −), clove (+ + +), geranium (+/−), jasmine (+ +), lavender (− −), lemon (− −), lemongrass (+), marjoram (− −), neroli (+ + +), patchouli (+), peppermint (+ + +), rose (+ +), sage (+), sandalwood (− − −), valerian (+/−), and ylang ylang (+ + +).

This study generally supports the claims of stimulation and relaxation made about essential oils, with particular reference to jasmine as stimulating and lavender as relaxing (Tisserand 1988). Overstimulation from the oils was found to have a lowering effect on brain waves, which is suggested to be the same effect that oil would have in clinical use. If this is so, then dosage of essential oils may need closer examination through further trials.

Analgesic Effects

Analgesic properties are attributed to some oils, although the evidence for this is scarce. One study demonstrated that lemongrass leaves produced a dose-dependent analgesia in rats. Both subplantar and oral doses of the constituent myrcene were administered with similar effect. Myrcene, a constitu-

ent of oils including rosemary, lavender, juniper, and lemongrass to a lesser extent, was credited with the effect (Lorenzetti 1991). Undiluted lavender oil is well known as a first-aid remedy for minor burns, both removing pain and promoting healing, as in Gattefossé's laboratory accident.

Recent Clinical Research

Most of the recent aromatherapy research in the conventional health care settings in the United Kingdom has been undertaken by nurses with a particular interest in the field. There have been a number of studies performed in the intensive care setting, with others performed in the field of midwifery, palliative care, and care of the elderly. Some of these trials found psychological benefits to the patients from aromatherapy, in addition to massage. In a randomized controlled trial, 100 cardiac surgery patients in intensive care received the aromatherapy oil of neroli citrus (*aurantium ssp. aurantium*) in foot massage and found anxiety in particular to be further reduced than in patients who were massaged with a plain vegetable oil after four days (Stevensen 1994). Both groups who had the massage with or without the neroli oil scored significantly better statistically on a modified Spielberger state anxiety questionnaire than did the control groups on the day of massage. The only significant physiologic difference between the massage and non-massage groups were transient and related to respiratory rate immediately after the massage. Buckle massaged postcardiotomy patients with two different lavender essential oils, *Lavandula angustifolia* and *Lavandula latifolia,* hoping to show a difference between the effects of the two oils. Although the presentation of the trial lacked detail, and the results were insignificant, there was some difference between the two oils, somewhat supporting the conclusion than massage with essential oils proved more beneficial that massage without essential oils (Buckle 1993). In an unpublished study, Dunn used intensive care as a setting in a randomized trial to measure the effects of massage with lavender oil compared to plain oil massage, and rest in 122 patients. Physiological changes were not significant, but positive psychological changes were better for the essential oil over the plain oil massage, and that over the period of rest (Dunn 1992).

Anecdotal reports from mothers that lavender oil helped relieve perineal discomfort after childbirth were followed with a randomized trial involving 635 women. Each was given a bottle of either pure lavender oil, a synthetic lavender oil which smelled like the other, or an inert compound, with instructions to add 6 drops to their bath daily. Results were not significant, but pain was slightly reduced in the pure lavender group. That group also suffered the most infection (Dale & Cornwall 1994). This study may demonstrate that anecdotal reports from patients about essential oils are not reliable.

In a study of 51 patients attending a center for palliative care, the effects of three aromatherapy massages given weekly were examined with or without the essential oil of Roman chamomile, *Chamemalum nobile*. Using the Rotterdam Symptom checklist (RSCL) and State-trait anxiety inventory, post-test scores for all patients improved. These were statistically significant in the aromatherapy group on the RSCL physical symptom subscale, quality of life subscale, and state anxiety scale (Wilkinson 1995). In a small study of four patients on an long stay elderly care ward, researchers assessed sleep over three consecutive two week periods—the first period with night sedation, the second without, and the third with lavender diffused into the air at set intervals. Sleep was poorer in the second week, and in the third week, sleep was as good as in the first week (Hardy 1992). However, this trial was assessed only by observation.

Aromatherapy in clinical research is in its infancy. There are methodological problems with much of the clinical research presented that make results difficult to assess. In the absence of further clinical trials there also is the problem that aromatherapists are relying on many trials from animal and tissue models for the basis of their practice. There is no guarantee that these results can be replicated in humans. It is likely that, as more and better quality research is performed in the clinical use of aromatherapy, its appropriate place in the field of complementary medicine will become established.

Conclusion

This chapter has demonstrated the relatively recent development of aromatherapy compared to other areas of complementary medicine. While aromatic substances and oils have been used throughout his-

tory, there has been no sound system developed for their use, a fact especially evident when comparing aromatherapy to a system such as Chinese Medicine. Recent interest in essential oils by both aromatherapists and health care professionals should encourage more research into the science of aromatherapy, so that understanding may be gained as to the importance and worth of this natural therapy. Until a sound scientific base is ascertained, it is believed that aromatherapy will not take a full place beside the more established complementary health care systems.

Acknowledgments

I would like to acknowledge the information given by Andrew Vickers of the Research Council for Complementary Medicine, London, in completion of the research section in this chapter.

References

Arcier M. 1990. Aromatherapy. Hamlyn, London

Ashby N. 1993. Aromatherapy in the balance: aromatherapy in the UK and Europe—an overview by law. Aromatherapy Q 37:13–14

Bauer WC, Dracup KA. 1987. Physiologic effects of back massage in patients with acute myocardial infarction. Focus Crit Care 14(6):42–46

Baylier MF. 1979. Bacteriostatic activity of some Australian essential oils. Perfumer and Flavourist, 4(23):23–25

Boyd EM, Pearson GL. 1946. The Expectorant Action of Volatile Oils. Am J Med Sci 211:602–611

Bronough RL. 1990. In vivo percutaneous absorption of fragrance ingredients in rhesus monkeys and humans. Food Chem Toxicol 28(5):369–374

Buchbauer G. 1991. Aromatherapy: Evidence for the sedative effects of the essential oil of lavender after inhalation. Zeitschrift fur Naturforschung. 46 C 1067–1072

Buckle J. 1993. Aromatherapy: does it matter which lavender oil is used? Nurs Times 89(20)32–35

Chambers Dictionary. 1988. R and W Chambers Ltd and Cambridge University Press. Cambridge

Collins AJ, Notarianni LJ, Ring EF, Seed MP. 1984. Some observations on the pharmacology of 'deep-heat', a topical rubefacient. Ann Rheum Dis 43(3):411–415

Consumers' Association. 1992. Survey: Alternative medicine. Which? London. November. pp. 44–49

Dale A, Cornwall S. 1994. The role of lavender oil in relieving perineal discomfort following childbirth: a blind randomized clinical trial. J Adv Nurs 19:89–96

Davis P. 1990. Aromatherapy: A–Z. CW Daniel. Saffron Waldon

Dodd GH. 1991. The molecular dimension in perfumery. In Van Toller S, Dodd GH (eds). Perfumery: The Psychology and Biology of Fragrance. Chapman and Hall. London

Dodd GH, Van Toller S. 1983. The biology and psychology of perfumery. Perfumer and Flavorist 8, 1–14

Dunn C. 1992. A report on a randomized controlled trial to evaluate the use of massage and aromatherapy in an intensive care unit. unpublished paper Reading, Battle Hospital

Falk A. 1990. Uptake, distribution and elimination of alpha-pinene in man after exposure by inhalation. Scand J Work Environ Health 16:372–378

Falk-Filipsson A. 1993. d-limonene exposure to humans by inhalation: uptake distribution, elimination and effects on the pulmonary system. Toxicology Environ Health 38:77–88

Franchomme P, Pénoël D. 1990. L'aromatherapie exactement. Roger Jallois. Limoges

Freud S. 1929. The complete psychological works. Vol 21 Civilization and its discontents. Strachy J (ed). Hogath Press. London

Hardy M. 1992. Sweet scented dreams. International J Aromatherapy CW Daniels, Saffron Waldon

Hotchkiss S. 1994. How thin is your skin? New Scientist 141 (1910) 24–27

House of Commons Notices of motions 1672 No. 150 27. October 1994

Jäger W, Buckbauer, Jirovetz L, Fritzer M. 1992. Percutaneous absorption of lavender oil from a massage oil. J Soc Cosmetic Chem 43:49–54

Janssen AM, et al. 1987. Antimicrobial activity of essential oils: 1976–1986 literature review. Planta Med 53(5): 395–398

Kaufman MA. 1964. Autonomic responses as related to nursing comfort measures. Nurs Res 13:45–55

Kovar KA, Gropper B, Friess D, Ammon HP. 1987. Blood levels of 1,8-cineole and locomotor activity of mice after inhalation and oral administration of rosemary oil. Planta Med 53(4):315–318

Kusmirek J. 1992. Perspectives in aromatherapy. In Van Toller S, Dodd GH (eds). Fragrance: The psychology and biology of perfume. Elsevier Science Pub. Ltd., Barking

Longworth JCD. 1982. Psychophysiological effects of slow stroke back massage in normatensive females. Adv Nurs Sci July:44–61

Lorenzetti BB, Souza GE, Sarti SJ, et al. 1991. Myrcene mimics the peripheral analgesic activity of lemongrass tea. J Ethnopharmacol 34(1):43–48

Madison AS. 1973. Psychophysiological response of female nursing home residents to back massage: an investigation of one type of touch. Doctoral thesis. University of Maryland

Maury M. 1964. The Secret of Life and Youth. Macdonald, London

Moleyar V, Narasimham P. 1992. Antibacterial activity of essential oil components. Int J Food Microbiol 16(4): 337–342

Panizzi L, Flamini G, Cioni PL, Morelli I. 1993. Composition and antimicrobial properties of essential oils of four Mediterranean Lamiaceae. J Ethnopharmacol 39(3): 167–70

Price S. 1995. Aromatherapy for health care professionals. Churchill Livingstone, Edinburgh

Reed BV, Held JM. 1988. Effects of sequential tissue massage on autonomic nervous system of middle aged and elderly adults. Phys Ther 68(8):1231–1234

Shepherd GM. 1983. Neurobiology. Oxford University Press, Oxford

Steele JJ. 1992. The anthropology of smell and scent in ancient Egypt and South American Shamanism. In Van Toller S, Dodd GH (eds). Fragrance: The Psychology and Biology of Perfume. Elsevier Science Pub. Ltd, Barking

Stevensen CJ. 1994. The psychophysiological effects of aromatherapy massage following cardiac surgery. Comple Ther Med 2, 27–35

Stoddart DM. 1991. Human odour culture: a zoological perspective. In Van Toller S, Dodd GH (eds). Perfumery: The Psychology and Biology of Fragrance. Chapman and Hall, London

Taylor BA, Luscombe CK, Duthie HL. 1983. Inhibitory effect of peppermint oil on gastrointestinal smooth muscle. Gut 24:A992

Taylor BA, Luscombe DK, Duthie HL. 1984. Inhibitory effect of peppermint and menthol on human isolated coli. Gut 25:A1168

Tisserand R. 1988. The art of aromatherapy. Daniel Co Ltd, Saffron Waldon, United Kingdom

Tisserand R, Balacs T. 1995. Essential Oil Safety. Churchill Livingstone. Edinburgh

Torri S, Fukuda H, Kanemoto H, et al. 1988. Contingent negative variation (CNV) and the psychological effects of odour. In Van Toller S, Dodd GH (eds). Perfumery: The Psychology and Biology of Fragrance. Chapman and Hall, London, pp. 107–121

UKCC (1992) Code of Professional Practice. United Kingdom Central Council of Nursing, Midwifery and Health Visiting, London

Valnet J. 1990. The Practice of Aromatherapy. Daniel Co Ltd, Saffron Waldon, United Kingdom

Van Toller S, Dodd GH. 1992. Fragrance: the psychology and biology of perfume. Elsevier Science Pub. Ltd. Barking

Vickers AJ. 1996. Massage and aromatherapy: A Guide for Health Care Professionals. Chapman and Hall. London

Wade AE, et al. 1986. Alteration of drug metabolism in rats and mice by an environment of cedarwood. Pharmacology 1:317–328

Wilkinson S. 1995. International J Palliative Nurs 1(1)21–30

Williams D. 1989. Lecture notes on essential oils. Eve Taylor

11
Light Therapy

Michael Terman

The field of light therapy and chronobiology concentrates on processes that repeat themselves at regular intervals under control of oscillatory timing mechanisms internal to the organism. Neural clockwork also is responsive to periodic environmental events, and it is the interplay of internal and external timing signals that determines the rhythms of physiology and behavior. Circadian rhythms with periods matching the solar day, i.e., 24 hours, have been the most extensively studied.

Daily rhythmicity is ubiquitous to all living organisms. For example, cortisol secretion, systolic blood pressure, body temperature, and urinary potassium excretion are highest during the day, while plasma melatonin and circulating lymphocytes are highest at night. The transitions between low and high states tend to be gradual and differ for each variable. From the vantage point of medicine, knowledge of the rhythmic pattern or the momentary rhythmic state can be critical to interpreting a laboratory result or making a diagnosis. Target neurons and organs show rhythmic changes in susceptibility to particular drugs with therapeutic dose and toxicity varying throughout day and night. In cancer treatment, for example, the particular morning–evening sequence of drug administration significantly determines the maximum feasible dosages (Hrushhesky 1985).

On the one hand, chronotherapeutics views treatment in the context of temporal changes in cell and tissue receptivity, as described above. However, chronotherapy also can involve manipulations of the internal clock itself. Correcting the clock, as by reset-

ting its phase, can result in symptom remission. Certain neurochemical agents affect the clock, such as the hormone melatonin and related synthetic agonists, and, in recent years, a nonpharmacologic intervention has come to the fore: *appropriately timed exposure to light.*

Despite a long history of basic research in chronobiology (Campbell et al 1995b), the seminal clinical literature is approximately a decade old. This chapter explains the functional relation between internal and external clocks, illustrates how pathologic symptoms can arise from internal clock dysfunction, and shows how circadian rhythm phase resetting can be therapeutic.

The Internal Circadian Pacemaker

For many years, it was argued that daily rhythms of physiology and behavior were driven directly by the solar cycle or its geophysical correlates. The *temporal isolation* experiment was designed to prove this wrong. Animals living in a controlled environment chamber under constant temperature, constant darkness, or dim illumination, as well as isolation from magnetic field variations, continue to show approximate 24-hour cycles of activity and rest, feeding and drinking, and body temperature. Critically, though, the period of these cycles deviates from 24 hours, running slightly shorter or longer. The endogenous *circadian* period ("circa," meaning approximately;" "dies" meaning "day") varies with the individual, the species, and the level of ambient illumination. Under temporal isolation, the rhythms drift in and out of sync with the external day. When a 24-hour light–dark cycle is imposed, however, the period becomes entrained and its phase synchronized. For example, rats are active at night, and sparrows during the day. Thus, the environment influences the internal, self-sustaining, free-running timing process.

The same experimental design has been applied to subjects living alone in an isolation bunker for several weeks, protected from outside time cues. Continuous records of sleep–wake cycles, ingestive activity, body temperature, and other measures were maintained for humans, with similar results. When external daily cues become available, the rhythms entrain to the 24-hour day (Fig. 11-1). However, under temporal isolation they free-run at a longer period.

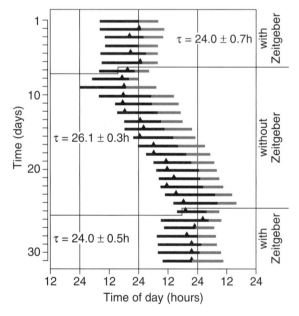

Figure 11-1. Daily cycles of wakefulness (black bars) and sleep (gray bars). Triangles indicate maxima of rectal temperature. τ, the mean circadian period for each sampling interval. Zeitgeber ("time-giver," German); the external signals of the 24-hour day, prominently including the light–dark cycle and social cues. When the Zeitgeber is removed, the rhythms show a free-running period of 26.1 hours. (From Aschoff J, Wever R. 1976. Human circadian rhythms: a multioscillatory system. Fed Proc 35:2326, with permission.)

The physical reality of the internal clock was established during the 1970s through a combination of neuroanatomic and behavioral experiments. Under temporal isolation, animals lost circadian rhythmicity after they received radio-frequency lesions of the suprachiasmatic nuclei (SCN) in the anterior hypothalamus. The distribution of behavior became random or highly fractionated (Moore-Ede et al 1982, Schwartz 1993). No other brain lesion produced this effect. When a light–dark cycle was imposed daily, however, some animals would resume a low-amplitude 24-hour rhythm (e.g., water intake mostly at night). Thus, two separate sources of biologic rhythmicity were identified: the internal clock or "master pacemaker," and a direct "masking" effect of the light–dark cycle that does not operate through the clock.

The intimate link between the external light–dark cycle and the internal clock was demonstrated in the discovery of a monosynaptic pathway between the retina and the SCN—the retinohypothalamic tract (RHT). Light stimulation of the retina results in electrical evoked potentials, activation of gene expression, and neurosecretory responses in the SCN. Although the intergeniculate leaflet of the lateral geniculate nucleus feeds back into the SCN, the classical visual sensory pathways are not involved. Indeed, an animal made cortically and perceptually blind by destruction of the ascending sensory pathways still transduces light to the SCN, allowing day–night cycles to entrain the internal clock. Furthermore, some retinally blind humans retain the capacity to transduce light to the SCN, as evidenced by light suppression of pineal melatonin secretory activity through SCN projection to the pineal gland (Czeisler et al 1995).

Since the discovery of the SCN's circadian pacemaking function (Klein et al 1991), experiments have succeeded in maintaining in vitro electrophysiologic and neurosecretory activity of SCN slices, and even transplanting SCN tissue into arrhythmic host animals bearing SCN lesions, with resumption of rhythmicity. The output routes of the SCNs to the many effector systems that drive end point behaviors—such as sleeping and waking, ingestion, body temperature, and hormonal cycles—have yet to be described in detail and may involve a diffusible signal above and beyond direct neural efferents.

Two Hands of the Clock: Body Temperature and Melatonin Rhythms

In humans and in vivo, the inner workings of the circadian pacemaker cannot be determined directly. Rather, they have to be inferred by end point markers, that is, physiologic functions that are driven by the SCN output signal. Two such phase markers are provided in the cyclic minimum of core body temperature (T_{min}) and the peak of pineal melatonin secretory activity, both of which occur normally at night within a few hours before the habitual time of awakening (Fig. 11-2).

Body temperature can be measured using a rectal thermistor probe connected to an ambulatory datalogger worn by the subject. However, core body temperature is masked partially by activity level and sleep state, among other factors. Behavioral restrictions (as in the "constant routine" described below) and mathematical transformations of raw data are used to determine internal clock phase precisely.

Melatonin provides a less confounded measure than body temperature because it is far less vulnerable to behavioral state. Further, melatonin might regulate the temperature rhythm directly (Cagniacci et al 1992). However, because exposure to bright light directly inhibits pineal activity, subjects must remain under dim light or darkness in order to examine the nocturnal melatonin cycle. Plasma or serum samples are taken throughout the night using an indwelling venous catheter, and a radioimmunoassay or gas chromatography/mass spectrophotometry is used to determine momentary concentration of the hormone.

Ideally, such results would be available quickly and provide a diagnostic basis for scheduling light administration, but that is rarely feasible. With the recent development of increasingly sensitive assays, saliva samples have been substituted successfully for blood; a restricted pre-sleep sampling interval is sufficient to determine the time of onset of the secretory episode, which can replace the nocturnal peak as a circadian phase marker. In the near future, one hopes, the physician will be able to order a melatonin onset profile, receive a prompt laboratory analysis, and prescribe treatment based on each patient's unique circadian phase.

The Circadian Phase Response Curve for Light

When we say that the light–dark cycle entrains a rhythm, we refer to the correction it imposes on the underlying clock, which would otherwise free-run at

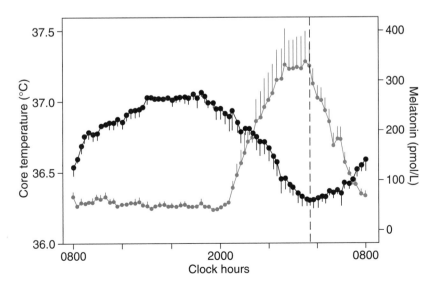

Figure 11-2. Covariation of core body temperature (black curve) and serum melatonin (blue curve) secretion. Average data for 12 women in the early follicular phase. (From Cagniacci A, Elliott J, Yen S. 1992. Melatonin: a major regulator of the circadian rhythm of core temperature in humans. J Clin Endocrinol Metab 75:447, with permission.)

a non-24-hour period. This action of light is very specific: light presented at certain points of the circadian cycle phase-shifts, or "pushes" the internal clock to an earlier, advanced position; at other points in the cycle, the very same light serves to phase-delay the clock; and at still other points it has no effect on the clock (the "dead zone"). In a human whose underlying free-running period is 24.5 hours, for example, a 30-minute phase advance is needed every day to achieve synchrony with the external world. This is achieved by light presentation during early morning hours. Light exposure earlier in the night would have the opposite effect: it would phase-delay the clock and thus might displace the rhythm further from its synchronized position. And light in the midday dead zone fails to make contact with the clock.

This bidirectional influence of light—described as the phase-response curve (PRC)—is the cardinal principle of the internal/external clock interface. The clinical application of light therapy requires a working knowledge of the PRC; otherwise the treatment might exacerbate the very symptoms it is designed to correct.

PRCs have been derived for humans by two strategies (Dijk et al 1995). In one paradigm, light pulses are presented to a subject who is free-running in a temporal-isolation environment (Minors et al. 1991). A continuous record of body temperature provides an index of underlying clock phase, against which the effect of the bright light can be measured. A single bright light exposure (e.g., 3 hours at 5000 lux) is sufficient to reset the internal pacemaker as much as 2 hours in either direction. Phase delays are obtained when light exposure is centered 1 to 3 hours before T_{min}; phase advances are obtained with light centered 1 to 4 hours after T_{min}.

In the second PRC paradigm, light pulses are presented to a subject who has been entrained to the external day–night cycle. To assess internal clock phase, the subject is released into a "constant routine"—remaining awake, supine, under constant low illumination, and eating frequent even-spaced isocaloric snacks for up to 40 hours (Czeisler et al 1989). This arduous procedure eliminates confounding thermoregulatory influences and yields an on-line temperature pattern determined primarily by the circadian clock. A series of light exposures is then administered at a standard time of day (e.g., 5 hours at 10,000 lux, for 3 days), after which the constant routine is repeated for a reassessment of circadian phase. Although the shape of the PRC is similar to that obtained in the free-running experiment—with the greatest delays before T_{min} and the greatest advances following it—the multiple pulse paradigm can produce phase shifts of up to 12 hours, essentially reversing circadian clock phase (Fig. 11-3). It is as if there were near-instantaneous physiologic adjustment to geographic displacement halfway around the world, an adjustment of magnitude that might take several weeks after jet travel.

An important feature of the human PRC is that the largest phase shifts are obtained when light coincides with the nocturnal sleep phase under entrainment—"when light invades the subjective night" (Pittendrigh 1988). Because of the system's capacity for large phase shifts in either direction, close attention to scheduling and monitoring is a sine qua non of light treatment. Clinically, it would be rare that 12-hour shifts are desired; the potential adverse effects of such sudden, large shifts have yet to be studied. Rather, subtler corrections of a few hours or less are sought using a long-term re-entrainment schedule of daily light exposures at the low-amplitude edges of the PRC, not too close to T_{min}.

The PRC for Exogenous Melatonin

Melatonin is high in the bloodstream at night, and absent during daylight hours (see Fig. 11-2). Melatonin may serve as the body's signal of darkness or night, guiding cycles of physiologic activity—indeed, driving core body temperature downward. Moreover, endogenous melatonin—secreted by the pineal gland in response to circadian signalling from the SCN—feeds back on the SCN, which is rich in melatonin receptors.

Just as the PRC for light shows its major activity during the hours of darkness, exogenously administered melatonin elicits phase shifts of the circadian clock during daylight hours (Lewy et al 1992). The melatonin PRC sits in antiphase to the light PRC (see Fig. 11-3). Thus, when subjects are given 0.5-mg doses of melatonin in the late afternoon and early

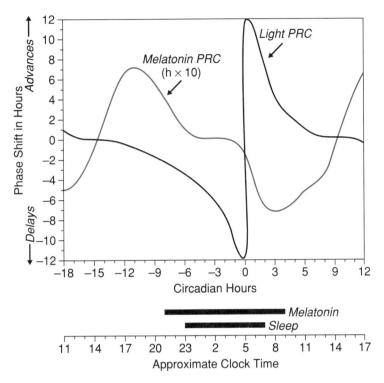

Figure 11-3. Phase response curves for light and melatonin, abstracted from group data (light, Czeisler et al 1989; melatonin, Lewy et al 1992). Circadian time on the abscissa indicates proportional hours within the cycle relative to the nocturnal core body temperature minimum (T_{min}). Lower axis shows typical corresponding sleep and melatonin secretion intervals in external clock time. Melatonin onset precedes sleep onset by about 2 hours, and T_{min} precedes awakening by about 2 hours.

evening, the pineal melatonin secretion rhythm responds with phase advances, and when the dose is given in the morning, the rhythm delays. (Melatonin capsules and tablets currently are available over the counter, but often in pharmacologic, sedating doses such as 5mg—far higher than the physiologic doses appropriate for phase shifting.)

Although the maximum phase shifts to exogenous melatonin are smaller than to light pulses, the hormone may prove useful as a chronotherapeutic agent in substitution for, or as an adjunct to light. Appropriately timed melatonin administration can facilitate 24-hour entrainment in blind people whose rhythms free-run (Sack et al. 1991). The use of melatonin in combination with lights—but at opposite times of day, according to the two PRCs—may potentiate and stabilize circadian phase adjustments,

and facilitate treatment of the sleep phase disorders (see below).

Artificial Bright Light Therapy

Artificial light therapy was developed at the National Institute of Mental Health in the early 1980s. A bank of fluorescent lamps mounted in a metal box behind a diffusing screen was placed on a table approximately three feet from the user, and provided illumination of 2500 lux—the lowest level of full natural daylight, found outdoors a few minutes after sunrise and before sunset. The lamps were of the commercial "full-spectrum" type, chosen to mimic the color distribution of skylight, with enhanced output of short-wavelength blue and near-ultraviolet (UV) light (see *Safety of Light Therapy*).

> Bright light therapy utilizes broad-spectrum white light that is distinct quantitatively and qualitatively from the traditional "color therapies" of alternative medicine, although the salutary effects of some color therapies may share a common mechanism. When narrow spectral ranges have been applied in bright light therapy, clinical efficacy has been greatest in the green wavelength range of 505 to 555 nm, which corresponds with the region of greatest retinal spectral sensitivity (Oren et al 1991). The putative mediation of color therapies by receptors in the skin provides an unlikely substrate for chronotherapeutic or antidepressant response (Wehr et al 1987).

The method first was applied to patients suffering winter depression (see *Seasonal Affective Disorder*) for whom daily exposures of 2 to 6 hours were required to achieve the therapeutic effect. Although clinical improvement was dramatic, the time required was infeasible for people on a normal work schedule, limiting widespread use of the treatment.

My group at Columbia University modified the lighting arrangement to present 10,000 lux illumination—a level found outdoors about 40 minutes after sunrise or before sunset—using lamps that minimize emission of UV and short visual wavelengths, resulting in a softer hue. At this increased light level, therapeutic response is obtained in daily sessions of 30 to 45 minutes, allowing for convenient breakfast-time treatments. In order to avoid the disturbing glare of straight-on illumination, the light box, positioned about 1 foot from the eyes, is raised on a tilted stand, providing downward illumination toward the eyes in a workstation arrangement (Fig. 11-4).

Taken together, the factors of illuminance (lux), exposure duration (minutes), and time of day of exposure trade-off with one another to produce a given light dose. The optimum combination needs to be determined individually for the patient. However, 10,000 lux exposure for 30 minutes at 7:00 AM is a good starting point, and often suffices for patients suffering from winter depression, those who show difficulty awakening, or who experience morning drowsiness. Some patients will find this dose excessive, causing symptoms of subjective speediness, irritability, or terminal insomnia (early-morning awakening). The insomnia can be interpreted as an excessive circadian phase-advance. In such cases, dose reductions—in the form of shorter sessions, sitting further from the lights, or treatment at a later hour—often eliminate such side effects. Other patients will require dose increases, that is, longer sessions (though rarely more than 1 hour), or light exposure at an earlier hour, to achieve the therapeutic response (Terman 1993a).

For practical purposes of clinical assessment, circadian phase can be approximately inferred from a person's spontaneous, habitual sleep–wake pattern. I have found in my laboratory that melatonin onsets vary among individuals across 5 hours, from about 7:30 PM to 12:30 AM, averaging around 9:30 PM. There is a strong correlation of melatonin onset with the sleep midpoint, as measured from log records of "steady-state" sleep onset and awakening for about 10 days. The time of melatonin onset is best predicted by the sleep midpoint, using the following equation:

$$Y_{\text{est. melatonin onset}} = 0.91\,X_{\text{sleep midpoint}} + 18.73,$$

where sleep midpoint is expressed as time of day in decimal hours (e.g., 3.81 AM). Using this indirect measure of internal clock phase, it becomes possible to estimate when in "circadian time" light exposure would yield phase advances or delays (by reference to the phase-response curve in Fig. 11-3), and thus to optimize the timing of treatment. If one wanted to maximize phase advances, for example, light therapy might be scheduled about 8 hours after melatonin onset (but not earlier, at the risk of obtaining phase delays).

Safety of Bright Light Therapy

From the start of our work with high-intensity light exposure, we have been concerned about potential ocular side effects and hazards. A structured eye examination is recommended for identifying patients at risk (Gallin et al 1995). Although, at this time, there are no known ocular contraindications for light treatment, patients with progressive retinal dis-

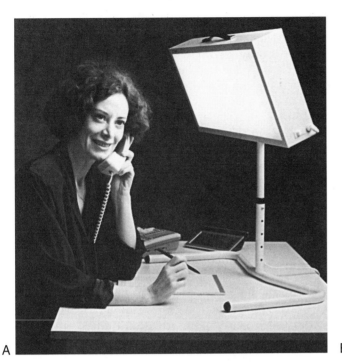

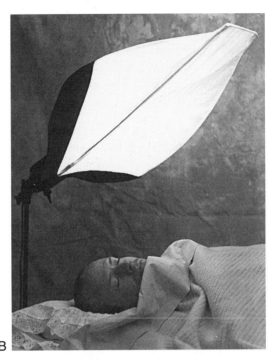

A   B

Figure 11-4. **(A)** Bright light therapy box for 10,000 lux exposure. (Courtesy of DayLight Technologies, Inc., Halifax, Nova Scotia, Canada.) **(B)** Light diffusion box for dawn/dusk simulation in the bedroom. (Courtesy of SphereOne, Inc., Silver Plume, CO.)

eases, e.g., macular degeneration, are excluded as a precaution. Periodic ophthalmologic monitoring is advised for patients using photosensitizing medications such as tricyclic antidepressants and lithium; however, no adverse drug-light ocular interactions have been detected. Patients have received cumulative irradiant doses as high as 40 J/cm^2 (corresponding to 1250 hours of 10,000 lux exposure over 5 years), without adverse ocular effect. Several mild ocular side effects such as eye irritation and headaches have been noted upon initiation of treatment, but these tend to wane quickly or can be controlled by dose reductions. Statistically, for each such side effect, a greater proportion of subjects has shown improvement under treatment relative to the pretreatment baseline.

Dawn/Dusk Simulation

Circadian research on animals has long suggested that behavior (or sleep onset) is triggered by the subtle, graded changes of low-intensity dawn and dusk

twilights in the outside world (Terman et al 1991). These are the very hours in which the PRC is active, at the edges of the "subjective night." Humans often miss these natural signals in the darkness of the bedroom, especially during the long winter nights at northerly latitudes, which can promote oversleeping and depressive symptoms (see Seasonal Affective Disorder). To rectify this putative deficit, we designed a computerized simulator of dawn and dusk transitions, allowing presentation of any naturally occurring light pattern as a function of latitude, longitude, and day of the year. In midwinter, a springtime lighting profile can be presented in the bedroom to the sleeping subject, and therapeutic adjustments obtained. A light diffusion fixture is mounted on a stand above the pillow (see Fig. 11-4) and the bulb power is varied to provide a precise mimic of dawn, dusk, or both dawn and dusk.

One of my patients became severely depressed in winter, showed hypersomnolence and irregular sleep hours, and often could not fall asleep till after 1 AM. She received a May 5 lighting profile at 45° N latitude, with sunrise anchored to 6 AM. Within 1 week, her sleep coalesced within the interval between dusk and dawn; she awakened refreshed approximately at the time of simulated sunrise, and depressive symptoms remitted (Terman & Schlager 1990).

Such treatment differs from bright light therapy in two major respects: the light levels are far lower (with maxima at 250 to 400 lux) and most exposure occurs during sleep with the light signal penetrating closed eyelids. Given retinal dark adaptation during sleeping hours, lower levels of photon energy appear sufficient to activate the therapeutic response, and elicit phase shifts of the endogenous melatonin rhythm. Dawn/dusk simulation provides an automatic alternative to post-awakening bright light therapy, without requiring daytime treatment sessions.

Advanced and Delayed Sleep Phase Syndromes, and Their Associated Insomnias

Advanced sleep phase syndrome (ASPS) is characterized by premature sleep onset and early morning awakening (Terman et al 1995). Patients experience difficulty staying awake in the evening, and maintaining sleep past a predawn hour (e.g., 3 AM). Delayed sleep phase syndrome (DSPS) is characterized by difficulty in initiating sleep before 1 AM, sometimes later. Patients with DSPS often adopt professional or social schedules with intense nighttime activity. Although DSPS predominates in younger people and ASPS in the elderly (Campbell et al 1995c), these syndromes tend to be chronic and can pose difficulties throughout one's life, especially to occupations and marriages. Milder forms of these disorders are highly prevalent, such as sleep-onset insomnia lasting about 1 hour and accompanied by difficulty awakening, a condition that often leads to dependence on sedatives such as benzodiazepines, that only provide limited long-term effectiveness.

The insomnia noted in sleep phase disorders often is associated with altered circadian timing of body temperature or melatonin secretion (ASPS showing phase advances and DSPS showing delays). However, pathogenesis of these disorders does not necessarily imply abnormal functioning of the internal clock. The displaced sleep pattern might result from inadequate light exposure in the evening (for ASPS) or morning (DSPS). For example, a person might choose a late bedtime and thus the opportunity for a corrective phase advance to morning light because of extended sleep after T_{min}. In another case, a person may initially awaken normally, but choose to remain in a dimly-lit bedroom or work environment, allowing the circadian pacemaker to drift later. For similar reasons, a shift worker may develop DSPS following shift rotations. Once the delay has occurred, it can be difficult or even impossible to resume an earlier sleep schedule solely by force of will.

Well before the advent of light therapy for sleep phase disorders, chronotherapy for DSPS was applied by gradually shifting the sleep episode later in daily steps of 3 hours until the desired phase was reached (Czeisler et al 1981) in order to awake at 7 AM rather than 1 PM, for example. The method derived from temporal isolation studies, in which humans free-ran at periods greater than 24 hours (see Fig. 11-1), suggests that patients would find progressive phase delays easier, or more natural, than phase advances. The procedure requires reserving approximately 1 week for sleeping during daylight hours as the progression moves around the clock. Maintaining the effect is difficult, however, with continual risk of relapse if the target sleep schedule is not maintained strictly.

Explicit bright light therapy presents an alternate strategy based on experiments that confined light exposure to the morning or evening, in order to advance or delay circadian rhythms, respectively (Terman et al 1995). Patients with DSPS have received progressive daily 1-hour advances of light exposure upon awakening; sleep phase often normalizes within less than a week. Similarly, patients with ASPS have been able to eliminate the urge to sleep in the evening by using evening light, and as a result, awaken later.

Although treatment with light is simple in concept, case management often is complicated (Terman 1993a). Despite social pressures to the contrary, many patients with DSPS are reluctant to shift earlier and find excuses to discontinue treatment, even after achieving a normalized pattern; this attitude results in relapse. Some use the treatment intermittently, for example, when a work assignment requires morning activity. Long-term treatment compliance might be facilitated by the use of automated dawn/dusk simulation in the bedroom, which would eliminate the schedule burden of daytime treatment sessions. Clinical trials of dawn/dusk simulation for the sleep phase disorders are still lacking, however, although the method has been used successfully for patients with seasonal affective disorder (see below) who show delayed sleep patterns.

Non-24-Hour Sleep–Wake Syndrome

An extreme and relatively rare sleep–wake disorder, the non-24-hour sleep–wake syndrome is characterized by progressive phase delays of sleep onset and awakening relative to the 24-hour day, even when living in normal social environments (Terman et al 1995). At one point in a month the patient cannot resist sleep during the day, while at another point the pattern drifts into a normal nocturnal phase. The circadian pacemaker—as indexed by the body temperature rhythm—might drift in and out of synchrony with the sleep cycle. When desynchronized, there are increased complaints of insomnia, fatigue, and impaired functioning. Indeed, as with DSPS, this syndrome might result from a patient's self-selected pattern of light–dark exposure; sleep extends through the phase-advancing portion of the PRC, facilitating phase delays. If so, appropriately timed light treatment should halt the pattern. Although cases have been reported in which sleep was stabilized within the nocturnal interval, or the drifting pattern was greatly decelerated given bright light exposure immediately upon awakening, other attempts at treatment have failed. Timing and dosing studies are a priority.

Seasonal Affective Disorder

At middle and extreme latitudes many people are vulnerable to the decreased light availability during winter months. As much as half of the population in these areas notes one or more symptoms of increased sleep, daytime fatigue, appetite (especially for carbohydrates), and weight gain. In a smaller proportion of the population, averaging about 6 percent in the United States, a winter-depressive syndrome develops, characterized by dysphoric mood, anxiety, and diminished work performance, social interaction, and sexual interest (Terman 1993a). Known as seasonal affective disorder (SAD) symptoms reliably remit in spring and summer. Most patients become calm and euthymic—"normal," without any signs of depression. A minority, however, experiences a bipolar switch to hypomania, with excessive energy, rapid thoughts and speech, euphoric mood, and occasional impulsive, irresponsible, high-risk behavior.

The efficacy of bright light therapy has been established for this clinical population (Rosenthal et al 1984, Terman et al 1989). Hundreds of patients have been studied in controlled trials to determine optimum timing and dosing, and thousands have received open clinical treatment. Several hypotheses have been advanced to explain the antidepressant mechanism of action of light (Terman 1993a). Following the hypothesis of a seasonal effect of photoperiod change, light was presented in dual early-morning and evening sessions in an attempt to extend the short winter day artificially. A related hypothesis suggested that circadian rhythms phase-delay in winter in response to the later dawn hour, and trials soon focussed on single morning sessions, which showed equal efficacy. Following a week of early-morning light exposures, symptom remission was accompanied by melatonin phase advances of up to several hours. However, there were patients who received evening light and showed clinical improvement without phase advances, suggesting that the timing of light exposure is not critical and that the mechanism of action is unrelated to adjustments of the circadian pacemaker. For example, it has been hypothesized that light potentiates a serotonergic response like that obtained with specific serotonin reuptake inhibitors; indeed, the drug fluoxetine also appears to ameliorate winter depression.

Despite the remarkably rapid and persistent improvement with bright light therapy for SAD, and the relapses observed when treatment is withdrawn, the hypothesis of a strong placebo effect has not been rejected (Terman 1993b). Conventional double-blind placebo controls are impossible because subjects can detect the presence or absence of the active agent. Dim light has yielded lower response rates than bright light, but this placebo control is problematic for two reasons: the difference between bright and dim light is obvious, and those responding to dim light may have a lower therapeutic threshold on a dose-response curve. Current trials are investigating a nonphotic, inert placebo—a deactivated negative ion generator at which the subject sits for the same duration at the same time of day as for light therapy (Eastman 1993). Response rate has been similar to that for light, although a difference may yet be found upon completion of the trials. In a related study, subjects were randomized into light and high- and low-density negative ion treatments (Terman & Terman 1995). Response rate to low-density ions was distinctly inferior to that for light or high-density ions, and subjects were unable to distinguish between ion doses. By that assessment, both light and high-density negative ions appear to be specifically active antidepressant agents.

Future Applications of Light Therapy

Perhaps it is fortuitous that light therapy was developed within psychiatry and has been applied mainly for depressive and sleep disorders. Future applications in other medical specialties are likely: one might hypothesize that if a syndrome or disease recurs seasonally, shows winter exacerbation, or plausibly is related to insufficient or ill-timed outdoor light exposure regardless of the season, light therapy might prove beneficial, whether or not a circadian mechanism is involved. Examples of this active research area include light treatment for bulimia nervosa (Lam et al 1994), premenstrual syndrome (Parry 1993), and behavioral disruptions of Alzheimer's disease including sleep (Campbell et al 1995c) and daytime agitation (Lovell et al 1995).

In a case of chronic fatigue syndrome (CFS) coupled with DSPS, I worked with a teenage patient who slept till midday, could not maintain classwork even in the afternoon, and despite a sense of continued fatigue could not fall asleep before 3 AM. Multiple attempts to regulate sleep with drugs had failed. With 10,000 lux light therapy upon spontaneous awakening, immediately she reported her "head clearing," and increased daytime energy and ability to concentrate, although still below normal. By relying on an alarm clock she was able to track the schedule as daily treatments were edged earlier toward 7 AM. When we added dawn simulation in the final hours of sleep, the alarm became unnecessary, but falling asleep remained a problem—no earlier than 1 AM. When we added a 0.5-mg dose of melatonin at 9 PM, however, her sleep length immediately increased to 8 hours, from 11 PM to 7 AM. Except for periods of CFS-associated aches and infections, she was able to resume classwork. This case illustrates the potential benefit of combined chronotherapies.

Beyond clinical populations, light treatment is being explored for amelioration of the circadian rhythm disruptions of shift work (Eastman et al 1995) and jet lag (Boulos et al 1995). A nonchronobiologic area of investigation is the immediate alerting/activating effect of bright light, which may enhance performance and counteract sleepiness and fatigue (Campbell et al 1995a).

Acknowledgments

Preparation of this chapter was supported in part by National Institute of Mental Health Grant MH-42931. The author thanks J.S. Terman for her collaboration in this work. Parts of this chapter were based on a task force report, *Light Therapy for Sleep Disorders*, commissioned by the American Sleep Disorders Association and Society for Light Treatment and Biological Rhythms (*Journal of Biological Rhythms*, vol. 10, no. 2, 1995). The author, who serves as chair, acknowledges the contributions of task force members Z. Boulos, S. Campbell, D.-J. Dijk, C.I. Eastman, and A.J. Lewy.

References

Aschoff J, Wever R. 1976. Human circadian rhythms: a multioscillatory system. Fed Proc 35:2326

Boulos Z, Campbell SS, Lewy AJ, et al. 1995. Light treatment for sleep disorders: consensus report. VII. Jet Lag. J Biol Rhythms 10:167

Cagniacci A, Elliott J, Yen S. 1992. Melatonin: a major regulator of the circadian rhythm of core temperature in humans. J Clin Endocrinol Metab 75:447

Campbell SS, Dijk D-J, Boulos Z, et al. 1995a. Light treatment for sleep disorders: consensus report. III. Alerting and activating effects. J Biol Rhythms 10:129

Campbell SS, Eastman CI, Terman M, et al. 1995b. Light treatment for sleep disorders: consensus report. I. Chronology of Seminal Studies in Humans. J Biol Rhythms 10:105

Campbell SS, Terman M, Lewy AJ, et al. 1995c. Light treatment for sleep disorders: consensus report. V. Age-related disturbances. J Biol Rhythms 10:151

Czeisler CA, Kronauer RE, Allan JS, et al. 1989. Bright light induction of strong (type 0) resetting of the human circadian pacemaker. Science 244:1328

Czeisler CA, Richardson G, Coleman R, et al. 1981. Chronotherapy: resetting the circadian clocks of patients with delayed sleep phase insomnia. Sleep 4:1

Czeisler CA, Shanahan TL, Klerman EB, et al. 1995. Suppression of melatonin secretion in some blind patients by exposure to bright light. N Engl J Med 332:6

Dijk D-J, Boulos Z, Eastman CI, et al. 1995. Light treatment for sleep disorders: consensus report. II. Basic properties of circadian physiology and sleep regulation. J Biol Rhythms 10:113

Eastman CI, Young MA, Fogg LF. 1993. A comparison of two different placebo-controlled SAD light treatment studies. In Wetterberg L (ed). Light and Biological Rhythms in Man. Pergamon Press, Oxford, p. 371

Eastman CI, Boulos Z, Terman M, et al. 1995. Light treatment for sleep disorders: consensus report. VI. Shift work. J Biol Rhythms 10:157

Gallin PF, Terman M, Remé CE, et al. 1995. Ophthalmologic examination of patients with seasonal affective disorder, before and after light therapy. Am J Ophthalmol 119:202

Hrushesky WJM. 1985. Circadian timing of cancer chemotherapy. Science 228:73

Klein DC, Moore RY, Reppert SM (eds). 1991. Suprachiasmatic Nucleus: The Mind's Clock. Oxford University Press. New York

Lam RW, Goldner EM, Solyom L, Remick RA. 1994. A controlled study of light therapy for bulimia nervosa. Am J Psychiatry 151:744

Lewy AJ, Ahmed S, Latham-Jackson JM, Sack RL. 1992. Melatonin phase shifts human circadian rhythms according to a phase-response curve. Chronobiol Int 9:380

Lovell BB, Ancoli-Israel S, Gevirtz R. 1995. The effect of bright light treatment on agitated behavior in institutionalized elderly. Psychiatry Res 57:7

Minors DS, Waterhouse JM, Wirz-Justice A. 1991. A human phase-response curve to light. Neurosci Lett 133:36

Moore-Ede MM, Sulzman FM, Fuller CA. 1982. The Clocks that Time Us: Physiology of the Circadian Timing System. Harvard University Press. Cambridge, Massachusetts

Oren DA, Brainard GC, Johnston SH, et al. 1991. Treatment of seasonal affective disorder with green or red light. Am J Psychiatry 148:509

Parry B. 1993. Light therapy of premenstrual depression. In Wetterberg L (ed). Light and Biological Rhythms in Man. Pergamon Press. Oxford, p. 401

Pittendrigh CS. 1988. The photoperiodic phenomena: seasonal modulation of the "day within." J Biol Rhythms 3:173

Rosenthal NE, Sack DA, Gillin JC, et al. 1984. Seasonal affective disorder: a description of the syndrome and preliminary findings with light therapy. Arch Gen Psychiatry 41:72

Sack RL, Lewy AJ, Blood ML, et al. 1991. Melatonin administration to blind people: phase advances and entrainment. J Biol Rhythms 6:249

Schwartz WJ. 1993. A clinician's primer on the circadian clock: Its localization, function, and resetting. Adv Intern Med 38:81

Terman M. 1993a. Light treatment. In Kryger MH, Roth T, Dement WC (eds). Principles and Practice of Sleep Medicine, 2nd Ed. WB Saunders. Philadelphia, p. 1012

Terman M. 1993b. Problems and prospects for use of bright light as a therapeutic intervention. In Wetterberg L (ed). Light and Biological Rhythms in Man. Pergamon Press. Oxford, p. 421

Terman M, Lewy AJ, Dijk D-J, et al. 1995. Light treatment for sleep disorders: consensus report. IV. Sleep phase and duration disturbances. J Biol Rhythms 10:135

Terman M, Remé CE, Wirz-Justice A. 1991. The visual input stage of the mammalian circadian pacemaking system: II. The effect of light and drugs on retinal function. J Biol Rhythms 6:31

Terman M, Schlager DS. 1990. Twilight therapeutics, winter depression, melatonin, and sleep. In Montplaisir J, Godbout R (eds). Sleep and Biological Rhythms. Oxford University Press. New York, p. 113

Terman M, Terman JS. 1995. Treatment of seasonal affective disorder with a high-output negative ionizer. J Altern Comp Med 1:87

Terman M, Terman JS, Quitkin FM, et al. 1989. Light therapy for seasonal affective disorder: a review of efficacy. Neuropsychopharmacology 2:1

Wehr TA, Skwerer RG, Jacobsen FM, et al. 1987. Eye versus skin phototherapy of seasonal affective disorder. Am J Psychiatry 144:753

*I*ntegrated and Traditional Systems

This section provides a survey of the fundamentals of global health traditions that form integrated systems of thought and practice, following from an explanation of their relevant world views. While this book aims to present a unified body of the theories and practices of alternatives, many world healing traditions are marked by a significant degree of heterogeneity, consistent with their historical evolution as well as their underlying philosophies.

12
Naturopathic Medicine

Joseph E. Pizzorno, Jr.

Naturopathic medicine is more than a system of health care; it is a way of life. Although the term naturopathy was coined in the late nineteenth century, its philosophical roots can be traced back to Hippocrates and the folk medicines of all peoples of the earth. It is a distinct system of medicine that stresses health maintenance, disease prevention, patient education, and patient responsibility—in contrast to the currently dominant system that emphasizes treatment of disease.

Unlike most other health care systems, naturopathy is not identified with any particular therapy, but rather with a philosophy of life, health, and disease. Fundamental to the practice of naturopathic medicine is a profound belief in the ability of the body to heal itself—the *Vis Medicatrix Naturae* (the healing power of nature)—given the proper opportunity, and the importance of living within the laws of nature.

Naturopathic medicine is vitalistic in its approach: Life amounts to more than the sum of biochemical processes, and the body has an innate intelligence that strives constantly for health. Vitalism maintains that the symptoms accompanying disease typically are not caused by the morbific agent (e.g., bacteria); rather, they result from the organism's intrinsic reaction to the agent, and the organism's attempt to defend and heal itself. Symptoms, then, represent a constructive phenomenon that is the best response the organism can muster, given the circumstances. The role of the physician is to understand and aid the body's efforts, not to take over the functions of the body.

> The doctor of the future will give no medicine, but will interest his patient in the care of the human frame, in diet, and in the cause and prevention of disease.
>
> —*Thomas Edison*

Naturopathy views health as more than the absence of disease; it is considered a vital dynamic state that enables a person to thrive in a wide range of environments despite various stresses. Health and disease are points on a continuum, with death at one end and optimal function at the other. The naturopath believes that a person who lives an unhealthy lifestyle will drift away from optimal function towards progressively greater dysfunction. Although our society endorses such deterioration as "normal aging," this degeneration does not occur to animals in the wild, or to people who live in an optimal environment, that is, one without pollution, with minimal stress, regular exercise, as well as abundant natural and nutritious food. Death is inevitable, but progressive disability is avoidable.

At times, even in the optimal environment, the body needs treatment, not just supportive help. The naturopathic physician uses the least invasive intervention to achieve the desired therapeutic effect or, when necessary, refers the patient to other health care professionals.

This approach necessitates a broad range of diagnostic and therapeutic skills accounting for the eclectic interests of naturopathic professionals. Since the goal of the Doctor of Naturopathic Medicine (ND) is restoration of normal body function, rather than the application of a particular therapy, virtually every natural medical therapy is utilized. In addition, to fulfill their role as primary care physicians, naturopaths also employ therapies such as outpatient surgical procedures and acute prescription drugs.

This eclectic nature results in diverse styles. At one end of the spectrum are practitioners who adhere to the strict "nature cure" tradition, that focuses on diet, detoxification, lifestyle modification, and hydrotherapy. At the other end are those whose practices might appear to be similar to practitioners of conventional medicine, with the only apparent difference being the use of pharmaceutical-grade botanical medicines instead of synthetic drugs. However, fundamental to each of these styles of practice is a common philosophy of health and disease. This commonality distinguishes the profession, while its eclectism allows for the consideration and incorporation of new therapies.

Today's naturopathic doctor is an extensively trained and state-licensed family physician equipped with a broad range of conventional and unconventional diagnostic and therapeutic skills. The modern ND considers himself or herself to be an integral part of the health care system and takes full responsibility for concerns of public health issues.

History

Naturopathic medicine* grew out of alternative healing systems of the eighteenth and nineteenth centuries, but traces its philosophical roots to the Hippocratic school of medicine (circa 400 BC). Over the centuries, natural medicine and biomedicine or techno-medicine (a term coined to refer to the currently dominant school of medicine) have alternately diverged and converged, shaping each other, often

---

* The author expresses his appreciation to George Cody, whose chapter "History of Naturopathic Medicine," in *A Textbook of Natural Medicine* (Pizzorno 1995) provided the basis for much of this section.

in reaction. The term itself was coined in 1895 by Dr. John Scheel of New York City, to describe his method of health care. But earlier forerunners of these concepts already existed in the history of natural healing, both in America and in the Austro-Germanic European core. Naturopathy became a formal profession under the creation of Benedict Lust.

Phases of Naturopathy

- Latter part of the nineteenth century: *The Founding By Benedict Lust*; origin in the Germanic hydrotherapy and nature cure traditions.
- 1900 to 1917: *The Formative Years*; convergence of the American dietetic, hygienic, physical culture, spinal manipulation, mental and emotional healing, Thompsonian/eclectic, and homeopathic systems.
- 1918 to 1937: *The Halcyon Days*; during a period of great public interest and support, the philosophical basis and scope of therapies diversified to encompass botanical, homeopathic and environmental medicine.
- 1938 to 1970: *Suppression and Decline*; growing political and social dominance of allopathic medicine combined with the American infatuation with technology, and the emergence of "miracle" drugs and effective modern surgical techniques perfected in two world wars, resulted in legal and economic suppression.
- 1971 to present: *Naturopathic Medicine Reemerges*; Reawakened awareness by the American public of the importance of health promotion, prevention of disease, and concern for the environment and the establishment of modern, accredited, physician-level training reestablished public interest in naturopathic medicine resulting in rapid regrowth.

The Founding of Naturopathy

"Naturopathy," as a generally used term, began with the teachings and concepts of Benedict Lust. In 1892, at the age of 23, Lust came from Germany as a disciple of Father Kneipp (the great practitioner of hydrotherapy) to bring Kneipp's hydrotherapy practices to America. Exposure to a wide range of practitioners and practices of natural healing arts broadened Lust's perspective. Lust had suffered from a debilitating condition in his late teens while growing up in Michelbach, Baden, Germany, and had been sent by his father to undergo the Kneipp cure at Woerishofen. Not only was he "cured"of his condition, but he became a protégé of Father Kneipp. He emigrated to America in 1892, at the age of 23, to proselytize the principles of the Kneipp Water-Cure. In 1896, Lust entered the Universal Osteopathic College of New York and became licensed as an osteopathic physician in 1898. He also acquired a chiropractic education; changed the name of his Kneipp Store to "Health Food Store" (the first facility to utilize that name and concept in this country) specializing in providing organically-grown foods and the materials necessary for drugless cures; and founded the New York School of Massage and the American School of Chiropractic. In 1902, he purchased the term "naturopathy" from Dr. John Scheel of New York City (who coined the term in 1895) to describe the eclectic compilation of doctrines that he envisioned to be the future of natural medicine. Naturopathy, or "nature cure," was defined by Lust as both a way of life and a concept of healing that employed various natural means of treating human infirmities and disease states. The earliest therapies associated with the term involved a combination of American hygienics and Austro-Germanic nature cure and hydrotherapy.

Lust, who had been publishing the *Kneipp Water Cure Monthly* since 1896, changed the name of the journal to *The Naturopathic and Herald of Health* and began promoting his new philosophy of health care (Lust 1902).

In 1902, when he purchased and began using the term naturopathy and calling himself a "naturopath," Lust founded the American School of Naturopathy. By 1907, Lust's enterprises had grown sufficiently large that he moved them to a 55-room building. It housed the Naturopathic Institute, Clinic, and Hospital; the American Schools of Naturopathy and Chiropractic; the now entitled "Original Health Food Store"; Lust's publishing enterprises; and New York School of Massage. The operation remained in this four-story building, roughly twice the size of the original facility, from 1907 to 1915.

In the period of 1912 through 1914, Lust took a sabbatical from his operations to further his education. He attended the Homeopathic Medical College in New York, which, in 1913, granted him a degree in Homeopathic medicine and, in 1914, a degree in Eclectic medicine. In early 1914, he obtained an MD's license on the basis of his graduation from the Homeopathic Medical College.

In 1902, Lust had replaced the Kneipp Societies with the Naturopathic Society of America. In December 1919, the society was formally dissolved due to insolvency and Lust founded the American Naturopathic Association. The association was incorporated in 18 additional states. Lust invested a great deal of his funds and resources in an attempt to organize a naturopathic profession. He published the first "Yearbook of Drugless Therapy." Annual supplements were published either in *The Naturopath and the Herald of Health* or *Nature's Path*, which commenced publication in 1925.

Benedict Lust's principles of health are found in the introduction to the first volume of the *Universal Naturopathic Directory and Buyer's Guide*, a portion of which is reproduced below.

The Principles, Aim, and Program of the Nature Cure System—Benedict Lust, 1918

- Since the earliest ages, Medical Science has been of all sciences the most unscientific. Its professors, with few exceptions, have sought to cure disease by the magic of pills and potions and poisons that attacked the ailment with the idea of suppressing the symptoms instead of attacking the real cause of the ailment.

(Continues)

- Medical science has always believed in the superstition that the use of chemical substances which are harmful and destructive to human life will prove an efficient substitute for the violation of (natural) laws, and in this way encourages the belief that a man may go the limit in self indulgences that weaken and destroy his physical system, and then hope to be absolved from his physical ailments by swallowing a few pills, or submitting to an injection of a serum or vaccine, that are supposed to act as vicarious redeemers of the physical organism and counteract life-long practices that are poisonous and wholly destructive to the patient's well-being.
- The policy of expediency is at the basis of medical drug healing. It is along the lines of self-indulgence, indifference, ignorance and lack of self-control that drug medicine lives, moves and has its being.
- The natural system for curing disease is based on a return to nature in regulating the diet, breathing, exercising, bathing and the employment of various forces to eliminate the poisonous products in the system, and so raise the vitality of the patient to a proper standard of health.
- Official medicine has in all ages simply attacked the symptoms of disease without paying any attention to the causes thereof, but natural healing is concerned far more with removing the causes of disease, than merely curing its symptoms. This is the glory of this new school of medicine that it cures by removing the causes of the ailment, and is the only rational method of practicing medicine. It begins its cures by avoiding the uses of drugs and hence is styled the system of drugless healing.

(Continues)

The Program of Naturopathic Cure

- Elimination of evil habits. Over-eating, alcoholic drinks, drugs, the use of tea, coffee and cocoa that contain poisons, meat eating, improper hours of living, waste of vital forces, lowered vitality, sexual and social aberrations, worry.
- Corrective habits. Correct breathing, correct exercise, right mental attitude. Moderation in the pursuit of health and wealth.
- New principles of living. Proper fasting, selection of food, hydropathy, light and air baths, mud baths, osteopathy, chiropractic and other forms of mechano-therapy, mineral salts obtained in organic form, electropathy, heliopathy, steam or Turkish baths, sitz baths.
- Natural healing is the most desirable factor in the regeneration of the race. It is a return to nature in methods of living and treatment. It makes use of the elementary forces of nature, of chemical selection of foods that will constitute a correct medical dietary. The diet of civilized man is devitalized, is poor in essential organic salts. The fact that foods are cooked in so many ways and are salted, spiced, sweetened and otherwise made attractive to the palate, induces people to over-eat, and over eating does more harm than underfeeding. High protein food and lazy habits are the cause of cancer, Bright's disease, rheumatism and the poisons of auto-intoxication.
- There is really but one healing force in existence and that is Nature herself, which means the inherent restorative power of the organism to overcome disease. Now the question is, can this power be appropriated and guided more readily by extrinsic or intrinsic

(Continues)

methods? That is to say, is it more amenable to combat disease by irritating drugs, vaccines and serums employed by superstitious moderns, or by the bland intrinsic congenial forces of Natural Therapeutics, that are employed by this new school of medicine, that is Naturopathy, which is the only orthodox school of medicine? Are not these natural forces much more orthodox than the artificial resources of the druggist? (Lust 1918)

While the terminology is almost a century old, these profound concepts provide a powerful foundation that has endured almost a century.

Schools of Thought

The following presents the formative schools of Western thought in natural healing and some of their leading adherents. While the therapies differ, the philosophical thread of promoting health and supporting the body's own healing processes runs through them all. However, it was not until Benedict Lust that the many threads were woven together into a unified professional practice.

Hippocrates

Hippocrates regarded the body as a whole and instructed his students to only prescribe beneficial treatments and refrain from causing harm or hurt. Hippocratic practitioners assumed that everything in nature had a rational basis; therefore, the physician's role was to understand and follow the laws of the intelligible universe. They viewed disease as an effect and looked for its cause in such natural phenomena as air, water, and food. They first used the term *vis medicatrix naturae,* the healing power of nature, to denote the body's ability and drive to heal itself.

Hydrotherapy

The earliest philosophical origins of naturopathy were clearly in the Germanic hydrotherapy movement, the use of hot and cold water for the maintenance of health and the treatment of disease. One of the oldest known therapies—water was used ther-apeutically by the Romans and Greeks—the modern history of hydrotherapy includes the publication of *The History of Cold Bathing* in 1697 by Sir John Floyer. The strongest impetus for its use came from Central Europe, where it was advocated by such well known hydropaths as Vincent Priessnitz and Father Sebastian Kneipp. They were able to popularize specific water treatments that quickly became the vogue in Europe during the nineteenth century. The first sanitarium in this country, called the Kneipp and Nature Cure Sanitarium opened in Newark, New Jersey in 1891.

The best known American hydropath was John Harvey Kellogg, a medical doctor who approached hydrotherapy scientifically, and performed many experiments to determine the physiological effects of hot and cold water. In 1900, he published *Rational Hydrotherapy,* which is still considered a definitive treatise on the physiological and therapeutic effects of water, along with an extensive discussion of hydrotherapeutic techniques.

Nature Cure

Natural living, a vegetarian diet, and the use of light and air formed the basis of the Nature Cure movement founded by Dr. Arnold Rickli (1823–1926). In 1848, he established the first institution of light and air cure in Veldes, Krain, Austria. He was an ardent disciple of the vegetarian diet and the founder of the National Austrian Vegetarian Association. Louis Kuhne (circa 1823–1907) wrote, in 1891, the *New Science of Healing,* which presented the basic principles of "drugless methods." Dr. Henry Lahman (circa 1823–1907), who founded the largest Nature Cure institution in the world at Weisser Hirsch, near Dresden, Saxony constructed the first appliances for the administration of electric light treatment and baths. He was the author of several books on diet, nature cure, and heliotherapy. Professor F.E. Bilz (1823–1903) authored the first natural medicine encyclopedia, *The Natural Method of Healing,* which was translated into a dozen languages, and in German alone ran into 150 editions.

Nature Cure became popular in America through the efforts of Henry Linlahr, MD, ND (-1927) of Chicago, Illinois. Originally a rising businessman with all the bad habits of the "Gay Nineties" he became chronically ill in his 30s. After receiving no relief from the orthodox practitioners of his day, he tried

Nature Cure, and his health improved. He went to Germany to be cured in a sanitarium and to learn Nature Cure. He returned to Chicago and earned his degrees from the Homeopathic/Eclectic College of Illinois. In 1903, he opened a sanitarium, a health food store, and the Lindlahr College of Natural Therapeutics. In 1908, he began to publish *Nature Cure Magazine* and began publishing his six volume series of *Philosophy of Natural Therapeutics.*

The Hygienic System

The hygienic school amalgamated hydrotherapy and nature cure movements with vegetarianism. It originated as a lay movement of the 19th century. Sylvester Graham began preaching the doctrines of temperance and hygiene in 1830, and published *Lectures on the Science of Human Life* in 1839, two hefty volumes that prescribed healthy dietary habits. He emphasized a moderate lifestyle, a flesh-free diet, and bran bread as an alternative to bolted or white bread.

The earliest physician to significantly impact on the hygienic movement and the later philosophical growth of naturopathy was Russell Trall, MD. Trall founded the first school of natural healing arts in this country to have a four-year curriculum and the authorization to confer the degree of MD. It was founded in 1852 as a "hydropathic and physiological school" and was chartered by the New York State Legislature in 1857 under the name New York Hygio-Therapeutic College. He eventually published more than 25 books on such subjects as physiology, hydropathy, hygiene, vegetarianism, and temperance. The most valuable and enduring of these was his 1851 *Hydropathic Encyclopedia,* a nearly 1,000-page volume that covered the theory and practice of hydropathy and the philosophy and treatment of diseases advanced by older schools of medicine.

Martin Luther Holbrook expanded on the work of Graham, Alcott and Trall and, working with an awareness of the European concepts developed by Preissnitz and Kneipp, laid further groundwork for the concepts later advanced by Lust, Lindlahr, and others. He proposed that disease could thrive only in individuals inclined to hygienic carelessness. Tuberculosis is contagious, but "the degree of vital resistance is the real element of protection. When

there is no preparation of the soil by heredity, predisposition or, lowered health standard, the individual is amply guarded against the attack." He gave an account of watching a smartly dressed lady unwittingly drag her skirt "over some virulent, revolting looking sputum, which some unfortunate consumptive had expectorated." (Whorton 1982)

Trall and Holbrook both advanced the idea that physicians should teach the maintenance of health rather than simply provide a last resort in times of health crisis. Besides providing a strong editorial voice denouncing the evils of tobacco and drugs, they strongly advanced the value of vegetarianism, bathing and exercise, and dietetics and nutrition along with personal hygiene.

Auto-Toxicity

Lust also was greatly influenced by the writings of John H. Tilden, MD. Tilden became disenchanted with orthodox medicine and began to rely heavily on dietetics and nutrition, formulating his theories of "auto-intoxication"—the effect of fecal matter remaining too long in the digestive process—and "toxemia." His 200-page dissertation entitled *Constipation* contained an entire chapter devoted to the evils of not responding to nature's call.

Elie Metchnikoff, director of the prestigious Pasteur Institute and winner of the 1908 Nobel Prize for a contribution to immunology, wrote prolifically on the theory of auto-intoxication. Kellogg felt that humans produced a variety of intestinal self-poisons in the process of digesting meat that contributed to auto-intoxication. As a result, he proselytized widely that man must return to a more healthy natural state by allowing the naturally designed usage of the colon. The average modern colon was devitalized by the combination of a low fiber diet, sedentary living, the custom of sitting rather than squatting to defecate, and the modern civilized habit of ignoring nature's call out of an undue concern for politeness.

Thomsonianism

In 1822, Samuel Thomson published his *New Guide to Health,* a compilation of his personal view of medical theory and Native American herbal and medical botanical lore. Thomson espoused the belief that disease had one general cause—derangement of the vital fluids from "cold" influences on the human body. Therefore, disease had one general remedy—animal warmth, or "heat." The name of the complaint depended upon the part of the body that was affected. Conventional American medical tradition advocated "heroic" procedures such as bloodletting, leeching, and the substantial use of mineral-based purgatives such as antimony and mercury. Thomson believed that minerals were sources of "cold" because they come from the ground; vegetation, which grows toward the sun, represents "heat."

Thomson believed that individuals could self-treat if they had an adequate understanding of his philosophy and a copy of his book the *New Guide to Health*. The right to sell "family franchises" for utilization of the Thomsonian method of healing was the basis of a profound lay movement until his death in 1843. Thomson adamantly believed that no professional medical class should exist and that democratic medicine was best practiced by laypersons within a Thomsonian "family" unit. By 1839, Thomson claimed to have sold some 100,000 of these family franchises called "friendly botanic societies."

Despite his criticism of the early medical movement for their heroic tendencies, Thomson's medical theories were heroic in their own fashion. Botanic purgatives—particularly *Lobelia inflata* (Indian tobacco)—were a substantial part of the therapy.

The Eclectic School of Medicine

Some of the doctors practicing Thomsonian, also called "botanics," separated themselves from the lay movement. They established a broader range of therapeutic applications of botanical medicines and were later absorbed into the Eclectic School, which originated with Wooster Beach of New York.

Wooster Beach started his medical studies at an early age, apprenticing under an old German herbal doctor, Jacob Tidd. Beach then enrolled in the Barclay Street Medical University in New York. After opening his own practice in New York, Beach set out to win over fellow members of the New York Medical Society to his point of view that heroic medicine was inherently dangerous to mankind and should be reduced to the gentler theories of herbal medicine. He was summarily ostracized. He soon founded his own school in New York, The United States Infirmary.

However, due to political pressure from the medical society, he was unable to obtain charter authority to issue legitimate diplomas. He located a financially ailing, but legally chartered school, Worthington College, in Worthington, Ohio. There he created the Eclectic School of Medical Theory, based on the European, native American, and American traditions. The most enduring eclectic herbal textbook is *King's American Dispensary* by Harvey Wickes Felter and John Uri Lloyd. Published in 1898, this two volume 2,500 page treatise describes the identification, preparation, pharmacognosy, history of use, and clinical application of over 1,000 botanical medicines. The eclectic herbal lore formed an integral core of the therapeutic armamentarium of the naturopathic doctor.

Homeopathy

Homeopathy, the creation of an early German physician, Samuel Hahnemann (1755–1843), had three central doctrines: the "law of similars" (that like cures like); the effect of a medication could be heightened by its administration in minute doses (the more diluted the dose the greater the "dynamic" effect); and nearly all diseases are the result of a suppressed itch, or *psora*.

Originally, most homeopaths in this country were converted orthodox medical doctors, or allopaths. The high rate of conversion made this particular medical sect the archenemy of the rising orthodox medical profession. The first American homeopathic medical school was founded in 1850 in Cleveland; the last purely homeopathic medical school, based in Philadelphia, survived into the early 1930s.

The Manipulative Therapies

In Missouri, Andrew Taylor Still, originally trained as an orthodox practitioner, founded osteopathy. He conceived a system of healing that emphasized the primary importance of the structural integrity of the body in the maintenance of health, especially as it affects the vascular system. In 1892, he opened the American School of Osteopathy in Kirksville, Missouri.

In 1895, Daniel David Palmer (originally a magnetic healer from Davenport, Iowa) performed the first spinal manipulation, which gave rise to the school he termed "chiropractic." His philosophy was similar to Still's, except for a greater emphasis on the importance of proper neurological function. He formally published his findings in 1910, after having founded a chiropractic school in Davenport, Iowa.

Less well known is "zone therapy," originated by Joe Shelby Riley, DC, a chiropractor based in Washington, DC. Zone therapy was an early forerunner of acupressure as it related . . . "pressures and manipulations of the fingers and tongue, and percussion on the spinal column, according to the relation of the fingers to certain zones of the body."

Christian Science and the Role of Belief and Spirituality

Christian Science, formulated by Mary Baker Eddy in 1879, comprises a profound belief in the role of systematic religious study (hence the widespread Christian Science Reading Rooms), spirituality and prayer in the treatment of disease. In 1875, she published *Science and Health with Key to the Scriptures,* the definitive textbook for the study of Christian Science.

Lust also was influenced by the works of Sidney Weltmer, the founder of "suggestive therapeutics." Weltmer's work dealt specifically with the psychological process of desiring to be healthy. Whether it was the mind or the body that first lost its grip on health, the two were inseparably related. When the problem originated in the body, the mind nonetheless lost its ability and desire to overcome the disease because the patient "felt" sick, and consequently slid further into the diseased state. Alternatively, if the mind first lost its ability and desire to be healthy and some physical infirmity followed, the patient was susceptible to disease.

Physical Culture

Bernarr McFadden, a close friend of Lust's, founded the "physical culture" school of health and healing, also known as "physcultopathy." This school of healing gave birth to gymnasiums nationwide, at which exercise programs designed to allow individuals to establish and maintain optimal physical health, were developed and taught.

Many theories explain the rapid dissolution of these diverse healing arts—which at one time comprised over 25 percent of practitioners—in the early part of the twentieth century; low ratings in the fa-mous Flexner Report which rated all these schools of medical thought amongst the lowest; the application of the term "scientific" on allopathic medicine; and the growing sophistication of the medical establishment clearly played the most significant role.

The Halcyon Years of Naturopathy

In the early 1920s, the "health fad" movement was reaching its peak in terms of public awareness and interest. Conventions nationwide were well attended by professionals, the public (over 10,000 flocked to the 1924 convention in Los Angeles), and even several members of Congress. This interest culminated in full legalization of naturopathy as a healing art in the District of Columbia.

The naturopathic journals of the 1920s and 1930s provide much valuable insight into the prevention of disease and the promotion of health. Much of the dietary advice focused on correcting poor eating habits including the lack of fiber in the diet and an over-reliance upon red meat as a protein source. In the 1990s, the National Institutes of Health and the National Cancer Institute confirmed the early assertions of the naturopaths that such dietary habits could lead to degenerative diseases, including cancers associated with the digestive tract and the colon.

The December 1928 volume of *Nature's Path* was the first American publication of the works of Herman J. DeWolff, a Dutch epidemiologist who was one of the first researchers to assert, based on studies of the incidence of cancer in the Netherlands, that there was a correlation between exposure to petrochemicals and various types of cancerous conditions. He saw a connection between chemical fertilizers and their usage in some soils (principally clay) that led to their remaining in vegetables after they had arrived at the market and were purchased for consumption. It was almost 50 years before orthodox medicine began to see the wisdom of such assertions.

Suppression and Decline

By 1937, however, the popularity of naturopathy began to decline. From the introduction of sulfa drugs in 1937 to the Salk vaccine's release in 1955, the American public became used to annual developments of miracle vaccines and antibiotics.

In the mid 1920s, Morris Fishbein, editor of the *Journal of the American Medical Association* (JAMA), took on a personal vendetta against what he characterized as "quackery." Lust, MacFadden, and others, became Fishbein's epitome of quackery. He proved to be particularly effective.

Just before his death in September 1945, Benedict Lust noted his concerns for the future, especially his frustration with blocking the efforts of the naturopaths to establish state licensing laws that would not only establish appropriate practice rights for NDs, but also protect the public from pretenders, i.e., those who chose to call themselves naturopaths without bothering to attain formal training:

> "Now let us see the type of men and women who are the Naturopaths of today. Many of them are fine, upstanding individuals, believing fully in the effectiveness of their chosen profession—willing to give their all for the sake of alleviating human suffering and ready to fight for their rights to the last ditch. More power to them! But there are others who claim to be Naturopaths who are woeful misfits. Yes, and there are outright fakers and cheats masking as Naturopaths. That is the fate of any science—any profession—which the unjust laws have placed beyond the pale. Where there is no official recognition and regulation, you will find the plotters, the thieves, the charlatans operating on the same basis as the conscientious practitioners. And these riff-raff opportunists bring the whole art into disrepute. Frankly such conditions cannot be remedied until suitable safeguards are erected by law, or by the profession itself, around the practice of Naturopathy. That will come in time." (Lust, 1945)

The public infatuation with technology, introduction of "miracle medicine," World War II's stimulation of the development of surgery, the Flexner Report, growing political sophistication of the AMA through the leadership of Fishbein, and the death of Benedict Lust in 1945, all combined to cause the decline of naturopathic medicine and natural healing in the United States.

American courts began to take the view that naturopaths were not true doctors, as they espoused doctrines from "the dark ages of medicine." Drugless healers were intended by law to operate without "drugs," which became defined as anything a person would ingest or apply externally for any medical purpose. Lack of insurance coverage, lost court battles, and a hostile legislative perspective progressively restricted practice until the core naturopathic therapies became essentially illegal and practices were financially nonviable.

Although under considerable public pressure the American Naturopathic Association undertook some of its most scholarly work in those years, coordinating all the systems of naturopathy under commission. This resulted in the 1948 publication of a formal textbook *Basic Naturopathy* by Spitler, and a compilation of all the known theories of botanical medicine, *Naturae Medicina,* by Kuts-Cheraux in 1953.

Naturopathic medicine splintered when Lust's ANA was succeeded by six different organizations in the mid 1950s. By the early 1970s, the profession's educational institutions had dwindled to one, the National College of Naturopathic Medicine (with branches in Seattle, Washington and Portland, Oregon).

Naturopathic Medicine Reemerges

The counter-culture of the late 1960s, the public's growing awareness of the importance of nutrition and the environment, and America's disenchantment with organized institutional medicine (when its limitations and prohibitive expense became apparent) resulted in increasing respect for alternative medicine and the rejuvenation of naturopathic medicine. A new wave of students were attracted to the philosophical precepts of the profession, bringing an appreciation for the appropriate use of science, a modern college education, and matching expectations.

In order for the naturopathic profession to move back into the mainstream, it needed to establish accredited institutions, perform credible research, and establish itself as an integral part of the health care system. In 1978, the John Bastyr College of Naturopathic Medicine (later renamed Bastyr University) was formed in Seattle, Washington, by Joseph E. Pizzorno, Jr, ND, Lester E. Griffith, ND, William Mitchell, ND, and Sheila Quinn to teach science-based natural medicine. Bastyr became the first naturopathic college to become accredited. In Fall 1993,

Michael Cronnin, ND and Conrad Kail, ND founded the Southwest College of Naturopathic Medicine and Health Science in Scottsdale, Arizona.

With three credible colleges, active research, and an appreciation of the appropriate application of science to natural medicine education and clinical practice, naturopathic medicine began its journey on the road to recovery.

Recent Influences

While the naturopaths of the past century were astute clinical observers, they lacked the scientific tools to assess the validity of their concepts. They also seemed to have little inclination for the application of laboratory research, especially as "science" was often utilized to suppress their profession. In the past few decades, a considerable amount of research is now providing the scientific documentation for most concepts of naturopathic medicine, and the new breed of scientifically-trained naturopaths is utilizing this research to continue developing the profession. The following are a few of the most important trends.

Therapeutic Nutrition

The discovery of vitamins, minerals, and deficiency diseases in the early part of the 20th century began to provide a scientific understanding of clinical nutrition. The realization that enzyme systems were dependent on essential nutrients provided the naturopathic profession with great insights into the importance of an organically grown, whole foods diet for health. Nutritional biochemist Roger Williams' formulation of the concept of "biochemical individuality" in 1955 further developed insights into the unique nutritional needs of each individual, how to correct in-born errors of metabolism, and even how to treat specific diseases through the use nutrient-rich foods or large dosages of specific nutrients. Linus Pauling, two-time Nobel Prize winner, coined the concept of orthomolecular medicine, and provided further theoretical substantiation for the use of nutrients as therapeutic agents.

Environmental Medicine/Clinical Ecology

Although the clinical impact of environmental toxicity and endogenous toxicity was recognized from the earliest days of naturopathy, it wasn't until the environmental movement and the seminal work of Rachel Carson and others that the scientific basis was established. Clinical research and the development of laboratory methods for assessing toxic load have provided objective tools that have greatly increased the sophistication of clinical practice. Clinical and laboratory methods were developed to evaluate idiosyncratic reactions to environmental factors and foods.

Laboratory Methodologies

The final influence of great significance is the development of laboratory methodologies for the objective assessment of nutritional status, metabolic dysfunction, digestive function, bowel flora, endogenous and exogenous toxic load, and liver detoxification function. Each of these tools has provided for ever more effective and accurate assessment of patient health status, as well as application of naturopathic principles.

Principles

While most health care professions are defined by the therapies used, the philosophical principles that guide practitioners are of far greater significance. Seven powerful concepts provide the foundation for naturopathic medicine and pave the way for a unique group of professionals to practice a form of medicine that fundamentally changes the way we think about health.

The Principles of Naturopathic Medicine*

- The Healing Power of Nature (*Vis Medicatrix Naturae*): Nature acts powerfully through healing mechanisms in the body

(Continues)

* The author expresses his appreciation to Drs. Pamela Snider and Jared Zeff for their leadership in establishing a profession-wide process to ensure broad input and agreement in establishing contemporary language for these age-old principles.

and mind to maintain and restore health. When these inherent systems are dysfunctional, naturopathic physicians work to restore and support them by using methods, medicines, and techniques that are in harmony with the natural processes

- First Do No Harm (*Primum Non Nocere*): Naturopathic physicians prefer noninvasive treatments that minimize the risk of harmful side effects. They are trained to know which patients they can treat safely, and which should be referred to other health care practitioners
- Find the Cause (*Tolle Causam*): Every illness has an underlying cause, often found in aspects of the lifestyle, diet, or habits of the individual. A naturopathic physician is trained to find and remove this cause
- Treat the Whole Person: Health or disease arises from a complex interaction of mental, emotional, spiritual, physical, dietary, genetic, environmental, lifestyle, and other factors. Naturopathic physicians treat the whole person, taking all these factors into account
- Preventive Medicine: The naturopathic approach to health care helps avoid disease altogether, as well as prevent minor illness from developing into more serious or chronic degenerative diseases. Patients are taught the principles by which to live a healthful life and prevent major illness
- Wellness: Establishing and maintaining optimal health and balance is vital to cure. Wellness is a state of being healthy, characterized by positive emotion, thought, and action. Wellness is inherent in everyone, no matter what "disease" is present. If wellness is truly recognized and experienced, the individual will heal more quickly than

(Continues)

through direct treatment of the "disease" alone
- Doctor as Teacher (*Doctore*): The original meaning of the word "doctore" is teacher. A principle objective of naturopathic medicine is to educate the patient and emphasize self-responsibility for health. Naturopathic physicians also recognize the therapeutic potential of the doctor-patient relationship

Translation of the Principles Into Clinical Practice

As eclectic physicians of natural medicine, naturopathic doctors use virtually any therapy that is consistent with these guiding principles. In other words, the naturopathic physician uses therapies that support the body's inherent healing processes, rather than therapies that damage or take over these processes. These family physicians focus more on promoting health than simply relieving the symptoms of disease.

In the naturopathic medicine program at Bastyr University, these principles are translated into a series of questions that drive curriculum development and guide students as they learn the art and science of naturopathy.

Diagnostic Issues Arising from the Principles of Naturopathy

- The healing power of nature
  How is the healing power of Nature supported in the case?
    Is the person in balance with Nature?
    What does it mean to be "in balance with Nature"?

(Continues)

Is this person in balance with his/her environment?

How are you assessing the healing powers of this individual?

What is the prognosis for this individual?

• First do no harm

What is the potential for harm with this particular treatment plan?

Are you doing no harm? How?

What is the appropriate course of action? Is a delay in treatment appropriate?

• Find the cause

What level of healing are you seeking, for example, suppression, palliation, or cure?

Considering that health is freedom from limitations, where and/or what are the limiting factors in this person's life?

Is the center of this person's disease physical, mental, or emotional?

What are the causative factors contributing to "dis-ease" in this individual? Of these causative factors, which are avoidable or preventable?

• Treat the whole person

How are you employing the holistic approach?

Can you see the person beyond the disease?

What aspects of the person are you addressing?

What aspects of the person are you not addressing?

Would a referral to another health care practitioner assist your holistic efforts? When? To whom?

What are the patient's goals and expectations in regard to health and treatment? What are your goals and expectations for the patient? How do these goals and expectations differ? How are they similar?

(Continues)

How will the treatment plan help the patient take more responsibility for his or her own health and healing?

Are you empowering the patient? How?

What is the vitality level of this patient?

• Preventive medicine

What is being done or planned in regard to prevention?

What are you teaching this person about his or her own health?

Have you assessed risk factors for this patient?

Does this patient do health screening self-examinations on a regular basis?

• Wellness

What is being done to cultivate wellness?

How are you contributing to optimal health in this individual? How can you contribute to optimal health in this individual?

What are the patient's goals and expectations in relationship to their own wellness, for example, creativity, energy, enjoyment, health, and balance?

Are the expectations realistic? How can these goals be achieved?

How can achievement of these goals be maintained and measured?

Are you stimulating wellness, treating disease, or both?

Is the patient demonstrating positive emotion, thought, and action? If not, why?

Can the patient recall or imagine a state of wellness?

Is the patient able to participate in his or her own process towards a state of wellness?

• Doctor as teacher

What type of patient education are you providing?

How can you determine the level of a patient's responsibility?

In what ways do you cultivate and enhance your role as teacher?

Vis Medicatrix Naturae

The foundation of naturopathic medicine is the vitalistic philosophy of *Vis Medicatrix Naturae*, "the healing power of nature." Naturopathic physicians assert that all true healing results from this principle. The application of *Vis Medicatrix Naturae* depends upon the patient's needs. Ideally, it involves only the use of therapies that support the organism and encourage intrinsic healing process to work effectively. It avoids the use of medicines and procedures that interfere with natural functions or that cause harmful side effects. Natural medicines and therapies are preferred; when used properly, they are the least harmful, least invasive, and best able to work in harmony with the natural healing process.

Since the total organism is involved in healing, the most effective diagnostic and treatment approach is to consider the whole person. In addition to physical and laboratory findings, important consideration is given to the patient's mental, emotional, and spiritual history, attitude, lifestyle, diet, environment, and family life. Careful attention to each person's individuality and susceptibility to disease is critical to the proper evaluation and treatment of any health problem.

Naturopathic physicians believe that most disease is the direct result of ignoring or violating "Natural Living Laws," which include: the consumption of natural, unrefined, organically-grown foods; ensuring adequate amounts of exercise and rest; living a moderately paced lifestyle; having constructive and creative thoughts and emotions; avoiding environmental toxins; and maintaining proper elimination. It is important to control these areas during illness, in order to remove as many unnecessary stresses as possible, and to optimize the success of the organism's healing attempt. Therefore, patient education and responsibility, lifestyle modification, preventive medicine, and wellness promotion are fundamental to naturopathic practice.

While the practice of naturopathic medicine is grounded in *Vis Medicatrix Naturae*, intervention in the disease process sometimes is efficacious, and possibly necessary. Naturopathic physicians have a long-standing tradition of integrating the best aspects of traditional, alternative, and conventional medicine in the interest of the patient. When appropriate, patients are referred to specialists and other health care practitioners. Every effort is made to use all treatment techniques in a manner that is harmonious with the naturopathic philosophy.

Naturopathy often is called holistic medicine, in reference to the term "holism," coined by philosopher Jan Christian Smuts in 1926 to describe the gestalt of a system as greater than the sum of its parts. Naturopathically, the body is viewed as a whole. A change in one part causes a change in every part; therefore, the study of one part must be integrated into the whole. This contrasts the high degree of specialization in the present medical system, which reflects a mechanistic orientation to single organs. The holistic model relegates specialists to an ancillary role. Emphasis is placed on the physical, emotional, social, and spiritual integration of the whole person.

Therapeutic Modalities

Naturopathic medicine is a vitalistic system of health care that uses natural medicines and interventionistic therapies as needed. Natural medicines and therapies, when properly used, generally have low invasiveness and rarely cause suppression or side effects. They generally support the body's healing mechanisms, rather than take over the body's processes.

Clinical nutrition, or the use of diet as a therapy, serves as the foundation for naturopathic medicine. An increasing body of knowledge supports the use of whole foods and nutritional supplements in health maintenance and disease treatment. The recognition of unique nutritional requirements due to biochemical individuality has provided a strong theoretical and practical basis for the appropriate use of nutritional therapy, and even controlled fasting.

Plants have been used as medicines since antiquity. The technology now exists to understand the physiological activities of herbs, and a tremendous amount of research worldwide, especially in Europe, is demonstrating clinical efficacy.

The term *homeopathy* is derived from the Greek word *homeos*, meaning similar, and *pathos*, meaning disease. Homeopathy is a system of medicine that treats a disease with a dilute, potentized agent, or drug, that will produce symptoms similar to disease when given to a healthy individual. The fundamental principle being that *like cures like*. This principle actually was first recognized by Hippocrates, who noticed that herbs given in low doses tended to cure the same symptoms that they themselves produced when given in toxic doses. Homeopathic medicines are derived from a variety of plant, mineral, and chemical substances, and are prepared according to the specifications of the Homeopathic Pharmacopeia of the United States. Approximately 100 clinical studies have demonstrated the clinical efficacy of these therapies.

Acupuncture is an ancient Chinese system of medicine involving the stimulation of certain specific points on the body to enhance the flow of vital energy (Qi) along pathways called meridians. Acupuncture points can be stimulated by the insertion and withdrawing of needles, the application of heat (moxibustion), massage, laser, electrical means, or by a combination of these methods. Traditional Chinese acupuncture implies a specific acupuncture technique and a knowledge of the Oriental system of medicine, which includes yin-yang, the Five Elements, acupuncture points and meridians, as well as a method diagnosis and differentiation of syndromes quite different from that of Western medicine. Although the majority of research in this country has focused on its use for relief of pain and the treatment of addictions, it is a complete system of medicine that effectively treats most diseases.

Hydrotherapy is the use of water in any of its forms (hot, cold, ice, steam) and methods of application (sitz bath, douche, spa and hot tub, whirlpool, sauna, shower, immersion bath, pack, poultice, foot bath, fomentation, wrap, colonic irrigations) in the maintenance of health or treatment of disease. It is one of the most ancient methods of treatment, and has been used to treat disease and injury by many different cultures, including the Egyptians, Assyrians, Persians, Greeks, Hebrews, Hindus, and Chinese. Its most sophisticated applications were developed in eighteenth century Germany.

Physical medicine refers to the therapeutic use of touch, heat, cold, electricity, and sound. This includes the use of physiotherapy equipment such as ultrasound, diathermy, and other electromagnetic energy agents; therapeutic exercise; massage; joint mobilization (manipulative) and immobilization techniques; and hydrotherapy.

An important theme in naturopathic medicine is recognition and correction of endogenous and exogenous toxicity. Liver and bowel detoxification, elimination of environmental toxins, correcting the metabolic dysfunction that causes the buildup of non-endproduct metabolites—all are important ways of decreasing toxic load.

Counseling and lifestyle modification techniques are essential modalities for the naturopathic physician. A naturopath is a holistic-minded physician formally trained in mental, emotional, and family counseling. Various treatment measures including hypnosis and guided imagery, counseling correcting underlying organic factors, and family therapy.

Therapeutic Approach

The therapeutic approach of the naturopathic doctor is basically two-fold: to help patients heal themselves, and to use this opportunity to guide and educate the patient in developing a more healthy lifestyle. Many supposedly incurable conditions respond very well to naturopathic approaches.

A typical first office visit with a naturopathic doctor takes 1 hour. The goal is to learn as much as possible about the patient through physical examination, laboratory tests, radiology, and other standard diagnostic procedures; also, a thorough history is taken, including assessments of the patient's diet, environment, toxic load, exercise, stress, and other aspects of lifestyle; and laboratory tests determine physiologic function. Diagnosis of a disease is only one part of this process; once a good understanding of the patient's health and disease status is established, the doctor and patient work together to establish a treatment and health promoting program.

Although every effort is made to treat the whole person, not just his or her disease, the limits of this chapter necessitate a simplified description of typical naturopathic therapies of specific conditions. Following are a few examples of how the person's health can be improved, resulting in alleviation of the disease.

Cervical Dysplasia

The allopathic medical approach to treating cervical dysplasia, a precancerous condition of the cervix, is surgical resection. The typical naturopathic treatment includes the following:

1. Education about factors that increase the relative risk of cervical cancer, such as smoking (risk = 3.0), multiple sex partners (risk = 3.4), and the use of oral contraceptives (risk = 3.6) (Clarke 1985).
2. Prevention: 67 percent of patients with cervical cancer are deficient in one or more nutrients (Orr 1985); serum beta-carotene level is only one-half that of normal women (Dawson 1984); the woman's nutritional status would be optimized through diet and supplementation, particularly in regard to those nutrients known to be deficient (often a result of oral contraceptive use) in women with cervical dysplasia and the deficiencies of which may promote cellular abnormalities: folic acid (Van Niekerk 1966), beta-carotene (Dawson 1985), vitamin C (Romney 1985), vitamin B_6 (Ramaswamy 1984), and selenium (Dawson 1985).
3. Treatment: The vaginal depletion pack (a traditional mixture of botanical medicines placed against the cervix) would be used to promote sloughing of the abnormal cells.

This approach provides for many advantages: the causes of the cervical dysplasia are identified and resolved, preventing recurrence; no surgery is used, so no scar tissue is formed; and the cost—particularly considering that many women with cervical dysplasia have recurrences when treated with standard surgery—is reasonable. Most important, the woman's health has been improved and other conditions which could have been caused by the identified nutritional deficiencies now have been helped.

Migraine Headache

The standard allopathic medical treatment primarily is to use drugs to relieve symptoms, a costly and recurrent practice. By contrast, the naturopath recognizes that migraine headache may be due to food allergies, and that abnormal prostaglandin metabolism due to nutritional abnormalities results in excessive platelet aggregation. The approach is straightforward:

1. Identify and avoid the allergic foods, as 50 percent or more have migraines in reaction to foods to which they are intolerant (Natero 1989).
2. Supplement with magnesium, as migraine sufferers have significantly lowered serum and salivary magnesium levels that sink even lower during an attack (Sarchielli 1992).
3. Re-establish normal prostaglandin balance by decreasing animals fats (high in platelet-aggregating arachadonic acid) and supplementing with essential fatty acids such as fish-oils (Woodcock 1984).

Hypertension

Patients with so-called idiopathic or essential hypertension can be effectively treated, if they are willing to make the necessary lifestyle changes.

1. Numerous studies have shown that excessive dietary salt in conjunction with inadequate dietary potassium may be a major contributor to hypertension (Meneely 1976, Fries 1976, Khaw 1984); that dietary deficiencies in calcium (McCarron 1982, Belizan 1983), magnesium (Resnick 1984, Dyckner 1983), essential fatty acids (Vergroesen 1978, Rhua 1981), and vitamin C (Yoshioka 1981) may contribute to increased blood pressure; and that increased consumption of sugar (Hodges 1983), caffeine (Lang 1983), and alcohol (Gruchow 1985), are associated with hypertension.
2. Smoking (Kershbaum 1968), obesity (Havlik 1983), stress (Ford 1982), and a sedentary lifestyle may contribute to the development of high blood pressure.
3. Exposure to heavy metals such as lead (Pruess 1992) and cadmium (Glauser 1976) may increase blood pressure.
4. Many herbal medicines are used when necessary for the patient's safety to initially lower his/her blood pressure rapidly until the slower, but

more curative dietary and lifestyle treatments take effect. Age-old favorites include *Allium sativa* garlic, and *Viscum album* mistletoe (Petkov 1979). Many causes of high blood pressure are not unknown, they simply are unheeded!

Lifestyle modification is crucial to the successful implementation of naturopathic techniques. Health does not come from a doctor, pills, or surgery, but rather from the patient's own efforts to take proper care of themselves. Unfortunately, our consumer society expends considerable talent, energy, and resources to induce disease-promoting habits. While it is relatively easy to tell a patient to stop smoking, get more exercise, and reduce stress, such lifestyle changes are difficult in the context of habit, and peer and commercial pressure. The naturopathic doctor is specifically trained to assist the patient in making the needed changes. This involves helping the patient to acknowledge the need; setting realistic and progressive goals; establishing a support group of family, friends, and others with similar problems; identifying the stimuli that reinforce unhealthy behavior; and giving the patient positive reinforcement for their gains.

Scope of Practice, Licensing, and Professional Organization

Naturopathic physicians practice as primary care providers. They see patients of all ages, from all walks of life, suffering from every known disease. They make a conventional Western diagnosis using standard diagnostic procedures such as physical examination, laboratory tests, and radiology. However, they also make a pathophysiologic diagnosis using physical and laboratory procedures to assess nutritional status, metabolic function, and toxic load. In addition, a considerable amount of time is spent assessing the patient's mental, emotional, social, and spiritual status. Therapeutically, NDs use virtually every known natural therapy: dietetics, therapeutic nutrition, botanical medicine (primarily the European, native American, and Chinese), physical therapy, spinal manipulation, lifestyle counseling, exercise therapy, homeopathy, acupuncture, psychological and family counseling, and hydrotherapy. In addition, according to state law, naturopaths

perform outpatient surgery, administer vaccinations, and prescribe a limited range of drugs. Naturopaths meet public health requirements and work with a referral network of specialists, just like a family practice medical doctor.

NDs (or NMDs) are licensed in Alaska, Arizona, Connecticut, Hawaii, Montana, New Hampshire, Oregon, and Washington, and have a legal right to practice in Idaho and the District of Columbia. Naturopaths also practice in other states without official government sanction; however, without licensing standards, individuals with little or no formal education may proclaim themselves naturopaths, to the possibly significant detriment of the public and the profession.

The scope of naturopathic practice is stipulated by state law, and typically allows standard diagnostic privileges including venipuncture and radiology. Therapeutic scope ranges from restricted to only natural therapies to natural therapies, vaccinations, and limited prescriptive rights. In addition, some states allow the practice of natural childbirth.

In addition to the Council on Naturopathic Medical Education (CNME), two key organizations provide leadership and standardization for the naturopathic profession. The American Association of Naturopathic Physicians (AANP), founded in 1985 by James Sensenig, ND, and others, was established to provide consistent educational and practice standards for the profession and a unified voice for public relations and political activity. The Naturopathic Physicians Licensing Examination (NPLEx) was founded under the auspices of the AANP in 1986 by Ed Hoffman-Smith, PhD, ND, to establish a nationally-recognized standardized test for licensing. NPLEx is recognized by all states that license NDs.

Education

The education of the naturopathic physician is extensive and incorporates much of the diversity that typifies the natural health care movement. The training program is very similar to conventional medical education, with the primary differences being in the therapeutic sciences. Prospective students first must successfully complete a conventional premedicine program including a college degree in a biological science. The naturopathic curriculum then takes an additional four years to complete.

The first two years concentrate on the standard human biologic sciences, basic diagnostic sciences, and an introduction to the various treatment modalities. The conventional basic medical sciences include anatomy, human dissection, histology, physiology, biochemistry, pathology, microbiology, public health, pharmacology, and biostatistics. The development of diagnostic skills is initiated with courses in physical diagnosis, laboratory diagnosis, and clinical assessment. Finally, introductory natural medicine subjects such as environmental health, pharmacognosy (pharmacology of herbal medicines), naturopathic philosophy, Chinese medicine, Ayurvedic medicine, homeopathy, counseling, spinal manipulation, nutrition, and hydrotherapy are covered.

The second two years are oriented toward the clinical sciences of diagnosis and treatment, including the standard diagnostic techniques of physical, laboratory, and radiologic examination. However, unique is its emphasis on preventive diagnosis, such as diet analysis, recognition of the early physical signs of nutritional deficiencies, laboratory methods for assessing physiologic dysfunction before it progresses to cellular pathology and end-stage disease, and methods of assessing toxic load and liver detoxification efficacy. The natural therapies, such as nutrition, botanical medicines, homeopathy, acupuncture, natural childbirth, hydrotherapy, fasting, physical therapy, exercise therapy, counseling, and lifestyle modification are studied extensively.

During the last 2 years, students also work in clinical settings. They see patients first as observers, and later as primary care providers under the supervision of licensed NDs. A limited number of optional residencies are available.

Currently, three schools exist in the United States: National College of Naturopathic Medicine (NCNM), Bastyr University (Bastyr), and the Southwest College of Naturopathic Medicine and Health Science (Southwest).

Naturopathic education is accredited by the U.S. Department of Education recognized Council on Naturopathic Medical Education (CNME), located in Portland, Oregon. The CNME has granted institutional accreditation to NCNM, accreditation of the naturopathic program at Bastyr (Bastyr is also re-gionally accredited by the Northwest Association of Schools and Colleges), and preaccredited status to Southwest. All states licensing naturopathic physicians recognize the CNME as the official accrediting agency for naturopathic medicine.

Research

Original research at naturopathic institutions has, until recently, been quite limited. The profession has relied on its clinical traditions and internationally published health care research. The most comprehensive compilation of the scientific documentation of naturopathic philosophy and therapies can be found in *A Textbook of Natural Medicine* (Pizzorno & Murray 1985). This two volume set is updated on a regular basis and now comprises over 200 chapters and references over 10,000 citations from the peer-reviewed scientific literature.

In the past decade, both National College of Naturopathic Medicine and Bastyr University have developed active research departments which have resulted in the publication of original research in several peer-reviewed journals, both alternative and mainstream. In October 1994, Bastyr University was awarded a three-year, $840,000 grant by the U.S. National Institutes of Health Office of Alternative Medicine to establish a research center to study alternative therapies for HIV/AIDS. A peer-reviewed journal, the *Journal of Naturopathic Medicine,* was founded in 1990 by Peter D'Adamo, ND of Norwalk, Connecticut.

Future

Naturopathic medicine, as well as the entire concept of natural medicine, might appear to be an unscientific fad that will soon pass away. To the informed, it is clear that naturopathic medicine is at the forefront of the future of medicine. The scientific tools now exist to assess and appreciate many aspects of natural medicine. It is now common for conventional medical organizations that in the past have spoken out strongly against naturopathic medicine to endorse such naturopathic techniques as lifestyle modification, stress reduction, exercise, consuming a high fiber diet rich in whole foods and other dietary measures, supplemental nutrients, toxin reduction, and many others.

This illustrates the paradigm shift that is occurring in medicine. What was once disregarded is now becoming more generally accepted as effective. In fact, in many instances, the naturopathic alternative offers significant benefit with standard medical practices. In the future, the concepts, philosophies, and practices of naturopathy should become accepted.

The naturopathic profession is growing rapidly; its therapeutic and diagnostic skills are becoming more sophisticated; licensing is being established in new states; and public interest is strong. Key to the profession's future is becoming an integral part of the health care system.

References

Belizan J, Villar J, Pineda O, et al. 1983. Reduction of blood pressure with calcium supplementation in young adults. JAMA 249:1161–1165

Clarke E, Hatcher J, McKeown-Essyen G, Liekrish G. 1985. Cervical dysplasia: Association with sexual behavior, smoking, and oral contraceptive use. Am J Obstet Gyncol 151:612–616

Dawson E, Nosovitch J, Hannigan E. 1984. Serum vitamin and selenium changes in cervical dysplasia. Fed Proc 46:612

Dyckner T, Wester O. 1983. Effect of magnesium on blood pressure. BMJ 286:1847–1849

Ford M. 1982. Biofeedback treatment for headaches, Raynaud's disease, essential hypertension, and irritable bowel syndrome: a review of the long term follow-up literature. Biofeedback Self Regul 7:521–535

Fries E. 1976. Salt, volume and the prevention of hypertension. Circulation 53:589–595

Garlic has to smell bad to do some good. 1992. Fam Prac News 22:31

Glauser S, Bello C, Gauser E. 1976. Blood-cadmium levels in normotensive and untreated hypertensive humans. Lancet: 717–718

Gruchow HW, Sobocinski MS, Barboriak JJ. 1985. Alcohol, nutrient intake, and hypertension in US adults. JAMA 253:1567–1570

Havlik R, Hubert H, Fabsitz R, Feinleib M. 1983. Weight and hypertension. Ann Intern Med 98:855–859

Hodges R, Rebello T. 1983. Carbohydrates and blood pressure. Ann Intern Med 98:838–841

Kershbaum A, Pappajohn D, Bellet S, et al. 1968. Effect of smoking and nicotine on adrenocortical secretion. JAMA 203:113–116

Khaw KT, Barrett-Connor. 1984. Dietary potassium and blood pressure in a population. Am J Clin Nutr 39:963–968

Lang T, Degoulet P, Aime F, et al. 1983. Relationship between coffee drinking and blood pressure: Analysis of 6,321 subjects in the Paris region. Am J Cardiol 52:1238–1242

Lust B. 1896. The naturopathic and herald of health

Lust B. 1918. Universal Directory of Neuropathy. Lust Publ, Butler, New Jersey

Lust B. 1945. Program of the 49th Congress of the American Naturopathy Association

McCarron D, Morris C, Cole C. 1982. Dietary calcium in human hypertension. Science 217:267–269

Meneely G, Battarbee. 1976. High sodium-low potassium environment and hypertension. Am J Cardiol 38:768–781

Natero R, et al. 1989. Dietary migraine: Fact or Fiction? Headache 29:315–316

Orr J, Wilson K, Bodiford C, et al. 1985. Nutritional status of patients with untreated cervical cancer, II. Vitamin assessment. Am J Obstet Gynecol 151:632–635

Petkov V. 1979. Plants with hypotensive, antiatheromatous and coronary dilating action. Am J Chin Med 7:197–236

Pruess HG. 1992. Overview of lead toxicity in early life, effects on intellect loss and hypertension. J Am Coll Nutr 11:608

Ramaswamy P, Natarajan R. 1984. Vitamin B6 status in patients with cancer of the uterine cervix. Nutr Cancer 6:176–180

Rao R, Rao U, Srikantia S. 1981. Effect of polyunsaturated vegetable oils on blood pressure in essential hypertension. Clin Exp Hyperten 3:27–38

Resnick LM, Gupta RK, Laragh JH. 1989. Intracellular free magnesium in erythrocytes of essential hypertension: Relationship to blood pressure and serum divalent cations. Proc Natl Acad Sci USA 81:6511–6515

Romney S, Duttagupta C, Basu J, et al. 1985. Plasma vitamin C and uterine dysplasia. Am J Obstet Gynecol 151:978–980

Sarchielli P, et al. 1992. Serum and salivary magnesium levels in migraine and tension-type headaches: Results in a group of adult patients. Cephalagia 12:21–27

Van Niekerk W. 1966. Cervical cytological abnormalities caused by folic acid deficiency. Acta Cytol 10:67–73

Vergroesen A, Fleischman A, Comberg H, et al. 1978. The influence of increased dietary linoleate on essential hypertension in man. Acta Biol Med Germ Band 37:879–883

Whorton J. 1982. Crusaders for Fitness. Princeton Press, New Jersey

Woodcock BE, Smith E, Lambert WH, et al. 1984. Beneficial effect of fish oil on blood viscosity in peripheral vascular disease. BMJ 288:592–594

Yoshioka M, Matsushita T, Chuman Y. 1981. Inverse association of serum ascorbic acid level and blood pressure or rate of hypertension in male adults aged 30–39 years. Int J Vitam Nutr Res 54:343–347

Suggested Readings

Beasley JD, Swift JJ. 1989. The Kellogg Report: The Impact of Nutrition, Environment and Lifestyle on the Health of Americans. Annadale-on-Hudson, New York

Benjamin H. 1981. Everybody's Guide to Nature Cure, 7th Ed. Thorsons Pub. England

Bilz FE. 1898. The Natural Method of Healing (2 vol). (English Translation) Bilz, Intl News Co. New York

Brown D. 1994. Quarterly Review of Natural Medicine. NPRC. Seattle

Coulter H. 1973. Divided Legacy, vol II. Wehawken Books. Washington, DC

Dejarnette MB. 1939. Technic & Practice of Bloodless Surgery. Private. Nebraska City, Nebraska

Filden JH. 1929. Impaired Health (Its Cause & Cure) 2nd Ed. Private. Denver

Graham RL. 1923. Hydro-hygiene. Thompson-Barlow Co. New York

Griggs B. 1981. Green Pharmacy. Jill, Norman, & Hobhouse. London

Johnson AC. 1996. Principles & Practice of Drugless Therapeutics. Chir Ed Extension Bureau, Los Angeles

Kellogg JF. 1901, 1902. Rational Hydrotherapy. Battle Creek, Michigan

Kellogg JH. 1923. New Dietetics. Modern Medical Publisher. Battle Creek, Michigan

Kuhne L. 1918. Neo-naturopathy (New Science of Healing). (Translated by B Lust), Lust Publisher. Butler, New Jersey

Kuts-Cheraux AW. 1953. Naturae Medicina. ANPSA. Des Moines, Iowa

Lindlahr H. 1914–1919. Philosophy Practice, and Dietetics of Natural Therapeutics, Vol I—II. Maidstone Osteopathic. Maidstone, England

Lust B. 1918. Universal Directory of Naturopathy. Lust Publisher. Butler, New Jersey

MacFadden B. 1904. Building of Vital Power. Phys Cult Publ. Physical Culture City. New Jersey

McKeown T. 1976. The Role of Medicine: Dream, Mirage, or Nemesis? Nuffield Provincial Hospitals Trust. London

Murray MT, Pizzorno JE. 1991. Encyclopedia of Natural Medicine, Prima Publications

Murray MT. 1994. Natural Alternatives to Over-the-Counter and Prescription Drugs. William Morrow. New York

Pizzorno JE, Murray MT. 1985–95. A Textbook of Natural Medicine, John Bastyr College Publications. Seattle

Richter JT. 1949. Nature—The Healer. Private, Los Angeles

Spitler. 1948. Basic Naturopathy. ANA, Des Moines, Iowa

Starr P. 1983. Social Transformation of American Medicine. Basic Books, New York, NY

Trall RT. 1880. Hydropathic Encyclopedia 3 vol. SR Wells. New York

Weltmer E. 1913. Practice of Suggestive Therapeutics. Weltmer Inst. Nevada, Missouri

Whorton J. 1982. Crusaders for Fitness. Princeton Press. Princeton, New Jersey

13
Chinese Medicine

China's Traditional Medicine

Kevin V. Ergil

China's Traditional Medicine in Cultural Perspective

Certain considerations are important to understanding ethnomedical systems in general and Chinese medicine in particular. Medicine is a human endeavor and as such is shaped by the considerations of the human beings using and practicing it. These considerations sometimes have very little to do with curing disease in the most simple and efficient way and a great deal to do with economics, politics, and culture. Ideology, belief, and even simple ignorance has influenced the practice of medicine more than rationality. A medical historian or a physician might perceive medicine to be a steady march from ignorance to the light, but these are typically revisionist histories. Medicine is a human enterprise embedded in and intersected by myriad other human projects. Even the choice of how to conduct a medical procedure or what kind of health care to choose may have more to do with habit or economics than with rationality or efficacy. For instance, American gynecologists position their patients for maximum visual exposure during routine examinations while physicians in the United Kingdom allow the patient to lie on their side, assuming a more relaxed posture during the examination (Payer 1988). An example closer to our subject is the case of a Chinese patient choosing traditional herbal medicine to manage painful and debilitating kidney stones. Although the treatment was ultimately efficacious, his choice was not motivated by a desire for efficacy. If he underwent surgery, the patient would have been classified as an invalid on his work papers and therefore barred from advancement in his job. Or, there is the example of a hospital in California which closes its doors to the practice of acupuncture despite the fact that acupuncturists in the state are licensed medical practitioners and their services are routinely requested by hospital patients. In each instance, considerations that are not directly linked to the rational and effective delivery of medical care influence medical choices.

Our own perspectives on medicine and our experience of our own medical systems provide us with ideas of what is normal or typical for medicine. We respond to aspects of a traditional system that correspond with our expectations. We imagine Chinese herbal medicine as a gentle therapy using nontoxic ingredients. Its use of highly toxic substances or drastic purgative therapies is easily overlooked. It is unlikely, for instance, that the traditional form of Tibetan therapeutic cautery applied with a hot iron will elicit substantial interest as a form of alternative therapy. Naturalistic and rational elements of systems intrigue us. Unfamiliar or magical diagnostic and therapeutic modes cause us concern.

It is easy to make intellectual errors when dealing with medical systems. We forget that our own perspectives may prevent us from understanding the meaning and utility of practices that have been developed within another culture. That failure to account for our own needs and biases also can lead to the overenthusiastic acceptance of ideas whose genesis and application we really do not understand.

If we want to avoid these errors, we must think about medical systems as being embedded in their respective cultures. Each system's structure and elements are vital to their practice in a particular cultural context. Culture, in this sense, does not imply an all-embracing system of meaning subscribed to by all members of a community, country, or ethnicity. Culture is a complex network of signification, elements of which might resonate only in a very local sense while other aspects have almost global relevance. This does not mean that the medical ideas and practices of one society cannot or will not be successfully appropriated by another, but rather that aspects of a system that are meaningful to one group of people might not be meaningful at all to another.

For example, the concept of neurasthenia (*sheng jin shuai ruo*) is an important syndrome in traditional Chinese medicine and Chinese psychiatry, despite the fact that this diagnosis has fallen into disrepute among Western psychiatrists and is no longer classified as a disease entity in diagnostic manuals. Neurasthenia was an exceptionally popular diagnosis in the nineteenth century, during periods of extensive medical exchange between the United States and China and Japan. The diagnosis has continued to be clinically important in China, because it fits well into certain traditional medical models and responds well to cultural and political concerns about mental illness (Kleinman 1986). Americans and Europeans who encounter neurasthenia within the corpus of Chinese medicine sometimes find it an unusual or obscure concept despite its relevance for Chinese medical practice.

Sometimes, upon encountering a new idea, we like to think about it in familiar terms. One example is the use of the word *energy* to express the idea of qi. An extension of this is the frequent translation of the therapeutic method of draining evil influences from channels as "sedation." Neither energy nor sedation have much to do with the concepts that underlie qi and draining, however, these terms are more familiar to us and make Chinese medicine more accessible. Unfortunately, this practice can obscure the breadth of meaning in these terms (Wiseman and Boss 1990).

We try to make sense of the world from our position in it, historically as well as culturally. We tend to view history as progressing, as if by design, to a specific end. Events of the past, viewed from the perspective of the present, offer tempting opportunities for reinterpretation in relation to current experience. For example, in the context of current perspectives on disease causation, Wu You Ke's statements that "miscellaneous qi" could cause epidemic disease, and his concept of "one disease, one qi" (Wiseman 1993) have led contemporary sources in China to suggest that coming prior to the invention of the microscope, such an insight is quite remarkable (Wiseman 1995). The implication that Wu You Ke's observation represented a precursor of germ theory is attractive to Chinese practitioners who are trying to find a place for traditional practices in an increasingly biomedicalized world. In fact, the concept of miscellaneous or pestilential qi has been used extensively in adapting traditional theory to the management of HIV infection. However, as Wiseman points out, it never was explored in relation to the causation of disease by microscopic organisms, nor was it ever conceived as a basis for such an exploration. Its relation to the concept is a retrospective interpretation.

The above points are generally relevant to almost any system or collection of medical practices. Some additional points are crucial to understanding the progression of medical thought in China. Although we tend to think that Chinese medicine has been practiced without any significant change for millennia, this is simply not true. Chinese medicine has undergone significant change and development over the centuries. Ideas that once were important are now almost invisible, and ideas that were left by the wayside for centuries found favor in later times. Recent ideas have been relatively significant in the organization of the system. Changes in technology, for instance, have broadened the clinical use of acupuncture and increased its safety. Ideas, substances, and medical practices have come to China from all over the world, some of which have become significant parts of traditional Chinese medicine and some of which remain only as observations in ancient texts.

Within China itself, many competing ideas have existed side-by-side. Old theories have been rejected, or discovered anew and accorded even more importance than they had at their conception. Some ideas found more fertile ground in other Asian countries, such as the transmission of acupuncture and Chinese herbal medicine to Japan.

Historian and anthropologist Paul Unschuld critiques the perspective of Chinese medicine as a homogenous monolithic structure.

> Proponents of this view depict "Chinese Medicine" as an identifiable, coherent system, the contents of which they attempt to characterize. Such an approach is both ahistorical and selective. It focuses on but one of the many distinctly conceptualized systems of therapy in Chinese history, that is the medicine of systematic correspondence, and it neglects both the changing interpretations of basic paradigms offered by Chinese authors through the ages and the synchronic plurality of differing opinions and ideas that existed for twenty centuries concerning even fundamental aspects of this therapy system such as pulse-diagnosis (Unschuld 1985).

This is a particularly important point because it is extremely tempting to encounter medical systems with the expectation that they be possessed of an internal logic that reconciles all of their aspects. Although many aspects of Chinese medicine can be applied with complete consistency, other aspects or concepts appear to be quite contradictory. This trait leads us to what has been probably the most important aspect of Chinese medicine throughout its history: it is a medical tradition that never threw anything away. Certain medical practices might have been relegated to the attic, but they were available if necessary. A striking example of this is the work of Zhang Zhong Jing, whose system of diagnosis and therapy did not attract much attention during his lifetime, but became highly influential centuries after his death. Later authors believed his theory to be incomplete and broadened its perspective, but his theories and these new theories that emerged in response to them are still important to the contemporary clinician. In the West, an incomplete theory is rejected and disappears. In the history of Chinese medicine, theories, practices, and concepts may fade, but they do not entirely disappear. A new theory can exist beside the one that it sought to correct. The clinician can choose to apply the perspective

that he feels is most applicable. In this way, conflicting concepts of etiology, and systems of diagnosis, and treatment have continued to exist side by side.

Unschuld considers this one of the basic characteristics distinguishing traditional Chinese thought from modern Western science (Unschuld 1985). It also is the aspect of Chinese medicine that is most challenging to Western students. The extent to which deductive reasoning and its necessary condition of "either this or that but not both" are pervasive in our society have made it difficult to approach a medical tradition that dispenses with what we view as a necessary precondition of valid human knowledge. Even European or American advocates of Chinese medical traditions sometimes err and insist that only certain theoretical perspectives or therapeutic methods are correct or authentic.

Years earlier, Lin Yutang wrote that systematic metaphysics or epistemology were alien to traditional Chinese thought.

> The temperament for systematic philosophy simply wasn't there, and will not be there so long as the Chinese remain Chinese. They have too much sense for that. The sea of human life forever laps upon the shores of Chinese thought, and the arrogance and absurdities of the logician, the assumption that "I am exclusively right and you are exclusively wrong," are not Chinese faults, whatever other faults they may have (Lin 1942).

Of course, the history of Chinese medical thought includes plenty of individuals who thought that they were exclusively right, but the breadth of traditional Chinese medical thought was sustained by an intellectual climate that retained all possible ideas for use and exploration. A given philosopher or clinician might reject an idea, but the idea itself would remain available for future use.

For example, during the Ming dynasty, Wu You Ke (c.a. 1644) was the leading exponent of the "offensive precipitation sect" (*gong xia pai*) of physicians whose tenets included a distinctive set of ideas concerning the management of epidemic disease and a wholehearted rejection of many established ideas in

Chinese medicine (Wong & Wu 1985). He was subsequently viewed alternatively as a contributor to Chinese medical thought; a proponent of a divergent and uninformed theory; and finally (as noted above) as the intellectual antecedent of Koch, the discoverer of the tuberculosis bacillus. At no point were his ideas discarded.

Interestingly enough, in modern China, where the sheer volume of information and the nation's health care needs makes it necessary to teach a standard curriculum to thousands of students each year, this tolerance for varying clinical perspectives continues. There are for instance, herbal physicians known as Minor Bupleurum Decoction (*Xiao Chai Hu Tang*) doctors because their prescriptions are organized around one formula from the *Treatise on Cold Damage (Shang Han Lun)*, an early text on diagnosis and herbal therapy written during the Han dynasty (206 BCE 220 CE). There also are herbal physicians who reject traditional formulas entirely and use contemporary perspectives on the Chinese pharmacopeia to organize their prescriptions.

There are acupuncturists whose clinical focus might be dedicated almost entirely to six acupuncture points and who use CT scans to plan clinical interventions. At the same time, two floors down in the same hospital, physicians base their selection of acupuncture points on obscure and complex aspects of traditional calendrics and systems such as the "Magic Turtle."

Once it is understood that Chinese medicine is a large and various tradition with many manifestations and philosophies, it is possible to begin its exploration.

History

Chinese medicine has an extensive history. As is the case with most medical traditions, this history can be approached from several perspectives. There is the ancient mythology of Chinese medicine, which attributes the birth of medicine to the legendary emperors Fu Xi, Shen Nong, and Huang Di. There is the history that can be deduced from the careful study of available ancient texts and records, which indicate, for example, that there is no reference to acupuncture as a therapeutic method in any Chinese

text before 90 BCE (Unschuld 1985) and that the oldest existing text to discuss medical practices that faintly resemble current Chinese medicine date from the end of the third century BCE (Unschuld 1985). Finally, there are the more extravagant interpretations of archeologic evidence and textual materials that seek to establish the ancient character of certain Chinese medical practices. An example would be the frequent assertion that the stone "needles" excavated at different times in various parts of China were remnants of ancient acupuncture (Wang 1986, Chuang 1982). This assertion is based on references to the ancient surgical application of sharp stones in texts from later periods and morphological similarities between the excavated stones and later metal needles.

Legendary Origins

The origins of Chinese medicine are mythically linked to three legendary emperors: Fu Xi, or the Ox Tamer, taught people how to domesticate animals and divined the *Ba Gua*, eight symbols that became the basis for the *Yi Jing*, or *Book of Changes*. Shen Nong, or the Divine Husbandman, also is known as the Fire Emperor. Shen Nong is said to have lived from 2698 to 2598 BCE, and is considered to be the founder of agriculture in China. He taught the Chinese people how to cultivate plants and raise livestock. He also is considered the originator of herbal medicine in China, having learned the therapeutic properties of herbs and substances by tasting them. Later authors would attribute their work to him to indicate the antiquity and importance of their text. The *Divine Husbandman's Classic of the Materia Medica (Shen Nong Ben Cao Jing)* is a case in point. The text probably was written in 220 CE and reconstructed in 500 CE by Tao Hong Jing. Given that all historical evidence points to the ancient character of herbal medicine in China, it is appropriate that Shen Nong is considered its originator (Fig. 13-1).

Huang Di, the Yellow Emperor (2697), is known as the originator of the traditional medicine of China. He also is seen as the "Father of the Chinese Nation." He is credited with teaching the Chinese how to make wooden houses, silk cloth, boats, carts, the bow and arrow, ceramics, and the art of writing. Legend has it that he gained his knowledge from visiting the immortals. Most important to our discussion is his work *Yellow Emperor's Inner Classic (Huang*

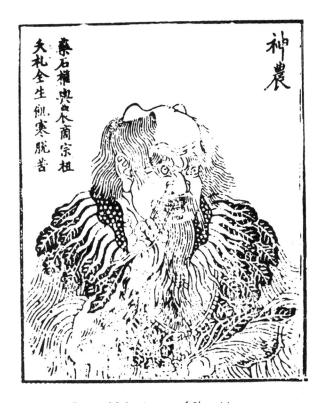

Figure 13-1. Image of Shen Nong.

Di Nei Jing), in which the traditional medicine of China is first expressed in a form that is familiar to us today. The text is divided into two books. *Simple Questions (Su Wen)* is concerned with medical theory, such as the principles of yin and yang, the five phases, and the effects of seasons. The *Spiritual Axis (Ling Shu)* deals predominantly with acupuncture and moxibustion. The texts are written as a series of dialogues between the Emperor and his ministers. Qi Bo, the most famous among the ministers, is said to have tested the actions of drugs, cured people's sickness, and written books on medicine and therapeutics.

> QI BO EXPLAINS THE ORDERLY LIFE OF TIMES PAST
>
> The first book of *Simple Questions* begins with the Yellow Emperor asking Qi Bo why peoples' life spans are now so short when in the past *(Continues)*

> they lived close to a hundred years. Qi Bo explains that in the past people maintained an orderly life. "In ancient times those people who understood Dao patterned themselves upon the yin and the yang and they lived in harmony with the arts of divination" (Veith 1972).

Today, it is generally agreed that the Yellow Emperor's Inner Classic was first compiled around 200 BCE. Both in terms of legend and practice, it remains a text that is critical to Chinese medicine.

Ancient Medicine 2205 to 206 BCE

Little is actually known about the practice of medicine in China before 200 BCE. The Shang Dynasty (1766 to 1121 BCE) is the first dynasty of which there exists clear archeologic evidence. It appears likely that prior to the Shang, nomadic cultures were scattered across Northern China. Interaction among these groups eventually led to the development of the Shang. This dynasty leaves us the first traces of some sort of therapeutic activity. In addition to developing the first Chinese scripts, the Shang had clearly defined social relations. There was a king and nobility and, perhaps most importantly, the people were no longer nomadic. The Shang response to illness is documented by archaeological finds and writings from the succeeding Zhou Dynasty (1122 to 221 BCE). During this period, ideas developed that would be central to Chinese culture, specifically, a relationship between the living and the dead that developed into a ritualized veneration of ancestors. Ancestors could be consulted concerning a variety of issues, including the cause of illness, through the use of oracle bones. Tortoise shells and the scapula of oxen were heated and rapidly cooled, causing them to crack. The resulting patterns would be used for guidance in resolving questions. Often, the question posed to the ancestors would be inscribed upon the bone itself. Bones could be used for more than one divination. One tomb has yielded more than 100,000 oracle bones, displaying questions such as "Swelling of the abdomen. Is there a curse? Does the deceased Chin-wu desire something of the king?" (Unschuld 1985). The ancestors were appropriately placated according to the response. Natural causes of illness also were encountered, but these appear to have been addressed through the intervention of ancestors as well.

The Zhou dynasty resulted from a political conflict with a group of Chinese-speaking descendants of the same neolithic peoples who had settled to form the Shang. The defeat of the Shang established one of China's longest dynasties, as well as a pattern of governance that would characterize Chinese society—a central government working in relation to smaller principalities.

The Zhou continued the practices of the Shang rulers, consulting tortoise shell oracles with the aid of *wu*, or shamans. The *wu* acted as intermediaries between the living and the dead, played important ritual roles in court activities and the weather, and were called upon to combat the demons who caused illness. During this period, the shamanic activity of chasing evil spirits away from towns and homes with spears might have been transferred to the human body, and the practice of acupuncture emerged. Later accounts (eighth century CE) describe the needling techniques used by the physician Bian Qu (fifth century BCE) to drive out demons. However, we have no clear evidence of this.

The Warring States period, toward the close of the Zhou, was marked by political strife and social upheaval. This era saw the emergence of two philosophers, Kong Fu Zi (Confucius) and Lao Zi, whose ideas about social and natural order were to have a lasting impact on Chinese culture. A similar trend occurred within medicine: the human body no longer was seen as subject only to the whims of spirits and demons, but as a part of nature, and subject to discernable natural relationships. Those ideas were elaborated upon during the Han Dynasty.

The Flowering of Chinese Medicine 206 BCE to 907 CE

In 206 BCE, the empire was reunited under the Han. The Han (206 BCE to 219 CE) created a stable aristocratic social order, expanded geographically and economically, and spread Chinese political influence throughout Vietnam and Korea. The Chinese people today refer to themselves as the Han. This dynasty was a period of great development for the Chinese, including the integration of the Confucian doctrine, elements of yin yang, and the five phase theory into the political picture. Textual evidence

reveals the emergence of a medicine that is similar to the Chinese medicine we know today.

The earliest texts available were recovered from three tombs dating to 168 BCE that were excavated at Ma Wang Dui in Hunan province (Unschuld 1985). These texts discuss magical and demonologic concepts, as well as some ideas about yin and yang in relation to the body. The texts present an early concept of channels in the body, but in a less developed fashion than the later *Yellow Emperor's Inner Classic*. Ma Wang Dui texts mention moxibustion and the use of heated stones, but they do not speak about acupuncture or specific points on the body, implying that the idea of acupuncture had not yet emerged at this time.

A biography written by a contemporary in 90 BCE describes Chun Yu Yi, the first known physician to record personal observations of clinical cases. Interestingly, he also was tried for malpractice due to his use of the apparently unfamiliar method of acupuncture to change the flow of qi (Unschuld 1985).

The *Divine Husbandman's Classic of Materia Medica (Shen Nong Ben Cao)* appears during this era as well. This text is the first known formal presentation of individual medicinal substances, the first in a long line of such texts.

The *Classic of Difficult Issues (Nan Jing)* was compiled sometime during the first or second century CE, although its authorship is attributed to the legendary physician Bian Qu. This text has had and continues to have a marked influence on the practice of Chinese medicine and, to an even greater extent, on the practice of Chinese medicine in Japan. It marks a drastic shift in medical thinking, systematically organizing the theory and practice of therapeutic acupuncture in terms of body structure, illness, diagnosis, and treatment. It is almost entirely devoid of magical elements. The author(s) of the *Classic of Difficult Issues* reconciled the contradictions of the *Inner Classic*, in addition to providing many new observations. It is thought to have been written as an independent text, but met with so much resistance as a result of its radical organization that it became known as a commentary on the *Inner Classic*.

The *Treatise on Cold Damage (Shang Han Lun)* and the *Survey of Important Elements from the Golden Cabinet and Jade Container (Jin Gui Yao Lue)* were published in the second century CE by Zhang Zhong Jing, also known as Zhang Ji (142 to 220 CE). Chinese medical texts of this period were primarily philosophical, but like the authors of the *Classic of Difficult Issues,* Zhang studied disease from a clinical standpoint, emphasizing the physical signs, symptoms, and course of disease, the method of treatment, and the action of the substances used. He was interested especially in fevers because most of his village was wiped out by fever epidemics (possibly typhoid). Although the texts were published during the Han, they remained relatively obscure until the Sung Dynasty (after 960 CE) when medical thinkers realized that the concepts of diagnosis and therapy presented reflected their own concerns. These texts enormously influenced the practice of herbal medicine in Japan (see page 213). We will examine an herbal formula derived from the Treatise on Cold Damage later in this chapter.

Hua Tou (110 to 207 CE), acupuncturist, herbalist, and surgeon, is an almost legendary figure in Chinese medicine. He is reported to have used acupuncture and herbs, and his adaptation of animal postures is one of the early forms of Qigong. He is said to have utilized the anesthetic properties of plants in order to render a patient insensible to pain, enabling him to successfully practice surgery.

Despite Hua Tou's reputation, his surgical innovations seem to have departed with him. Chinese medical history reveals the practice of a variety of minor surgical interventions for growth, hemorrhoids, and wound healing, but none of the significant abdominal surgeries attributed to Hua Tou. The surgical castration used to produce eunuchs for the imperial court was medically significant, and there is textual evidence of Chinese exposure to the surgical practices developed in India for the treatment of cataracts but these did not form surgical traditions *per se.*

Huang Pu Mi (215 to 286 CE) wrote the *Systematic Classic of Acupuncture (Zhen Jiu Jia Yi Jing),* which exercised substantial influence over the acupuncture traditions of China, Korea, and Japan. This text presented and reorganized material from the *Inner Classic* and earlier texts.

It is important to realize that the histories of individual physicians and the texts that have come down to us reflect the medicine of the literate elite of China more than the medical traditions of that nation as a whole. About 80 percent of the total population consisted of farmers, peasants, and farming villages. These people lived at a level of bare subsistence and worked extremely hard to stay there, entirely dependent on the soil and the weather. They were not exposed to formal education and typically were illiterate. Very little is known of what these people knew or thought at any particular time. Their traditions were regionally oriented, full of folk superstition, historical legend, and aspirations dominated by the hope of survival.

Some authors, especially compilers of materia medica texts, would explore the nonliterate traditions of the Chinese people, but the first systematic publication of this material did not occur until late in the Qing dynasty (Unschuld 1985). Folk herbal and medical traditions were most systematically explored under the guidance of the postrevolutionary government of China. Texts such as *The Barefoot Doctor's Manual* reflect the inclusion of this type of material.

In 220 CE, after approximately 30 years of strife and religious rebellion by Daoist sects, the Han dynasty fell. After the Han, there was another long period of division in China, although not as violent nor as divisive as the Warring States period after the Zhou dynasty. In 589 CE, the Sui dynasty reunified China, and soon was succeeded by the Tang dynasty, considered by many to be the height of China's cultural development. The Tang dynasty spread China's influence as far as Mongolia, Vietnam, Central Asia, Korea, and Japan. During this period, both Buddhism and Daoism strongly influenced medical thought.

Sun Si Miao (581 to 682), a famous physician of the period, was a prolific author and a productive scholar who was well versed in both Daoist and Buddhist practice. His *Thousand Ducat Prescriptions (Qian Jin Yao Fang),* a text on eye disorders, and *The Classic of Spells,* a guide to magic in medicine, are some of the texts he authored. The *Thousand Ducat Prescriptions* contains a section entitled "On the absolute sincerity of great physicians" that established him as China's first medical ethicist. He addresses the need for diligent scholarship, compassion towards the patient and high moral standards in the physician, that remain pertinent and seem to speak directly to issues in medicine today.

SUN SI MIAO EXPLAINS THE INCURABLE NATURE OF PHYSICIANS

Finally, it is inappropriate to emphasize one's reputation, to belittle the rest of the physicians and to praise only one's own virtue. Indeed, in actual life someone who has accidentally healed a disease, then stalks around with his head raised, shows conceit and announces that no one in the entire world could measure up to him. In this respect all physicians are evidently incurable (Unschuld 1979).

Academic Medicine and Systematic Therapeutics 960 CE–1368 CE

By the time of the Sung dynasty, the practice of medicine had become more specialized, and efforts were made to systematically integrate past insights. The number of texts published in this dynasty may have exceeded the number written during all of the previous dynasties put together. In 1027, Wang Wei Yi designed and oversaw the casting of two bronze figures designed to illustrate the location of acupuncture points. One of these was used in the imperial medical college. The bronzes were pierced at the location of the acupuncture points, covered with wax, and filled with water. When a student found the hole under the wax with a needle, water would drip out, indicating it to be the correct spot.

During the Sung dynasty, there was a huge advance in herbal therapeutics and the publication, under imperial decree, of several complete herbal texts that contained illustrations. It was during this time that tastes and properties were assigned to herbs according to their yin or yang nature, and functions were assigned that were a result of the herb's nature and its ability to treat specific symptoms. Efforts were made to systematize herbal therapeutics. The writings of Zhang Zhong Jing received great interest because of his systematic application of traditional theoretical principles to the use of herbal medicine. The revival of the *Treatise on Cold Damage* influenced medicine for the next several hundred years as it precipitated warm induced disease theory (*wen bing xue*) during the Ming Dynasty.

During the Sung dynasty, the education of physicians became more formal. The Imperial College, which had provided for the training of the emperor's physicians, was expanded. In 1076, an Imperial Medical College was founded with an enrollment of 300 students. There were regional schools as well.

The Jin and the Yuan dynasties saw the continuation of specialized medical thought and independent inquiry. Much of what we recognize as Chinese medicine today—and what we shall discuss in the section on fundamental concepts—stems from the Sung, Jin, and Yuan dynasties. Physicians of this period developed ideas involving the elaboration of therapeutic approaches on the basis of early theory. They espoused the application of five phase theory in relation to seasonal influences, supplementing the body, purging the body to eliminate evil influences, and supplementing the yin.

Medicine in the Ming and Qing Dynasties 1368 to 1911

Physicians continued to pursue lines of inquiry pursued in preceding dynasties, such as the far reaching naturalistic explorations of Li Shi Zhen (1518 to 1593). His *Grand Materia Medica (Ben Cao Gang Mu)* included discussions of 1892 substances and, among its topics, described the use of kelp and deer thyroid to treat goiter.

The exploration of more precise linkages between factors in disease causation and therapeutics continued, and a number of medical sects emerged. During a virulent epidemic that struck from 1641 to 1644 Wu You Ke (Xing) (1592 to 1672) used an unorthodox method that was highly successful. His text, *Discussion of Warm Epidemics (Wen Yi Lun)* explored the theoretical basis for his treatment.

Some authors consider the Ming dynasty to be the peak of the cultural expression of acupuncture and moxibustion in China (Qiu 1993). This period saw the production of numerous texts on the subject. One of the most influential acupuncture texts, *The Great Compendium of Acupuncture and Moxibustion (Zhen Jiu Da Cheng)*, was written by Yang Ji Zhou toward the end of the dynasty.

Intellectual trends of the Ming continued into the Qing dynasty. *The Discussion of Warm Disease (Wen Re Lun)* by Ye Tian Shi complemented Zhang Zhong Jing's method of diagnosing and treating diseases caused by cold with an equally systematic method of diagnosing and treating those caused by heat.

Political, economic, and social trends during the Qing exacerbated the isolation of the Manchu rulers of the time and exposed the Chinese to the power of Western knowledge, technology, and science. The broadening of cultural horizons and the broadening of medical inquiry combined to shake the classical underpinnings of Chinese medical thought. In 1822, acupuncture was formally eliminated from the Imperial Medical College (Qiu 1993).

By the close of the Qing dynasty in 1911, political and cultural institutions were in a state of decline. The scattered practitioners of traditional Chinese medicine found themselves increasingly under fire from the advocates of a new and modern China and a new and modern medicine.

The collapse of the Qing and the formation of the Republic laid traditional medicine open to the conquering influence of Western medicine. The Imperial College of Physicians was eliminated (Wong & Wu 1985) and the Western-educated proponents of reform began to work towards the elimination of the traditional medicine of China and the establishment of Western medicine as the dominant medical system.

From 1914 through 1936 a series of encounters and clashes over the regulation, establishment, or elimination of practitioners of Chinese medicine occurred (Wong & Wu 1985). The traditional medicine of China, or "medicine" (*yi*) as it had been known, came to be termed "Chinese Medicine" (*Zhong Yi*). Both nationalist and marxist reformers disliked Chinese medicine with a passion.

SO-CALLED CHINESE MEDICINE

Initially, the external threat reduced the internal spectrum of competing Chinese interpretations of the classics. The great diversity of individual efforts to reconcile insights from personal experience with the ancient theories of yin yang and the Five Phases, as well as with other older views about the structure of the body, disappeared behind the illusion of a so-called Chinese medicine (*chung-I*) [*zhong yi*], suppos-

(Continues)

edly well-defined and with theory easily converted into practice. This situation, in turn, has given rise to the historically misleading impression that these diverse elements, like the concepts and practices of Western medicine, constituted a unified, coherent system (Unschuld 1985).

A critical feature of this new Chinese medicine was its rejection of practices that were manifestly "unscientific," represented in the creation of *Zhong Yi*. This disciplined form of medicine has emerged today as traditional Chinese medicine.

The aspects of the traditional medicine of China that were secured in *Zhong Yi* were later appropriated by the Chinese Marxists in an effort to build a strong medical infrastructure for substantial populations in the face of economic and technical limitations. Chairman Mao's declaration, in 1958, that "Chinese medicine is a great treasure house! We must uncover it and raise its standards!" (Unschuld 1985), inspired efforts to rehabilitate the traditional medicine of China and to "discover" a primitive dialectic within the theoretical underpinnings of the system. The *Revised Outline of Chinese Medicine* stated that "Yin-yang and the five phases (*wu-hsing [wu xing]*) are ancient Chinese philosophical ideas. They are spontaneous, naive materialist theories that also contain elementary dialectic ideas" (Sivin 1987).

The development of Chinese medicine as a system parallel to Western medicine was under way by the time of Mao's declaration. In 1956, four colleges of Chinese medicine were created, with many more to follow. Today, *Zhong Yi* exists as a parallel medical system, integrating necessary biomedical elements while retaining fidelity to the traditional concepts of Chinese medicine. Educational programs emphasize acupuncture and herbal medicine and range from an undergraduate technical certificate to PhD programs. Most independent practitioners enter the field with a five year medical baccalaureate degree (MB/BS) that is earned following high school (Ergil 1994). In this system both inpatient and outpatient medical care is delivered from large, well-equipped hospitals, as well as private clinics and pharmacies.

Fundamental Concepts

Yin and Yang

The philosophy of Chinese medicine begins with yin and yang. These two terms can be used to express the broadest philosophical concepts, as well as the most focused perceptions of the natural world. Yin and yang express the idea of opposing, but complementary phenomena that exist in a state of dynamic equilibrium. The most ancient expression of this idea seems to have been that of the shady and sunny sides of a hill (Wilhelm 1967, p. 297, Unschuld 1985, p. 55). The sunlit southern side was the yang and the shaded northern side was the yin. The contrast between the bright and dark sides of a single hill portrayed the yang and the yin respectively. If you imagine, for a moment, the different environments that exist on either side of this one hill you can begin to get an idea of yin and yang. On the bright, sunny side, plants and animals that enjoy light are more prevalent, the air is drier, and the rocks are warm. On the dim, shaded side, the air seems moist and cool.

Yin and yang are always present simultaneously. The paired opposites observed in the world gave tangible expression to the otherwise uncontemplatable Dao, of ancient Chinese thought.

ORIGINS OF YIN AND YANG

Out of Tao, One is born;
Out of One, Two;
Out of Two, Three;
Out of Three, the created universe.
The created universe carries the yin at its back and the yang in front;
Through the union of the pervading principles it reaches harmony (Laozi in Lin 1942).

The *Book of Changes (Yi Jing)*, which sought to explore the myriad manifestations of yin and yang, expressed the idea thusly, "That which lets now the dark, now the light appear is tao" (Wilhelm 1967).

The *Yellow Emperor's Inner Classic*, the oldest text to discuss the medical application of yin and yang in a comprehensive way (Unschuld 1985, p. 56), tells us that "yin and yang are the way of heaven and earth" (Wiseman 1985). This text showed how yin and yang were to be used to correlate the body and other phenomena to the human experience of health and disease.

THE *INNER CLASSIC* ON YIN AND YANG

As to the yin and yang of the human body, the outer part is yang and the inner part is yin. As to the trunk, the back is yang and the abdomen is yin. As to the organs, the viscera are yin whereas the bowels are yang. The liver, heart, spleen, lung, and kidney yin; the gallbladder, stomach, intestines, bladder, and triple burner are yang (Wiseman et al 1993).

It is important to note that the above quote is taken from the translation of an important contemporary textbook of Chinese medicine. Many ideas expressed in the *Yellow Emperor's Inner Classic* are taught and applied routinely in the contemporary clinical practice of Chinese medicine.

Yin and yang were used to express ideas about both normal physiology and pathological processes. They were applied to the organization of phenomena in many ways, for example, to organize phenomena in terms of the emergence of its dominant yin or yang character. Summer was yang within yang, fall was yin within yang, winter was yin within yin, and spring was yang within yin. Thus the coldest, darkest, and most yin period was yin within yin, while spring, when the yang began to emerge from the yin, was yang within yin.

There is a distinctly ecological orientation to the world view that is supported by yin and yang; each phenomenon is seen in relation to its surroundings. And it is expected that each phenomenon will exert an influence on its surroundings that is balanced by an equal, but opposing influence. Just as the language of ecology is the language of interrelation and interdependence, the language of Chinese medicine is a language of interrelation and interdependence. The external landscape, or human environment, is understood to be in profound and dynamic relationship with the internal landscape, or human organism. We will see this idea even more clearly when we explore the idea of disease causation.

The ancient Chinese understood human beings to have a nature and structure inseparable from yin and yang, and as such, inseparable from the world around us—a structure which is to be understood by the same rules that guide us in understanding the world in which we live. Life on the shaded side of a mountain has characteristics that differ from those on the sunny side. Finally, the comprehension and adjustment of life in relation to yin and yang would support life itself. Thus it was said "To follow (the laws of) yin and yang means life; to act contrary to (the laws of yin and yang) means death" (Unschuld 1985).

Yang and Yin Correspondences

Yang	Yin
Light	Dark
Heaven	Earth
Sun	Moon
Day	Night
Spring	Autumn
Summer	Winter
Hot	Cold
Male	Female
Fast	Slow
Up	Down
Outside	Inside
Fire	Water
Wood	Metal

Within the traditional medical community of contemporary China, there is debate over the actual nature of yin and yang. Some exponents of a more scientific, less traditional, perspective on Chinese medicine would like yin and yang to be used as concepts to organize phenomena. Others who express a less modern perspective will emphatically state that yin and yang are actually tangible phenomena (Farquhar 1987). While it is probably easiest for us to think about yin and yang as descriptive terms that help the Chinese physician to organize information,

it should be remembered—and this is especially true in traditional pharmaceutics—that the yin and yang constituents of the body are actual things that can be reinforced by specific substances or actions.

An analogy that is useful for thinking about yin and yang in this way is that of a candle. If one considers the yin aspect of the candle to be the wax and the yang aspect to be the flame, we can see how the yin nourishes and supports the yang, how the yang consumes the yin and, in doing so, burns brightly. When the wax is gone, so is the flame. Yin and yang exist in dependence on each other.

The Five Phases

Another idea that has played a significant part in the development of some aspects of Chinese medicine is that of the five phases (*wu xing*). The five phases are earth, metal, water, wood, and fire. In Chinese, *wu* means five and *xing* expresses the idea of movement, to go. For a period of time, the *wu xing* were translated as the five elements. This translation conveys little of the dynamism of the Chinese concept, instead focusing on the apparent similarities between the *wu xing* and the elements of medieval alchemy. This is an example of the translation problem in which we use the familiar to understand the new. However useful this method may be at first, it can lead to some confusion in the long run. *Wu xing* may include the implication of material elements, but, in general, the five phases speak to a set of dynamic relations occurring among phenomena that are organized in terms of the five phases. This philosophy can cover almost every aspect of phenomena from seasons to the weather (Table 13-1).

Qi, and the Essential Substances of the Body

Apart from the ideas of yin and yang and the five phases, there is no concept more crucial to Chinese medicine than qi—the idea that the body is pervaded by subtle material and mobile influences that cause most physiological functions and maintain the health and vitality of the individual. This idea is not common to biomedical thinking about the body. It is not unusual to see the idea of qi translated with the term energy, but this translation conceals its distinctly material attributes. Furthermore, while en-

Table 13-1. **Five Phase Correspondences**

Category	Wood	Fire	Earth	Metal	Water
Viscus	Liver	Heart	Spleen	Lungs	Kidney
Bowel	Gallbladder	Small Intestine	Stomach	Large Intestine	Urinary Bladder
Season	Spring	Summer	Late Summer	Autumn	Winter
Time of Day	Before Sunrise	Forenoon	Afternoon	Late Afternoon	Midnight
Climate	Wind	Heat	Damp	Dryness	Cold
Direction	East	South	Center	West	North
Development	Birth	Growth	Maturity	Withdrawal	Dormancy
Color	Cyan	Red	Yellow	White	Black
Taste	Sour	Bitter	Sweet	Pungent	Salty
Sense Organ	Eyes	Tongue	Mouth	Nose	Ears
Odor	Goatish	Scorched	Fragrant	Raw Fish	Putrid
Vocalization	Shouting	Laughing	Singing	Weeping	Sighing
Tissue	Sinews	Vessels	Flesh	Body Hair	Bones
Mind	Anger	Joy	Thought	Sorrow	Fear

ergy is defined as the capacity of a system to do work, the character of qi extends considerably further.

The Chinese character for qi is traditionally composed of two radicals; the radical which symbolizes breath or rising vapor is placed above the radical for rice (Fig. 13-2). Qi is linked with the concept of "vapors arising from food" (Unschuld 1985). Over time, this concept broadened, but never lost its distinctively material aspect. Unschuld favors the use of the phrase "finest matter influences" or "influences" to translate this concept. Wiseman points out that some phenomena labeled as qi do not fit conventional definitions of substance or matter, further confusing the issue (Wiseman et al 1995). It is for this reason that many authors prefer to leave the term qi untranslated.

The idea of qi is extremely broad, encompassing almost every variety of natural phenomena. There are many different types of qi in the body. In general, the features that distinguish each type derive from its source, location, and function. There is considerable room for debate in this area, and exploration of a wide range of materials can suggest a variety of different ideas about categories of qi. In general, qi has the functions of activation, warming, defense, transformation, and containment.

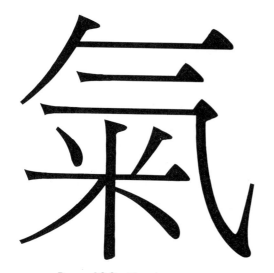

Figure 13-2. **The character qi.**

Types of Qi

Ying qi	Construction qi	Supports and nourishes the body
Wei qi	Defense qi	Protects and warms the body
Jing qi	Channel qi	Flows in the channels (felt during acupuncture)
Zang qi	Organ qi	Flows in the organs (physiological function of organs)
Zong qi	Ancestral qi	Responsible for respiration and circulation

The qi concept is important to many aspects of Chinese medicine. Organ and channel qi are influenced by acupuncture. In fact, one characteristic feature of acupuncture treatment is the sensation of obtaining the qi or *de qi*. Qigong is a general term for the many systems of meditation, exercise, and therapeutics that are rooted in the concept of mobilizing and regulating the movement of qi in the body. Qi is sometimes compared to wind captured in a sail; we cannot observe the wind directly, but we can infer its presence as it fills the sail. In a similar fashion, the movements of the body and the movement of substances within the body are all signs of the action of qi.

In relation to qi, blood and fluids constitute the yin aspects of the body. Blood is produced by the construction qi, which in turn is derived from food and water. Blood nourishes the body. Blood is understood to have a slightly broader and less definite range of actions in Chinese medicine than it does in biomedicine. Within the body, qi and blood are closely linked, as blood is considered to flow with qi and to be conveyed by it. This relationship often is expressed by the Chinese saying "qi is the commander of blood and blood is the mother of qi," and it has been suggested that qi and blood are linked in the manner of a person and their shadow.

Fluids are a general category of thin and viscous substances that serve to moisten and lubricate the body. Fluids can be conceptually separated into humor and liquid. Humor is thick and related to the body's organs; among its functions is the lubrication of the joints. Liquid is thin and is responsible for moistening the surface areas of the body, including the skin, eyes, and mouth.

Essence and Spirit

Together with qi, essence and spirit make up what are known in Chinese medicine as the three treasures. In brief, essence is the gift of one's parents and spirit is the gift of heaven. Essence is the most fundamental source of human physiologic processes, the bodily reserves that support human life and that must be replenished by food and rest, and the actual reproductive substances of the body. Spirit is the alert and radiant aspect of human life. We encounter it in the luster of the eyes and face in a healthy person, as well as in their ability to think and respond appropriately to the world around them. The idea expressed by

spirit or *shen* in Chinese encompasses consciousness and healthy mental and physical function.

The relation of the mind to the body in Chinese medicine does not include the notion of a distinct separation. It is understood that the psyche and soma interact with each other and that aspects of mental and emotional experience can impact the body, and vice versa. In this sense, spirit is linked both to the health of the body and to the health of the mind. Similarly, aspects of human experience that are understood as predominantly mental in a biomedical frame of reference are linked to specific organs in Chinese medicine. Anger is related to the liver, obsessive thought is related to the spleen, and joy to the heart.

Viscera and Bowels (*Zang* and *Fu*)

The anatomy of human beings was understood by the ancient Chinese in ways that are not too distant from their European contemporaries, up to the seventeenth century. There are instances of systematic dissection in Chinese history, but none of these reached the extensive explorations into the structure of the body that characterized European medicine by the fifteenth century. Instead the Chinese medical perspective of the body, although rooted in familiar anatomic structures, represented a system in which organs serve as markers of associated physiologic functions rather than actual physical structures.

The physician of Chinese medicine encounters a body in which 12 organs function. These organs are divided into the viscera, which includes six *zang* or solid organs and the bowels, including six *fu* or hollow organs. These organs often are related to the physical structures that we associate with conventional biomedical anatomy. The heart, lungs, liver, spleen, kidneys, and pericardium are the six viscera. The six bowels are the small intestine, large intestine, gallbladder, stomach, urinary bladder, and the "triple burner" (*san jiao*). These organs have physiologic functions that often are similar to those associated with them in biomedicine, but that also might be very different. The liver is said to store blood and to distribute it to the extremities as needed. The spleen is understood as an organ of digestion. The Chinese understood the physical structure and location of most of the organs, but as systematic dissection was not extensively pursued, the close observation of physiologic function was more often the basis of medical thought.

For example, circulation and elimination of fluids was observed and attributed to an organ that was said to have a name, but no form was established. This organ, the "triple burner," is considered alternatively to be the combined expression of the activity of other organs in the body, or a group of spaces in the body. This example clearly expresses the idea that physiologic function, rather than substance, establishes an organ in Chinese medicine. At the same time, the "triple burner" has always been surrounded by debate because it does not have a clear anatomic structure.

The organs of viscera and bowel are paired in what is known as the yin and yang, or interior/exterior relationship. The heart is linked with the small intestine, the spleen with the stomach, and so on. Each viscera and each bowel have an associated channel that runs through the organ, the paired organ, within the body, and across the body's surface, and then connects with the channel of the related organ.

Historical evidence suggests that the idea of channels is more ancient than the idea of specific acupuncture points. There has been disagreement about the locations of specific points and efforts have been made to systematize knowledge of them. Recent research in the People's Republic of China has led to the publication of a number of texts dedicated to resolving historical, philological, and anatomic questions about acupuncture points. At this time, there are understood to be 12 primary channels and 8 extraordinary vessels. The 12 channels are classically organized in terms of a six-fold yin and yang organizational scheme, although they can also be organized in terms of five phase theory. Qi is understood to flow in these channels, making a rhythmic circuit.

Along the pathways of 14 of these channels (the 12 regular channels and 2 of the extra channels) lie 361 specific points. In addition, there are a large number of "extra" points that have been derived from clinical experience but are not traditionally considered part of the major channel systems. Beyond this, various individual elaborations of acupuncture theory suggest new points. There are also local micro systems of acupuncture points that have postulated numerous points on the ear, scalp, hand, foot, and other areas of the body.

Acupuncture points appear at many locations on the body. Most often, they are located where a gentle and sensitive hand can detect a declivity with slight pressure on the skin surface. Points are located at the margins or bellies of muscles, in between bones, and over distinctive bony features that can be detected through the skin. Methods used to locate points vary. In general, points are found by seeking anatomic landmarks, by proportionally measuring the body, and by using finger measurements. The first method is considered the most reliable. With time and clinical experience some practitioners can be less formal in their approach to locating acupuncture points, but this topic interests even advanced practitioners. In Japan, clinicians gather regularly to hone their point location skills, and in China, point location in relation to classical sources, anatomic study, and empirical evidence is an area of advanced study.

As with qi, the actual term and usage of the Chinese expression that we translate as "point" is important. The character *xue*, which has been translated as point, actually means "hole" in Chinese. A hole often is part of the clinician's subjective experience of the acupuncture point. *Xue* are holes where the qi of the channels can be influenced by inserting a needle or by other means. If one imagines the channel system as a vast subcutaneous waterway with caves and springs punctuating its course as it flows to the surface, one will have a concept of the holes that is not far from the way the Chinese thought of them for many centuries.

Leg Three Li

- *Location:* 3 cun (body inch) below the depression below the patella, one finger breadth from the anterior crest of the tibia.
- *Indications:* Stomach pain, vomiting, abdominal distension, indigestion, diarrhea, constipation, dizziness, mastitis, mental disorders, hemiplegia, pain in knee joint and leg.
- *Depth of needle insertion:* 0.5 to 1.3 inches.

Holes, or points along the channels, have been categorized and organized in myriad ways. One of the oldest and most well known is a system of categories based on the idea of *shu*, or transport points. This system of point categories applies exclusively to points on the forearm and lower leg, which embody the image of qi welling gently forth from a mountainous source at the finger tips and gradually gaining strength and depth as it reaches the seas located at the elbow and knee joints.

What has been presented above is a very brief discussion of the essential anatomy and physiology of Chinese medicine. It is important to remember that this anatomy forms a general reference for physiologic function, rather than an anatomy of direct links between discrete categories of tissue and specific physiologic processes. A strength of Chinese medicine is that its theory allows for generalizations about complex physical processes in addition to responding to signs and symptoms whose origins are obscure. Finally, the distinction between mind and body is not present in Chinese medicine. Although Chinese physicians may display a disconcerting lack of interest in contemporary psychotherapy or its patients, they are quick to posit a link between affect and physiologic process, in a manner that might intrigue a contemporary psychobiologist.

On this basis then we can proceed to examine how illness manifests in the body.

The Causes of Disease

Ultimately, all illness is a disturbance of qi within the body. Its expression as a pathologic process displaying specific signs and symptoms depends on the location of the disturbance. Contemporary formal discussions on the cause of disease make use of the ideas of Chen Yen (1161 to 1174), who wrote *Prescriptions Elucidated on the Premise That All Pathological Symptoms Have Only Three Primary Causes (San Yin Qi Yi Bing Cheng Fang Lun),* and an additional idea of Wu You Ke, that each disease has its own qi.

The three categories of disease are organized in terms of external causes of disease, internal causes, and causes that are neither external nor internal (Wiseman et al 1995). The first category includes six influences that are distinctly environmental: wind, cold, fire, dampness, summer heat, and dryness. When they cause disease, these six influences are

known as "evils." If the defense qi is not robust, or the correct qi is not strong, or if the evil is powerful—the evil may enter the surface of the body and, under certain conditions, penetrate to the interior.

The Three Causes of Disease (San Yin)

- External Causes, or "the six evils": wind, cold, fire, damp, summer heat, and dryness
- Internal Causes, or internal damage by the seven affects: joy, anger, anxiety, thought, sorrow, fear, and fright
- Nonexternal, noninternal causes: dietary irregularities, excessive sexual activity, taxation fatigue, trauma, and parasites.

The nature of the evil and its impact on the body was understood through the observation of nature and the observation of the body in illness. The clinical meaning of the causes of disease does not lie, for the most part, in the expression of a distinct etiology, but in the manifestation of a specific set of clinical signs. In this sense, the biomedical distinction between etiology and diagnosis is somewhat blurred in Chinese medical theory.

For example, the evils of wind and cold are frequently implicated in the sudden onset of symptoms that are associated with the common cold: headache, pronounced aversion to cold, aching muscles and bones, fever, and a scratchy throat. Wind is expressed in the sudden onset of the symptoms and in their manifestation in the upper part of the body, and cold is displayed in the pronounced aversion to cold and the aching muscles and bones. Whether the patient had a specific encounter with a cold wind shortly before the onset of the symptoms is not particularly relevant. Although it is not unusual for a patient to announce that they were abroad on a chilly and windy day prior to the onset of a cold, such exposure could easily result in signs of wind heat as well, that is, a less marked aversion to cold, a distinctly sore throat, and a dry mouth. The six evils are not agents of specific etiology, but agents of specific symptomatology. These ideas developed in a setting where the possibility of investigating a bacterial or viral cause was nonexistent. Rather, careful observation of the body's response to disease provided the information necessary for treatment.

Each of the evils affects the body in a fashion similar to its behavior in the environment. Images of these processes observed in nature and society were inscribed on the body to permit its processes to be readily understood. The human body stood between heaven and earth, and was subject to all their influences in a relationship of continuity with its environment. Although these six evils are identified as environmental influences that attack the body's surface, it also is clearly understood they may occur within the body, causing internal disruption.

Internal damage by the seven affects refers to the way in which mental states can influence body processes. However, such a statement expresses a separation not implied in Chinese medicine. Each of the seven affects can disturb the body if it is strongly or frequently expressed. As was discussed above each of the mental states—joy, anger, anxiety, thought, sorrow, fear, fright—is related to a specific organ.

Finally, nonexternal, noninternal causes encompass the causes of disease that do not arise specifically as a result of environmental influences or mental states. These include dietary irregularities, excessive sexual activity, taxation fatigue, trauma, and parasites. The role that most of these have in producing disease is obvious to us, with the exceptions of excessive sexual activity and taxation fatigue. Excessive sexual activity suggests the possibility that too frequent emission of semen by the male can cause illness. This can occur because semen is directly related to the concept of essence, which is considered to be vital to the body's function and difficult to replace. This category also includes possible damage that can occur to the essence through excessive childbearing or bearing a child at too young or too old an age.

Taxation fatigue is an intriguing category. This category expresses the dangers of engaging in a variety of activities for a prolonged period of time. This category includes both the idea of overexertion and the idea of inactivity as possible causes of disease. All of the concepts included within taxation fatigue reflect the essential thought of Chinese medicine that moderation is the key to health. Lying down for prolonged periods damages the qi and prolonged standing damages the bones. From the moment that the Yellow Emperor asks Qi Bo why people now die before their time and receives his answer, the images of balance, harmony, and moderation have informed Chinese medicine.

Each of the causes of disease—from prosaic ones, such as dietary irregularities, to somewhat exotic notions, such as wind evil—disrupt the balance of yang and yin within the body and disrupt the free movement of qi. The next step is to determine the precise pattern of imbalance.

Diagnosis

Diagnostics in Chinese medicine is traditionally expressed within four categories: inspection, listening and smelling, inquiry, and palpation. The fundamental goal is to collect information that reflects the status of physiological processes, and then to analyze this information to determine how that process has been impacted by a disorder.

The first of the four diagnostic methods, inspection (*wang*), refers to the visual assessment of the patient, particularly their spirit, form and bearing, the head and face, and substances excreted by the body. Inspection makes use of a large body of empirically derived information as well as theoretical considerations. The color, shape, markings, and coating of the tongue are inspected. In the case of our patient who had been attacked by wind and cold, one would expect to see a moist tongue with a thin white coating, signaling the presence of cold. If heat were present, we might expect a dry mouth and a red tongue. The observation of the spirit, which is considered very important in assessing the patient's prognosis, relies on assessing the overall appearance of the patient, especially the eyes, the complexion, and the quality of the patient's voice. Good spirit—even in the presence of serious illness—is thought to bode well for the patient.

The second aspect of diagnosis, listening and smelling (*wen*), refers to listening to the quality of speech, breath, and other sounds, as well as to being aware of the odors of breath, body, and excreta. As is the case with each aspect of diagnosis, five phase theory can be incorporated into the assessment of the patient's condition. Each phase and pair of viscera and bowel has a corresponding vocalization and smell.

The third aspect of diagnosis, inquiry (*wen*), is the process of taking a comprehensive medical history. This process has been presented in many ways, but perhaps best known is the system of ten questions described by Zhang Jie Bin in the Ming dynasty. The questions were presented as an outline of diagnostic inquiry and included querying the patient about sensations of hot and cold, perspiration, head and body, excreta, diet, chest, hearing, thirst, previous illnesses, and previous medications and their effects.

One might, for example, expect the patient suffering from wind and cold symptoms to report an aversion to any sort of exposure to cold, headache, body aches, and an absence of thirst.

This step is considered critical to a good diagnosis. Although pulse diagnosis is sometimes regarded as a central feature of Chinese medicine and is, rightly, regarded as an art, it should not form the sole basis of a complete diagnosis.

> The *Simple Questions* expresses the following idea: If, in conducting the examination, the practitioner neither inquires as to how and when the condition arose, nor asks about the nature of the patient's complaint, about dietary irregularities, excesses of sleeping and waking, and poisoning, but instead proceeds immediately to take the pulse, he will not succeed in identifying the disease (Wiseman et al 1995).

Contemporaries of Li Shi Zhen the author of *The Pulse Studies of Bin Hu (Bin Hu Mai Xue)*, placed tremendous emphasis on the pulse. He was considered an expert himself, but rejected the notion that one would place an unequal emphasis on any aspect of the diagnostic process.

Palpation (*qie*) is the fourth diagnostic method, and includes pulse examination, general palpation of the body, and palpation of the acupuncture points. Pulse diagnosis offers a range of approaches, and can provide a remarkable amount of information about the patient's condition. The process of pulse diagnosis is carried out on the radial arteries of the left and right wrists. The patient may be seated or lying down and should be calm. The pulse is divided into three parts: the middle part is adjacent to the styloid process of the radius, in what is called the "bar position." The inch is distal to it and the cubit is proximal. The inch position, which is nearest the wrist, can indicate the status of the body above the diaphragm; the bar indicates the status of the body between the diaphragm and the navel; and the cubit, the area below the navel. Beyond this simple conceptual structure, each pulse position can be interpreted to shed light on the status of the organs and the channels. Table 13-2 presents two models of what can be felt at each pulse position. The first chart is derived from the *Classic of Difficult Issues*, where this type of pulse diagnosis was first presented in a systematic way, and the second chart shows a less elaborate, contemporary pattern. Some authors have suggested that the pattern associated with the *Classic of Difficult Issues* is related more to the use of pulse diagnosis in the practice of acupuncture, while the later pattern is of more relevance to the herbalist (Maciocia 1989). Not all herbalists or acupuncturists make use of the pulse, but certain styles of acupuncture rely quite heavily on it. There are many possible approaches to the pulse, making it a very rich area for the clinician and a somewhat vexing one for the biomedically oriented researcher (Birch 1994).

The pulse allows the clinician to feel the quality of the qi and blood at different locations in the body. Table 13-3 provides a list of 29 pulse qualities and some possible associations (Wiseman 1994). Pulse qualities are organized on the basis of the size, rate, depth, force, and volume of the pulse. The overall quality of the pulse and the variations in quality at certain positions can, after several years of patient attention, become quite meaningful to the clinician. The patient who has been afflicted with a wind cold evil, might display a pulse that was floating and tight, signaling the presence of a cold evil on the surface of the body.

Once the practitioner of Chinese medicine has

Table 13-2. **Pulse Positions**

| | Position | Left | | Right | |
		Deep	Superficial	Deep	Superficial
Nan Jing	Inch	Heart	Small intestine	Lung	Large intestine
	Bar	Liver	Gallbladder	Spleen	Stomach
	Cubit	Kidney	Urinary bladder	Pericardium	Triple warmer
Contemporary Chinese sources	Inch	Heart		Lung	
	Bar	Liver	Gallbladder	Spleen	Stomach
	Cubit	Kidney	Urinary bladder	Kidney	Urinary bladder

Table 13-3. **Pulse Types**

English	Chinese	General Association
1 Normal	zheng chang mai	Normal pulse
2 Floating	fu mai	Exterior condition
3 Deep	chen mai	Interior condition
4 Slow	chi mai	Cold and yang vacuity
5 Rapid	shuo mai	Heat
6 Surging	hong mai	Exuberant heat, hemorrhage
7 Faint	wei mai	Qi and blood vacuity desertion
8 Fine	xi mai	Blood and yin vacuity
9 Scattered	san mai	Dissipation of qui and blood, critical
10 Vacuous	xu mai	Vacuity
11 Replete	shi mai	Exuberant evil with right qi strong
12 Slippery	hua mai	Pregnancy, phlegm, abundant qi and blood
13 Rough	se mai	Blood stasis, vacuity of qi and blood
14 Long	chang mai	Often normal
15 Short	duan mai	Vacuity of qi and blood
16 Stringlike	xian mai	Liver disorders, severe pain
17 Hollow	kou mai	Blood loss
18 Tight	jin mai	Cold, pain
19 Moderate	huan mai	Slower than normal not pathological
20 Drumskin	ge mai	Blood loss
21 Confined	lao mai	Cold, pain
22 Weak	ruo mai	Vacuity of qi and blood
23 Soggy	ru mai	Vacuity of qi and blood with dampness
24 Hidden	fu mai	Deep lying internal cold
25 Stirred	dong mai	High fever, pregnancy
26 Rapid, irregular	cu mai	Debility of visceral qi or emotional distress
27 Slow, irregular	jie mai	Debility of visceral qi or emotional distress
28 Regularly intermittent	dai mai	Debility of visceral qi or emotional distress
29 Racing	ji mai	Heat, possible vacuity

(Data from Wiseman N, Ellis A, Zmiewski P, Li C. 1995. In Wiseman N, Ellis A (trans) Fundamentals of Chinese Medicine. Paradigm. Brookline) carried out the diagnostic process, he or she must make sense of the information derived. The practitioner constructs an appropriate image of the configuration of the disease so that it can be addressed by effective therapy. Central to this process is the notion of pattern identification (*bian zheng*), the process of gathering signs and symptoms through the diagnostic process and using traditional theory to understand how the fundamental substances of the body, the organs, and the channels have been impacted. Many intellectual aspects of the diagnostic processes of Chinese medicine, especially when applied to the practice of herbal medicine, are as analytical as a biomedical clinical encounter. The physician must elicit signs and symptoms from the patient, and then use them to understand the disruption of underlying physiological processes.

The first step of pattern identification is the localization of the disorder and the assessment of its essential nature, using the eight principles that are an expansion of yin and yang correspondences: yin, yang, cold, hot, interior, exterior, vacuity, and repletion.*

Like many other aspect of contemporary Chinese medicine, the eight principles originated in the Sung dynasty. Kou Zong Shi proposed a structure that organized disease into eight essentials: cold, hot, interior, exterior, vacuity, repletion, evil qi, and right qi (Bensky & Barolet 1990). These were improved upon in 1732, in the text *Awakening the Mind in Medical Studies (Yi Xue Xin Wu)* (Sivin 1987). The original source was written, in the spirit of the times, to create a formal diagnostic structure for herbs that could be conceptually integrated with the ideas already in use for acupuncture. Today this formal structure is applied both to acupuncture and to herbal medicine.

The wind cold patient came to us with these symptoms: marked aversion to exposure to cold, headache, body aches, absence of thirst, a moist tongue with a thin white coating, and a floating and tight pulse. In terms of the eight principles, this would be an exterior, cold, repletion pattern. The principles of yin and yang would not directly apply.

What does this mean? The eight principles serve fundamentally to localize a condition. When the Chinese physician says that a condition is external, he means that it has not yet penetrated beyond the skin and channels to the deeper parts of the body. In this case a cold condition betrays itself through the body's expression of cold signs. To say a condition is replete is to say that the evil attacking the body is strong, or that the body itself is strong.

Typically, the eight principles are the first step in developing a clear pattern identification, especially if there is organ involvement. The eight principles are the application of a yin and yang based theoretic structure.

A single biomedical disease entity can be associated with a large number of Chinese diagnostic patterns. For example, viral hepatitis is associated with at least six distinctive diagnostic patterns, and lower urinary tract infection might be related to one of four distinct diagnostic patterns (Ergil 1995). Each of these patterns would be treated in different ways, as it is said, "one disease, different treatments." Our patient whose clinical pattern is wind cold has the common cold and a headache, but the same disease could manifest in other patterns.

Also many different diseases may be captured within one pattern, hence the saying, "different diseases, one treatment." One contemporary text lists such diverse entities as nephritis, dysfunctional uterine bleeding, pyelonephritis, and rheumatic heart disease under the diagnostic pattern of "disharmony between the heart and kidney" (Huang 1993, p. 79).

This comparatively precise diagnostic linkage begins to be broadly appreciated in the historical trends of the Sung, Jin, and Yuan dynasties. The six channel pattern identification proposed by Zhang Zhong Jing is one among many patterns currently used. The patient who has encountered a wind cold evil would, under Zhang Jong Jing's system, be categorized as having tai yang disease. There is considerable room for overlap within the available methods of pattern identification.

---

* Although many authors continue to use the terms "excess" and "deficiency" to express the Chinese expressions *shi* and *xu*, I prefer Wiseman's "repletion" and "vacuity" as a translation. The use of "excess" simply is incorrect, because of the existence of other Chinese terms that convey this idea exactly. "Deficiency" is problematic because it implies measurable quantity, which is not a consideration in the Chinese concept (Wiseman & Boss 1990). Unschuld uses "depletion" and "repletion" instead.

<table>
<tr><td>

Types of Diagnostic Patterns

- Eight principle
- Six evils
- Qi and blood and fluids
- Five phases
- Channel patterns
- Viscera and bowels
- Triple burner
- Six channels
- Four levels

</td><td>

Methods of Treatment

- Diaphoresis
- Clearing
- Ejection
- Precipitation
- Harmonization
- Warming
- Supplementation
- Dispersion
- Orifice opening
- Securing astriction
- Settling and absorption

</td></tr>
</table>

Therapeutic Concepts

Once a diagnosis has been determined and, where relevant, a pattern has been differentiated, therapy begins. Therapeutics in Chinese medicine is fundamentally allopathic, that is, it addresses the pathologic condition with opposing measures.

> Cold is treated with heat, heat is treated with cold, vacuity is treated by supplementation, and repletion is treated by drainage. [Inner Classic (Wiseman et al 1985)]

Within the realm of acupuncture and moxibustion and herbal medicine, three fundamental principles of therapy are understood: treating disease from its root; eliminating evil influences and supporting the right; and restoring the balance of yin and yang. These refer, respectively, to approaches that are appropriate to the patient's condition. It would be appropriate to eliminate the cold evil and support the right qi of the wind cold patient. In a patient where the symptomatology reflects a complex underlying pattern, one might attempt to treat the root of the patient's condition. For instance, functional uterine bleeding due to a disharmony of the heart and kidney would be addressed primarily by harmonizing the heart and kidney; treating the root of the condition would adjust its symptoms. Treatment methods vary widely. The simplest expression of their organization is given below.

Therapeutic Methods

Acupuncture and Moxibustion

These two clinical methods certainly can be used independently of each other, but are so deeply wedded to each other in Chinese medicine that the term for this therapy is *zhen jiu*, meaning "needle moxibustion." In order to capture the distinctively composite character of this phrase, some authors translate the expression as "acumoxa therapy." The basis of their close linkage lies in the ancient origins of these methods, and the fact that moxibustion appears to have been the form of therapy that first was applied to the channels and holes in order to treat problems on or within the body. Both techniques are used to provide a discrete stimulus to points that lie along channel pathways or to other appropriate sites. I will begin by discussing acupuncture, and then move on to moxibustion.

The therapeutic goal of acupuncture is to regulate the qi. Qi and blood flow through the body, its organs, and the channel pathways. When it flows unimpeded, the body is in a state of health. When some cause—such as an evil, mental state, or trauma—interrupts the flow of qi, illness results and pain can occur. Pain is directly linked to an injury or an interruption of the flow of qi. Acupuncture is employed to remove the obstruction. The technique may be

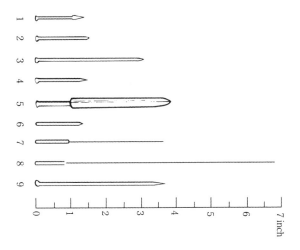

Figure 13-3. The nine needles according to the *Spiritual Pivot.* (From Qiu M-L. 1995. Chinese Acupuncture and Moxibustion. Churchill Livingstone. Edinburgh. p. 184, with permission.)

used to remove the evil, to direct qi to where it is insufficient, or to cause qi to flow where it previously had been obstructed.

The *Spiritual Axis* of the *Inner Classic* described nine needles (Fig. 13-3) for use in acupuncture. With the exception of one that appears to have had a specifically surgical application, the remaining needle types are still in use, either in original or adapted form. Acupuncture is performed today with a wider variety of tools and methods. The filiform or fine needle is the typical acupuncture tool, and it can vary significantly in terms of structure, diameter, and length.

A typical acupuncture needle has a body or shaft that is one inch long and a handle of approximately the same length (Fig. 13-4). The distinctive part of an acupuncture needle is its tip, which is rounded and moderately sharp, much like the tip of a pine needle. The acupuncture needle is solid and gently

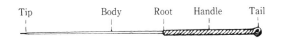

Figure 13-4. The structure of the filiform needle. (From Qiu M-L. 1995. Chinese Acupuncture and Moxibustion. Churchill Livingstone. Edinburgh. p. 186, with permission.)

tapered; it does not have the lumen or cutting edge of the hypodermic needle used for injection. Its diameter typically is 0.25 mm.

Once the site for insertion has been determined, the needle is inserted rapidly through the skin and then adjusted to an appropriate depth. Although a substantial number of considerations affect the angle and depth of insertion, methods of manipulation, and the length of retention, this is the basic procedure. A twelfth century text, *Ode of the Subtleties of Flow*, states, "Insert the needle with noble speed then proceed (to the point) slowly, withdraw the needle with noble slowness as haste will cause injury" (Shanghai College of Traditional Chinese Medicine 1981).

The essential aim of the acupuncturist is to obtain qi at the needling site. The physician seeks either an objective or subjective indication that the qi has arrived. Qi can become manifest to the practitioner through sensations experienced by the hands as the needle is manipulated, through observation, or through reports from the patient. The sensation of the arrival of qi often is felt by the practitioner as a gentle grasping of the needle at the site, as if one is fishing, and one's line has suddenly been seized by the fish. The patient senses the arrival of qi as a sensation of itching, numbness, soreness, or a swollen feeling. The patient might experience local temperature changes or a distinct "electrical" sensation. Acupuncture points in different areas of the body respond differently; these variations in response can be an important diagnostic indicator. It is not unusual for a clinician to retain a needle in an acupuncture point where the qi has not arrived until the characteristic sensation occurs.

Once a point has been correctly located, needled, and qi obtained, the clinician may choose to manipulate the needle to achieve a desired therapeutic effect. Styles of needle manipulation have inspired extensive discussions both in ancient and modern texts. Methods may range from simply putting the needle in place and leaving it there, to engaging in complex manipulations that involve slow or rapid insertion of the needle to greater or more shallow depths. These techniques might create a distinctive sensation along the channel pathway. This needle may be withdrawn promptly after qi arrives, or a short fine needle (known as an intradermal), may be retained in the site for several days. In all instances, the goal of the clinician is to influence the movement of qi.

One simple style of needle manipulation involves adjusting the direction of the needle to supplement or drain the qi at the particular channel point. If one thinks of the acupuncture point as a hole where the channel qi can be touched and moved, this operation can either cause the qi to become secure and increased in the channel (supplementing), or cause the qi to spill out (draining).

For our patient who is experiencing the symptoms of wind cold, an acupuncturist might choose to needle a number of acupuncture points including: Wind Pool (*Feng Chi* GB 20), located on the back of the neck below the occipital bone; Union Valley (*He Gu* LI 4), located in the fleshy area between the base of the thumb and forefinger; and Broken Sequence (*Lie Que* LU 7), on the forearm just above the styloid process of the radius. These particular points could all be treated with a draining method since, in this case, the channels are replete with the influences of the external evils of wind and cold. Wind Pool, as its name indicates, often is used to drain wind from the surface of the body and to relieve headache and neck pain. Union Valley is an important acupuncture point that is used frequently to influence the upper part of the body and to control pain. In this case, the point is used because of its ability to course wind, resolve the exterior, and to treat headache and sore throat. Broken Sequence is said to dispel cold and to diffuse the lung. It courses the channels and can be used to treat sore throat and headache.

Practitioners use various methods to select acupuncture points for treating a particular patient. One of the most traditional methods is an empirically derived understanding of what points work best for a given condition. Each acupuncture point has numerous indications associated with it, based on the accumulated experience of generations of acupuncture practitioners.

Ancient and contemporary texts abound with descriptions of specific sets of acupuncture points that may be used to treat a condition successfully. Broken Sequence and Leg Three Li (*Zu San Li* St 36) are described by the Song of Point Applications for Miscellaneous Disease as useful for rapid breathing and dyspnea (Ellis 1991, p. 84).

Besides choosing points based on their indications and the experience and descriptions accumulated in texts, acupuncturists also can apply specific theoretical considerations to traditional acupuncture point categories. For example, they can choose acupuncture points based on their theoretical associations with the five phases. An inference concerning the relative status of the five phases and the organs is made, based on the pulses and presenting symptoms. If the patient displayed signs of vacuity of the water phase, a choice of points could be made from the transport points along the kidney channel associated with water, in order to supplement the water phase.

Points also may be chosen on the basis of the actual trajectory of the channel upon which they lie. Union Valley is considered an important point for the head and face because the pathway of the large intestine channel on which it lies traverses that area of the body. Similarly, points on the lower extremity that lie on the urinary bladder channel, which traverses the entire back, frequently are used for back pain (Fig. 13-5).

Finally, points often are selected entirely on the basis of their sensitivity to palpation, or on the basis of a variation in texture that can be perceived by the practitioner. Often, a number of suitable acupuncture points in a specific area may be assessed to determine which would be most suitable for needling. In some cases, points that do not lie on specific channels or form part of the collection of recognized extra points can be identified by their tenderness. These points are known as *ah shi*, or "ouch, that's it," points, and are an important part of clinical acupuncture's traditional history and contemporary practice.

With many acupuncture points to choose from, and a multiplicity of methods on which to base that choice, it is not surprising that many clinicians focus on a few specific methods or a particular collection of points. Some clinicians restrict their approach so that they can focus on adjusting the application of treatment.

Moxibustion (*Jiu Fa*)

Moxibustion (*jiu*) refers to the burning of the dried and powdered leaves of artemesia vulgaris (*ai ye*), either on or in proximity to the skin, in order to

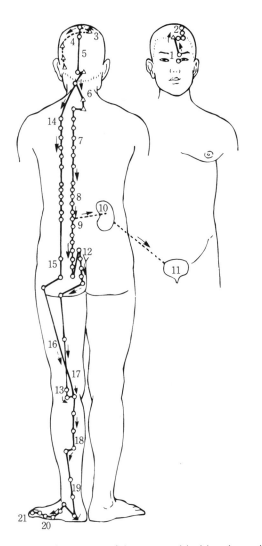

Figure 13-5. The course of the urinary bladder channel of the foot taiyang. (From Qiu M-L. 1995. Chinese Acupuncture and Moxibustion. Churchill Livingstone. p. 103, with permission.)

Moxibustion of the Eleven Vessels of Yin and Yang (Yin Yang Shi Yi Mai Jiu Jing) describes the application of moxa to treat illness by doing moxibustion on the channels (Auteroche et al 1992).

Moxibustion can be applied to the body in many ways—directly, indirectly, pole moxa, and the warm needle method. Direct moxa involves burning a small amount of moxa, perhaps the size of a grain of rice, directly on the skin. Depending on the desired effect, larger or smaller pieces of moxa can be used, and the moxa fluff can be allowed to burn directly to the skin causing a blister or a scar, or it can be removed before it has burnt down to the skin. Techniques such as these are used to stimulate acupuncture points where the action of moxibustion is traditionally indicated, or where warming the point seems to be the most appropriate response. Older texts described the use of direct moxibustion on Leg Three Li and other acupuncture points as a method of health maintenance and prevention.

Indirect moxibustion involves the insertion of a mediating substance between the moxa fluff and the patient's skin (Fig. 13-6). This gives the practitioner greater control over the amount of heat applied to the patient's body and offers the patient increased protection from burning, allowing for the treatment of delicate areas such as the face and back. Popular substances include ginger slices, garlic slices, and salt. The mediating substance often will be chosen on the basis of its own medicinal properties and how they combine with the properties of moxa. Ginger might be selected in cases where vacuity cold is present, while garlic is considered useful for treating hot and toxic conditions. The photo shows a patient being treated for facial paralysis with indirect moxibustion using ginger slices.

During pole moxa, a cigar-shaped roll of moxa wrapped in paper is used to gently warm the acupuncture points without touching the skin. This is a very safe method of moxibustion that can be taught to patients for self-application. The warm needle method is accomplished by first inserting an acupuncture needle into the point and then placing moxa fluff on its handle. After the moxa is ignited, it burns gradually, imparting a sensation of gentle warmth to the acupuncture point and channel. This method is useful especially for patients with arthritic joint pain.

affect the movement of qi in the channel, locally or at a distance. Artemesia is said to be acrid and bitter and, when used as moxa, to have the ability to warm and enter the channels. References to moxa appear in very early materials, such as the texts recovered from the excavated tombs at Ma Wang Dui (Unschuld 1985). These texts discuss a number of therapeutic methods including moxibustion, but do not mention acupuncture. One of them, the *Treatise on*

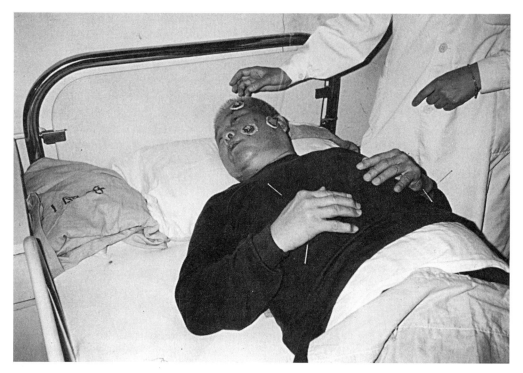

Figure 13-6. Patient receiving indirect moxa. (Photo credit Wind Horse, Marnae Ergil.)

Together, acupuncture and moxibustion are used to treat, or at least ameliorate, a wide range of conditions and symptoms. Based on the simple premise that all disease involves the disruption of the flow of qi and that acupuncture and moxibustion regulate the movement of qi, there is, at least theoretically, no disease that cannot benefit from these methods. A brief review of acupuncture texts will provide ample evidence of the range of conditions in which acupuncture is considered appropriate. The boxed list below reproduces a list of "diseases that lend themselves to acupuncture treatment" developed in the late 1970s by a World Health Organization Interregional Seminar (Bannerman 1972). The list is not based on controlled clinical research, and the specific disease names are not meant to indicate acupuncture's efficacy in treating them. The list is comparatively short if compared with a clinical manual or acupuncture textbook, but it is informative in terms of the routine application of acupuncture in China.

Diseases That Lend Themselves to Acupuncture

- Upper respiratory tract
  Acute sinusitis
  Acute rhinitis
  Common cold
  Acute tonsillitis
- Respiratory system
  Acute bronchitis
  Bronchial asthma
- Disorders of the eye
  Acute conjunctivitis
  Central retinitis
  Myopia (in children)
  Cataract (without complications)

(Continues)

- Disorders of the mouth
  Toothache, postextraction pain
  Gingivitis
  Acute and chronic pharyngitis
- Gastrointestinal disorders
  Spasms of oesophagus and cardia
  Hiccough
  Gastroptosis
  Acute and chronic gastritis
  Gastric hyperacidity
  Chronic duodenal ulcer (pain relief)
  Acute duodenal ulcer (without complications)
  Acute and chronic colitis
  Acute bacillary dysentery
  Constipation
  Diarrhea
  Paralytic ileus
- Neurologic and musculoskeletal disorders
  Headache and migraine
  Trigeminal neuralgia
  Facial palsy (early stage, i.e., within 3 to 6 months)
  Pareses following a stroke
  Peripheral neuropathies
  Sequelae of poliomyelitis (early stage, i.e., within 6 months)
  Meniere's disease
  Neurogenic bladder dysfunction
  Nocturnal enuresis
  Intercostal neuralgia
  Cervicobrachial syndrome
  Frozen shoulder, tennis elbow
  Sciatica
  Low back pain
  Osteoarthritis

Cupping and Bleeding

Two methods that are very important to the practice of Chinese medicine are cupping and bleeding. These may be used separately or together, and are often used in conjunction with other methods such as moxibustion and acupuncture. Cupping involves inducing a vacuum in a small glass or bamboo cup,

and promptly applying it to the skin surface. This therapy brings blood and lymph to the skin surface under the cup, increasing local circulation. The method is often used to drain or remove cold and damp evils from the body or to assist blood circulation. Bleeding is done to drain a channel or to remove heat from the body at a specific location. Unlike the bloodletting practiced by western physicians throughout the nineteenth century, this method expresses comparatively small amounts of blood, from a drop to a few centiliters. Figure 13-7 shows a pa-

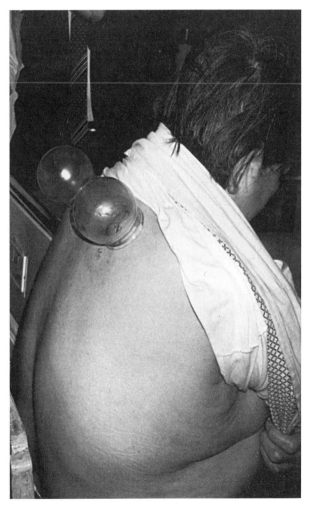

Figure 13-7. Cupping and Bleeding. (Photo credit Wind Horse, Marnae Ergil.)

tient receiving cupping and bleeding at an acupuncture point on the urinary bladder channel associated with the lungs.

Chinese Massage (*Tui Na*)

Tui Na, literally "pushing and pulling," refers to a system of massage, manual acupuncture point stimulation, and manipulation that is vast enough to warrant a chapter of its own. These methods have been practiced at least as long as moxibustion, if not longer, but the first massage training class was created in Shanghai in 1956 (Wang 1990, p. 16). Today, this field of study can serve as a minor component of a traditional medical education or an area of extensive clinical specialization.

A distinct aspect of Tui Na is the extensive training of the hands necessary for clinical practice. The practitioner's hands are trained to accomplish focused and forceful movements that can be applied to various areas of the body. Techniques such as pushing, rolling, kneading, rubbing, and grasping are practiced repetitively until they become second nature (Fig. 13-8). Students practice on a small bag of rice until their hands develop the necessary strength and dexterity.

Tui Na often is applied to limited areas of the body, and the techniques can be quite forceful and intense. Tui Na is applied routinely to orthopedic and neurologic conditions. It also is applied to conditions that might not be thought of as susceptible to treatment through manipulation, such as asthma, dysmenorrhea, chronic gastritis, and other conditions. Tui Na is used as an adjunct to acupuncture treatment, to increase the range of motion of a joint, or instead of acupuncture, when needles are uncomfortable or inappropriate, such as pediatric applications.

As with all aspects of Chinese medicine, regional styles and family lineages of practice abound. The formal curriculum available in Chinese programs is extensive, but probably not a complete expression of the range of possibilities.

Qi Cultivation (*Qigong*)

Qigong is a term that literally embraces almost every aspect of the manipulation of qi by means of exer-

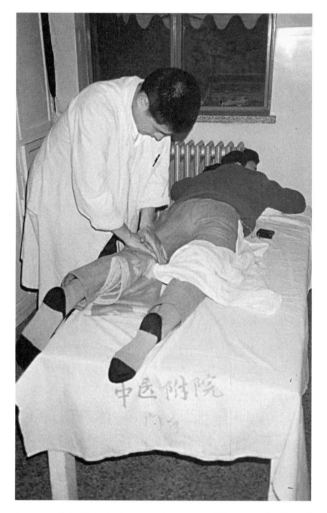

Figure 13-8. Tui Na in clinical practice. (Photo credit, Wind Horse, Marnae Ergil.)

cise, breathing, and the influence of the mind. The second part of this chapter is devoted to this topic, so only a few points need to be made here. Qigong includes practices ranging from the meditative systems of Daoist and Buddhist practitioners to the martial arts traditions of China. Qigong is relevant to medicine in three specific areas: The first is to allow the practitioner to cultivate demeanor and stamina to enable him or her to engage in performing the strenuous activities of tui na, to sustain the constant demands of clinical practice, and to quiet the mind to facilitate diagnostic perception. The second involves cultivating the practitioner's ability to safely transmit qi to the patient. Practitioners may direct qi to the patient either through the needles or directly through their hands. This activity may be the main focus of treatment or an adjunctive aspect, in which case the qi paradigm is expanded to include direct interaction between the patient's qi and that of the clinician. Finally, patients may be taught to do specific Qigong practices that are useful for their illness.

Chinese Herbal Medicine (*Zhong Yao*)

Since the legendary emperor Shen Nong tasted herbs and guided the Chinese people in their use, diet, and therapeutics, herbal medicine has been an integral part of Chinese culture and medical practice. The traditional Chinese materia medica includes far more than herbs: minerals and animal parts are listed as well. The number of substances currently identified numbers 5,767, as recorded in the *Encyclopedia of Traditional Chinese Medicinal Substances (Zhong Yao Da Ci Dian)* published in 1977 by the Jiangsu College of New Medicine (Bensky & Gamble 1986). This publication is the latest in a long line of definitive discussions of materia medica that have been produced in China over the millenia. The earliest known is the *Divine Husbandman's Classic of the Materia Medica,* which we obtained from its reconstruction by Tao Hong Jing (452 to 536 CE). This text classified upper, middle, and lower grade herbs, and discussed the tastes, temperatures, toxicities, and medicinal properties of 364 substances.

Today substances are categorized systematically as expansions of the eight methods of therapy discussed above. While a comprehensive discussion of the organization of the materia medica is beyond the scope of this paper, it should be mentioned that within the basic categories into which substances are organized, there are further subcategories. Beyond these are prescribing rules that take into account the compatibilities and incompatibilities of substances, the traditional pairings of substances, and their combination for specific symptoms.

Chinese Materia Medica Fundamental Categories

- Exterior-resolving
- Heat-clearing
- Ejection
- Precipitant
- Wind-dispelling
- Water-disinhibiting dampness-percolating
- Interior-warming
- Qi-rectifying
- Food-dispersing
- Worm-expelling
- Blood-rectifying
- Phlegm-transforming cough-suppressing panting-calming
- Spirit-quieting
- Liver-calming wind-extinguishing
- Orifice-opening
- Supplementing
- Securing and astringing
- External use

Recommendations for the therapeutic combination of substances are given by both the Ma Wan Dui texts and the *Inner Classic.* Zhang Zhong Jing's work in systematizing herbal prescriptions as therapeutic approaches to specific diagnostic patterns, based on the system of yin and yang correspondences, was unusual for its time. It was not until physicians of the Sung dynasty became interested in relating herbal practice to a systematic theory, and organizing diagnostics accordingly, that interest in the *Treatise on Cold Damage* picked up. Today, this book remains a significant resource for the practitioner of Chinese herbal medicine. One of the most comprehensive English language compilations of Chinese herbal prescriptions derives approximately 20 percent of its formula from this source (Bensky & Barolet 1990).

Not all herbal prescriptions or texts discussing their application followed the lead of Zhang Zhong Jing. Many texts offered herbs or prescriptions for specific symptoms without reference to distinct theoretic structures or diagnostic principles. Very likely, the masses applied herbs in exactly this fashion. Even today, despite the fact that the prescription of herbal formula is primarily driven by traditional diagnostic theory and pattern diagnosis, extensive compilations of empirically derived herbal formula with symptomatic indications are published.

Contemporary compilations of formula are organized in a fashion similar to substances. The result is that both substances and formula are organized in a fashion that makes them accessible in terms of traditional theories.

Formulas

- Exterior-resolving
- Heat-clearing
- Ejection
- Precipitant
- Harmonizing
- Dampness-dispelling
- Interior-warming
- Qi-rectifying
- Dispersing
- Blood-rectifying
- Phlegm-transforming cough-suppressing panting-calming
- Spirit-quieting
- Tetany-settling
- Orifice-opening
- Supplementing
- Securing and astringing
- Oral formulas for sores
- External use

Let us examine the formula and its constituent substances that might be provided to our patient who has encountered a wind cold evil or who, in the pattern identification system described in the *Treatise on Cold Damage,* would be said to have a tai yang stage pattern. In either case, ephedra decoction (*Ma Huang Tang*) would be an appropriate choice, particularly if the patient had a slight cough as well. The constituents and dosage of the formula are 9 g of ephedra (*ma huang*), 6 g of cinnamon twig (*gui zhi*), 9 g of apricot kernel (*xing ren*), and 3 g of licorice (*gan cao*). These ingredients are cooked together in water to make a slightly concentrated tea, which is drunk in successive doses. The tea is taken warm to induce sweating, a sign that the qi of the surface of the body that had been impeded by the cold evil is free to move and throw off the evil. The patient stops drinking the tea once sweat arrives.

A traditional system of organizing formula is to identify ingredients as the ruler, minister, adjutant, and emissary. In this case, the ruler of the formula is ephedra. The ruler sets the therapeutic direction of the formula. Acrid and warm, ephedra promotes sweating, dispels cold, and resolves the surface. (We will examine ephedra again in a discussion of herbal research.) Cinnamon twig is the minister, working to assist the ruler in carrying out its objectives. In addition to the effects described for ephedra, it also is said to warm the body. Apricot kernel is the adjutant, and so addresses the possible involvement of the lung and moderates the acrid flavor of the two other substances. Because the lung is the organ most immediately affected by wind cold or wind heat, the formula addresses the organ. Finally, licorice is the emissary, serving both to render the action of the other herbs harmonious and to distribute it through the body.

The foregoing example is brief and simple, but illustrates fundamental concepts. Chinese herbal therapeutics can be complex. Its practice is quite broad and the range of conditions addressed is more extensive than acupuncture. In terms of complexity and the diagnostic acumen required of the practitioner, it resembles the practice of internal medicine. Herbal therapy also encompasses the external applications of herbs and a variety of methods of preparation. Besides the traditional water decoction, or tea, substances may be powdered, or rendered into pills, pastes, or tinctures.

Dietetics

Traditional dietetics encompasses the practice of herbal therapy, but also addresses traditional Chinese foods in terms of the theoretical constructs of Chinese medicine. Five phase theory has been applied to foods since the time of the *Inner Classic.* It is not unusual to see a classroom in a college of Chinese medicine equipped as a kitchen. In larger cities, special restaurants prepare meals with specific medicinal purposes. The practices of this field are deeply rooted in the cultural practices of China and that culture's beliefs concerning diet. Many of the foods that are organized for use in therapy also are routinely prepared by families when seasons change, when illness strikes, to strengthen a woman after birth, to cause milk to fill the breasts of a new mother, or to nourish the elderly in their declining years.

Chinese Medicine in Other Countries

Today, China's traditional medicine is practiced, in various forms, all over the world. Sometimes its practice follows the contemporary patterns of traditional Chinese medicine (TCM or *zhong yi*). Sometimes its practice is deeply informed by local custom, preference, or regional elaborations.

Chinese Medicine in Korea

The relationship between China and Korea is a close one. Chinese medicine arrived in Korea during the Qin dynasty (221 to 207 BCE). However, the textual basis of Korean medicine in the literary tradition of Chinese medicine seems to have been established during the Han and Tang dynasties (Hsu & Peacher 1977), during a period of political domination by the Chinese. A close relationship between China and Korea during the Kingdom of Silla (400 to 700 CE) facilitated this exchange of ideas. Formal medical instruction by government-appointed physicians began in 693 CE. Texts such as the *Systematic Classic of Acupuncture* were important to the development of the tradition. With the formation of the Liao dynasty (907 to 1168), Korea established its independence from Chinese rule, but cultural and medical exchange continued. During the Li dynasty (1392 to 1910), many texts, including the *Illustrated Classic of Acupuncture Points as Found on the Bronze Model*, reached Korea (Chuang 1982). Widely-used techniques of acupuncture point selection based on five phase theory have emerged from Korea, including those of the Buddhist priest Sa-am (1544 to 1610).

At least two comparatively recent innovations

based on Chinese medicine have been developed in Korea, and have become well known in other parts of the world. Korean constitutional diagnosis was developed initially by Jhema Lee (1836 to 1900) and based a system of herbal therapeutics on a system of diagnostic patterning that employed the four divisions of yin and yang. It was elaborated subsequently by Dowon Kuan who, in 1965, expanded the system to an eightfold classification and applied it to acupuncture (Lee & Bac 1981, Hirsch 1985).

Another influential contemporary system is that of *Koryo Sooji Chim*, the system of Korean hand and finger acupuncture developed by Yoo Tae Woo and published in 1971. The system maps the channel pathways and acupuncture points of the entire body onto the hands, where they are stimulated using very short, fine needles and magnets. This system has gained a significant level of international exposure.

Chinese Medicine in Japan

The history of cultural exchange between China and Japan dates back to at least 57 CE. Kon Mu was the first physician to use Chinese methods to come to Japan. He was sent in 414 CE by the king of Silla, in southeast Korea, to treat the emperor Inkyo Tenno. This interaction continued. In 552, a Korean delegation brought a selection of Chinese medical texts to Japan (Bowers 1970). In 562, Zhi Cong came from southern China with more than 100 books on the practice of Chinese medicine (Huard & Wong 1968), including the *Systematic Classic of Acupuncture* (Chuang 1982). By the early eighth century, the influence of Chinese medicine was well established. With the adoption of the Taiho code in 702, provision was made for a ministry of health comprised of specialists, physicians, students, and researchers (Lock 1980). In 754, a Buddhist priest, Chien Chen, brought many medical texts from China to Japan. His influence was memorialized in a shrine in Nishinokyo (Chuang 1982).

Chinese influences on Japanese medicine were derived primarily from the *Classic of Difficult Issues* and *Systematic Classic of Acupuncture*. A revisionist movement in the late 17th century established *The Treatise on Cold Damage (Shokanron)* as the core text of herbal medicine, or *kanpo* (Chinese method), in Japan (Lock 1980).

Several factors have influenced the development

of Chinese medicine in Japan, giving it a somewhat unique appearance. The scarcity of ingredients for the preparation of Chinese herbal formula have led to an emphasis on lower doses in herbal prescription than are typical in China. An emphasis on palpatory diagnosis involving channel pathways and the abdomen also became well established. The use of somewhat finer gauge needles and shallow insertion became typical of Japanese acupuncture.

In the mid-seventeenth century, Waichi Sugiyama, a blind man, began to train the blind in acupuncture using very fine needles and guide tubes. Since it had become customary in the earlier part of the Edo period for the blind to do massage, both massage and acupuncture now became associated with blind practitioners. This contributed to a lower social position for acupuncture practitioners and to the specialization in medical practice. Kanpo physicians became primarily practitioners of herbal medicine (Lock 1980).

This trend toward specialization has continued to the present day with the division of acupuncture, moxibustion, and massage into separately licensed practices (although many individuals hold all three licenses), and the actual practice of herbal medicine being retained in the hands of medical doctors. Interestingly, a large number of Chinese herbal prescriptions are recognized as appropriate therapy for certain medical conditions according to regulations governing health care in Japan.

Japan has seen both focused specialization in and the innovative exploration and expansion of traditional acupuncture. The *Classic of Difficult Issues* often has been the focus for movements to revive the practices of traditional acupuncture. Its influence has contributed heavily to the comparatively recent development of groups of acupuncturists advocating meridian therapy (*keiraku chiryo*) based on the application of concepts in the *Classic of Difficult Issues* and their subsequent interpretation by later Chinese authors. A distinctive feature of meridian therapy is the application of five phase theory to the transport points, a practice that has influenced the perception and adoption of five phase theory by European practitioners (Kaptchuk 1983).

The pioneering work of Yoshio Manaka also has contributed dramatically to the practice of acupuncture. Manaka, a physician who experimented with

acupuncture principles during a period where medical supplies were absent during World War II, became convinced of the efficacy and physiological relevance of traditional theories and continued to experiment and develop them throughout his life.

The range of practices and interests of Japanese acupuncture practitioners is quite broad. Although some are particular partisans of specific schools of thought, including some based on contemporary Chinese medicine perspectives, many practitioners have adopted a comparatively eclectic approach.

Chinese Medicine in Europe

The history of Chinese medicine, particularly acupuncture, in Europe is both longstanding and broadly developed. The medical use of acupuncture in Europe dates from the middle of the sixteenth century (Peacher 1975). The work of Willem Ten Rhyne (1647 to 1690) in this area culminated in the publication in 1683 of *Dissertatio de Arthritide: Mantissa Schematica: de Acupunctura: et Orationes Tres,* based on information gathered during his service in Japan as a physician for the Dutch East India Company. The German physician Kampfer who also traveled with the Dutch East India Company and spent time in Japan, contributed his observations.

In France the Jesuit Du Halde published a text that included a detailed discussion of Chinese medicine in 1735 (Hsu 1989). Soulie de Morant's publication of *L'acupuncture Chinoise* was an extensive discussion of the practice of acupuncture based on direct translation, observation, and actual practice by the author. Published in 1939, the text was rooted in de Morant's exposure to the medicine of China in that country from 1901 to 1917.

England saw the publication of JM Churchill's *A Description of Surgical Operations Peculiar to Japanese and Chinese* in 1825. Among early notable English acupuncturists are Dr. Felix Mann and Dr. Sidney Rose-Neil, both of whom began their explorations of acupuncture in the late 1950s, and who have influenced its development substantially in English-speaking countries. JR Worsley, a physical therapist, who began his studies of acupuncture in 1962, came to have a substantial impact on the perceptions of many practitioners in England and the United States. He visited Hong Kong and Taiwan for a brief period and then became a part of the study group established by Rose-Neil (Hsu & Peacher 1977). Worsely went on to create the British College of Traditional Chinese Acupuncture as well as two schools in the United States.

Chinese Medicine in the United States

In 1826 Bache became one of the first American physicians to use acupuncture in his practice (Haller 1973). Ten Rhyne's text was a part of Sir William Osler's library (Peacher 1975) and in his *Principles and Practice of Medicine,* Osler prescribes acupuncture for lumbago (Osler 1913).

Apart from occasional explorations by the conventional medical community in the United States, the traditional medicine of China has been practiced in the United States since the middle of the 19th century. Herbal merchants, entrepreneurs, and physicians accompanied Chinese who sold their labor in the United States. The practice of the China Doctor of John Day Oregon, Doc Ing Hay probably is one of the most famous (Barlow & Richardson 1979). Ah Fong Chuck, who came to the United States in 1866, became the first licensed practitioner of that medicine in the United States in 1901, when he successfully won a medical license through legal action in Idaho (Muench 1984). With the strengthening of medical practice acts throughout the United States, the interruption of the herb supply from China, and the advent of World War II, these practices disappeared or retreated into Chinatowns nationwide.

Substantial attention was focused on acupuncture, the traditional medicine of China, and its regional variants, as a result of James Reston's highly publicized appendectomy and postoperative care in 1971 and the subsequent opening of China by Nixon. This caused varieties of medical practice that had been largely confined to Asia and the Chinatowns of America to gain visibility throughout the United States. Increased visibility led to substantial public interest in acupuncture and gradually to the licensure and development of training programs in many states. Today, 30 states (including the District of Columbia) license, certify, or register the practice of acupuncture and a range of other activities including herbal medicine by nonphysicians. There are at least 35 programs in the United States offering training in what is often understood as acupuncture and Oriental medicine.

In America, there has been a clear interest in the available range of expressions of the medical tradition of China. In the United States, European interpretations of the application of five phase theory, Korean constitutional acupuncture, traditional Chinese medicine (acupuncture, herbs, qigong, and tui na), Japanese meridian therapy, and special family lineages within the Chinese tradition all are taught and practiced. This willingness to accept and explore the traditional and contemporary interpretations of traditional Chinese medicine has led to the emergence of the concept of "Oriental medicine" as an umbrella term for the global domain of practice in this area.

Practice Settings

In general, traditional Chinese medicine is practiced in a range of clinical settings. Large hospitals entirely devoted to its practice are common in China. In this setting, acupuncture, herbal medicine, and tui na are provided both on an inpatient and outpatient basis. It is not unusual to see a large outpatient facility treating 20 patients simultaneously in the same space. Smaller practices and even roadside stands also are not unusual. Herbal prescriptions can be obtained from a Chinese herb store in almost any country that has a significant Chinese population. In Japan, small hospitals, large clinics, and private offices are typical settings.

Wherever the medicine is practiced, the settings in which it is delivered do not appear significantly different from the environment in which biomedical services are provided—unless the practitioner has a desire to emphasize the distinctive character of his or her practice, or if the practice is marginalized through lack of regulation. In the United States, record-keeping processes, insurance billing, the use of biomedical screening processes, and concerns surrounding office hygiene often produce a setting that—except for the presence of such peculiarities as acupuncture needles, moxa fluff, or herbs—looks very much like a typical physician's office.

Research and Evaluation

Many aspects of Chinese medicine have been the focus of concerted research efforts in China and Japan since the early part of this century. Recently, substantial research initiatives in this area have been undertaken in Europe and the United States as well.

The actual and perceived quality of such research, in both east and west, varies widely. As is the case for medical systems, research standards—even scientific research—are subject to cultural influences. Where the randomized, placebo controlled, and double blinded clinical trial is the definitive standard for an unambiguous biomedical recognition of efficacy, not all societies require or encourage their medical communities to secure knowledge in this fashion. Consequently, the simple accessibility of research data is influenced by the language and location of publication. These problems can inhibit the availability and use of information concerning research. Therefore, research that is meaningful to the scientific communities of China, Japan, Europe, or the United States does not have the same influence among other communities within that same group, and particularly on the biomedical communities of the United States or Europe.

Another problem that emerges in relation to clinical research in Chinese medicine is study design. Problems surrounding research methodology have come into focus as the Chinese medicine community within the United States and Europe has participated more in research, and as the biomedical community has become better educated about various modalities of Chinese medicine. Efforts by the Office of Alternative Medicine (OAM) under the National Institutes of Health in the United States have contributed to this process substantially. The OAM has hosted several conferences dealing with methodological considerations in the field of alternative medicine and each of these events has come to grips with aspects of traditional Chinese medicine.

Other projects supported by the OAM have included funding of numerous small research grants, many in the area of Chinese or Oriental medicine.

Office of Alternative Medicine Funded Studies

Medical Condition	Modality
Unipolar Depression	Acupuncture
Osteoarthritis	Acupuncture
Premenstrual Syndrome	Traditional Chinese Medicine
Common Warts	Chinese Herbal Therapy
Balance Disorders	Tai Ji
Menopausal Hot Flashes	Chinese Herbs
Postoperative Oral Surgery Pain	Acupuncture
Breech Version	Acupuncture and Moxibustion
Chronic Sinusitis in HIV Infection	Traditional Chinese Medicine
Hyperactivity	Acupuncture
Intractable Reflex Sympathetic Dystrophy	Qi Gong

The OAM also has sponsored a workshop on acupuncture in cooperation with the United States Food and Drug Administration. On April 21 and 22, 1994, members of the acupuncture, medical, and scientific community gave presentations detailing the safety and the apparent clinical efficacy of acupuncture needles. These presentations became the core of a petition that may lead to the reclassification of acupuncture needles in the United States.

Other organizations, such as the Society for Acupuncture Research (SAR), have emerged out of the broad-based community of acupuncturists, physicians, and researchers interested in the range of research issues posed by this field. The SAR holds annual meetings and publishes its proceedings. Among its objectives are scholarly exchange between researchers in the area of acupuncture, as well as other modalities related to Oriental medicine, the encouragement of research activities by acupuncturists, and the clarification of methodological issues related to research in these areas.

Research in Relation to Specific Areas of Chinese Medicine

Research on fundamental concepts, or what might be called fundamental theory, includes the exploration of whether concepts such as qi, the channels, acupuncture points, the diagnostic aspects of the pulse, and aspects of pattern diagnosis actually can refer to a reproducibly identifiable and quantifiable phenomenon. All of these areas have been or are being actively pursued in a number of countries. This research in these areas resembles basic research in physiology, and relies on the development of sophisticated models and the design of instrumentation to test those models.

Research questions formed by seeking the physiologic basis of Chinese medical concepts have been pursued for some time in China. One such study pursued the nature of kidney yang and reached the conclusion that patients displaying a diagnostic pattern associated with kidney yang vacuity showed low levels of 17-hydroxy cortical steriods in their urine, ultimately suggesting a relationship between the concept of kidney yang and the adrenal cortical system (Hao 1983).

Research on the correlation between the force and wave forms of the radial artery and the diagnostic perceptions of clinicians and the physical status of the patient has gone on for sometime now in China, the United States, Japan, and Korea (Broffman & McCulloch 1986, Takashima 1995, Zhu 1991). Typically, this research depends on the use of pressure sensors that are pressed against the skin overlying the radial artery, in a manner and location that replicates that of the finger position of the traditional clinician. Pulse patterns are recorded and correlated to observations made by the clinician in an effort to determine the physical basis that must be present for a diagnostic perception. Preliminary results are intriguing, but methodological questions concerning population size and standardization of measurement remain.

Research concerning channels and acupuncture points has relied on a variety of techniques, including the measurement of electrical resistance, ther-

mography, tracing the pathways of injected radioisotopes, and dissection. This last has not produced particularly interesting results. The so-called Bonghan corpuscles, identified on dissection by Kim Bong Han in Korea, once were proposed as the anatomical basis of acupuncture points. This research has not been replicated, and although reference is occasionally made to it in contemporary materials, (Burton Goldberg Group 1993), it generally is not perceived as credible.

More interesting are the discussions that propose or demonstrate an archaic or cellularly mediated signaling system utilizing the bioelectrical properties of the body to propagate information. Early contributors in this area include Robert O. Becker, an orthopedist whose interest in the body's bioelectric properties and bone healing led him to explore the electrical properties of acupuncture points and channel pathways (Reichmanis et al 1975, Becker 1985). A component of this hypothesis is the measurable, lowered electrical resistance of the skin at acupuncture points. This unusual electrical property is characteristic of many acupuncture points (Pomeranz 1988).

Yoshio Manaka, a Japanese surgeon and acupuncturist, hypothesized the presence of an archaic signaling system he called the X-signal System, based on information theory concepts of biological systems, his reading of texts such as the *Inner Classic* and the *Classic of Difficult Issues,* and experimental observations in his acupuncture clinic (Manaka & Itaya 1994). His perspective grew out of exploration of both Chinese and Japanese needling methods and the use of the gentler needling techniques associated with the school of meridian therapy that arose in Japan.

In his extensive discussion of the biophysical basis of acupuncture phenomena, James Oschman observes that the solid state phenomena and the piezo electric properties of the body's connective tissues provide a potential structure and mechanism that would allow for the existence of a signaling system similar to the role of the channels and points described in traditional literature (Oschman 1993). Oschman goes on to explore a rich range of topics, including the measurable emission of electromagnetic fields from the hands of qigong practitioners (Seto et al 1992).

All of these discussions are preliminary. Even in cases where research has been carried out and replicated, as in the case of lowered electrical resistance over acupuncture points, there is a need for continued exploration. It is unlikely that we will see a precise validation of the concepts of Chinese medicine in these areas, but rather a validation of the physiological basis for the existence of such concepts. It may be that the genius of Chinese medicine in these areas lies in its ability to generalize about the manifestations of incredibly complex biological phenomena in an articulate and useful fashion. Given the preliminary findings concerning the possible nature of acupuncture points and channels, or the variety of mechanisms that seem to be involved in acupuncture as a therapeutic phenomena, it seems increasingly likely that a concept such as "qi," or the therapeutic effects of an acupuncture point, must represent the action of many discrete and identifiable physiological processes. The likelihood is that aspects of these processes, observed as a whole, are the basis of the traditional concept.

Materia Medica and Traditional Pharmacology

Investigations of materia medica and traditional pharmacology have been ongoing since the early part of this century, in both China and Japan. This is an area where the quality of research work is generally high, and the availability of translated literature is comparatively extensive. This is because research in this area can be divided into two areas: the examination of the pharmacological properties of traditional materia medica and the clinical efficacy of traditional pharmacology. The first area does not differ from the typical concerns of pharmacological research. In vitro studies and exploration of traditional use can suggest the potential usefulness of certain substances. If one becomes aware of a substance that is alleged to have pharmacological properties, it is comparatively easy to conduct studies to assess the presence of these properties and to isolate apparently active compounds.

A famous case in point is the first herb listed in the Chinese materia medica: *Herba Ephedra,* known botanically as *Ephedra Sinica* Stapf (*ma huang*). Herba Ephedra is recorded in the *Divine Husbandman's Classic of Materia Medica*. Its chief active component was isolated in 1887 in Japan, but remained largely unexplored for 35 years, until CF Schmidt and KK Chen began to explore its pharmacological effects at the Peking Union Medical College, where the department of pharmacology was beginning a systematic exploration of the Chinese materia medica (Chen 1977).

These explorations revealed that ephedrine was a sympathomimetic with properties of epinephrine, causing an increase in blood pressure, vasoconstriction, and bronchodilation. Clinically, it had several distinct advantages over epinephrine: it could be used orally; it had a long duration of action; and it was less toxic. It also was found to be useful in the management of bronchial asthma and hay fever, and to support the patient's vital signs during the administration of spinal anesthesia. In subsequent years, it became possible to synthesize ephedrine. Today, we encounter this product of the Chinese materia medica in a number of pharmaceuticals, including over the counter products as Sudafed and Actifed.

Historically and clinically, Herba Ephedra has been applied in a similar fashion in Chinese medicine, excepting spinal anesthesia. As we saw above, it is a principle ingredient in the herbal formula Ephedra Decoction. This herb also figures prominently in formulae that are applied to presentations that relate to asthma and allergy. Herba Ephedra represents an early and impressive example of pharmacological research in the Chinese materia medica. Other examples where the traditional clinical applications of single herbs is supported in recent clinical experimentation include *Herba Artemisiae (yin chen hao)* for hepatitis and *Caulis Mu Tong (mu tong)* for urinary tract infections. Extensive compilations discussing identified active constituents, clinical studies, and toxicity of large numbers of substances have been prepared (Chang 1986).

Explorations of traditional pharmacology are somewhat more complex although, they too are amenable to the methods of double blinding and placebo control that are critical to recognition in the biomedical world. However, given the breadth of possible substances that may be applied clinically (over 5000), and the number of possible permutations for their combination in formula, the scope of the inquiry becomes quite large. In addition, there is the question of whether or not to include the traditional considerations that surround diagnosis and pattern identification in the process of prescription and selection of herbal formulas for investigation. Some contemporary studies are designed to take this into account, with the traditional clinician being able to assign individuals to specific treatment groups based on symptomatology, while still being blinded in relation to the actual constituents of the substances administered to the patient. Research in this area has been extensive both in China and Japan, and is beginning to emerge in the United States. As can be seen from the list of OAM funded studies, a number of research projects are beginning in these areas. In addition, other researchers are independently pursuing the investigation of traditionally organized compounds in the management of HIV-related symptomatology.

Acupuncture

> Disappointingly little has been achieved by literally hundreds of attempts to evaluate acupuncture. Major methodological flaws are apparent in the vast majority of studies (Vincent 1993).

Vincent was speaking to a concern that is shared by many individuals working in the area of acupuncture research. Despite the relatively early interest in acupuncture as a form of alternative or complementary medicine, comparatively few studies have been designed in a fashion that renders their results useful to other researchers, clinicians, or policy makers.

Despite general concerns among workers in the field, research on acupuncture in the west displays promising results in a number of areas. The Workshop on Acupuncture that was sponsored by the Office of Alternative Medicine presented results in areas that were thought to represent the best and most positive research related to acupuncture. These areas were pain management, substance abuse treatment, antiemesis treatment, the treatment of paralysis due to stroke, and the treatment of pulmonary disease.

The use of acupuncture for the treatment of pain is an area of long-standing medical interest. Pain control is the one application of acupuncture that has been used repeatedly by the traditional medical community in Europe and the United States for many years. This area became visible in the 1970s as a result of Chinese reports on acupuncture anesthesia. As a result, this is one of the most widely researched of acupuncture applications. However, it also is one of the most problematic.

Some of the problems that are typical of researching acupuncture treatments for pain, as well as acupuncture therapy in general, are exemplified by the results of two meta-analyses of studies examining acupuncture in the management of chronic pain. A meta-analysis is a research method that pools the results of many studies in an effort to try to reach a more powerful conclusion than an individual study might provide. The first was conducted by pooling data from 14 studies that used randomized and controlled trials of acupuncture to treat chronic pain, and that measured their outcomes in terms of the number of patients whose condition was improved (Patel 1989). This study reached a number of conclusions concerning the relationship of study design to research outcomes, and concluded that acupuncture compared favorably with placebo and conventional treatment.

A second meta-analysis reviewed 51 studies and compared the quality of published controlled clinical trials on the basis of research designs and specific factors including randomization, single and double blinding, and numbers of subjects. This meta-analysis concluded that of the studies reviewed those favorable to acupuncture were more poorly designed than those that associated negative results with acupuncture. The evidence suggested that the efficacy of acupuncture as a treatment for chronic pain is doubtful (ter Riet et al 1990).

A careful review of the ter Reit meta-analysis by Delis and Morris suggested that its authors had "included studies which did not meet their criteria," such as a study that was not controlled or where laser light was used instead of acupuncture needles (Delis 1993). This finding prompted them to conduct their own analysis and to reanalyze the studies examined by ter Riet in relation to a number of factors, including investigator training and the appropriateness of treatment. Their meta-analysis showed a trend towards improvement in study design over time, suggesting that many poorly designed acupuncture studies might be viewed best as preliminary efforts by investigators who were sufficiently familiar with the modality to design effective studies.

All three of these meta-analyses pointed out significant issues in relation to acupuncture study design. Besides questions concerning randomization, blinding, placebo control, and sample size, a variety of questions emerged pertinent to the practice of acupuncture as a distinct modality. Is the investigator trained in acupuncture? Is the acupuncture treatment appropriate for the condition? Does the study allow for adjusting the treatment to the individual patient's needs according to traditional diagnostics? Are outcome measures clear? Is placebo or sham acupuncture used and how will it be administered?

Of all the debated areas in acupuncture research, this last may receive the most attention. The problem of how to provide a sham treatment in acupuncture is a vexing one. In herbal studies, a capsule of inert material that appears similar to the capsule of the medication being investigated can be provided to the patient. Since the patient cannot tell the difference between the two capsules, he or she is effectively blind to the use of a placebo. In acupuncture, the problem is more complex, since patients receiving treatment definitely know whether they have been stuck with needles or not. Solutions that have been proposed vary from comparing real acupuncture to other modalities, to carefully selecting a treatment with few effects (Vincent 1993), or selecting acupuncture points that are entirely irrelevant (BRITS method) to the conditions being treated (Birch 1995).

The potential importance of traditional diagnostic and therapeutic considerations in trial design have been raised by a number of authors (Jobst 1995, Ergil 1995, Coan 1980). At the same time, some researchers and physicians reject the potential importance of these ideas. Vincent tells us that traditional ideas need to be understood in outline, but that questions about efficacy can be asked without considering them in detail. The treatment may be effective whether or not the theory is valid (Vincent 1993). Hans Agren attempted to make this distinction over 20 years ago, in order to identify suitable research agendas, arguing that only the simple empirical observations of Chinese medicine should be an object of medical inquiry (Agren 1975). The question emerging from some clinical researchers is whether some aspects of traditional theory are relevant to the delivery of effective treatment and, consequently, the inquiry.

Although the control of pain is considered to be a major area for the clinical application of acupuncture, research in this area has been problematic. However, a number of individual studies strongly suggest the clinical relevance of acupuncture to pain management. Among some of the more notable studies are a clinical trial involving 43 women with menstrual pain, in which women receiving acupuncture treatment had considerably less pain than the placebo and control groups (Helms 1987). A controlled trial of acupuncture in the management of migraines involved 30 patients suffering from chronic migraines. Acupuncture was significantly effective in controlling the pain of migraine headaches (Vincent 1989). Several studies of the management of various types of back pain with acupuncture also have shown it to be helpful. Arthritis pain seems to respond to acupuncture therapy (Christensen 1992).

Research in the area of antiemesis revolves around the use of the acupuncture point Inner Gate (*neiguan*, P6) to control nausea and vomiting. The use of this point in acupressure to control nausea and vomiting is well known, and its use to control the nausea of pregnancy with pressure bands has been determined to be effective (Aloysio & Penacchioni 1992). There even are consumer products available that exploit this effect. The point also has been investigated in relation to its use in controlling perioperative emesis that resulted from premedication and anesthetic agents (Ghaly et al 1987) and in relation to cancer chemotherapy (Dundee et al 1989).

Based on clinical experiences in China, acupuncture is used extensively in the United States for the management of symptomatology associated with withdrawal from a variety of substances, including alcohol and cocaine. The summary conclusion reached by presenters at the Workshop on Acupuncture panel on substance abuse suggested that early trial and empirical findings suggest positive treatment effects (Kiresuk & Culliton 1994).

Acupuncture has been studied clinically in the west in relation to the management of a variety of specific medical conditions, among them pulmonary disease and paralysis subsequent to stroke. An extensive review of acupuncture in pulmonary disease led the author to conclude that acupuncture produced favorable effects in the management of patients with bronchial asthma, chronic bronchitis, and chronic disabling breathlessness (Jobst 1995). A recent study involving 16 patients with right sided paralysis who had experienced an ischemic infarction of the left hemisphere showed acupuncture produced a good response in patients whose lesion affected no more than half the motor pathway areas (Naeser et al 1992).

It should be pointed out that while the volume of published research on acupuncture in the west is relatively low—by one count there are 200 randomized controlled trials, 42 review articles, and four meta-analyses (Foreman 1995)—the amount of research conducted in the areas discussed above and in many other areas is vast. Although study and publication quality can be a problem, and design issues are still present, acupuncture research in China must be regarded as a significant resource. One English compilation contains 117 Chinese studies on acupuncture and moxibustion (Research on Acupuncture, Moxibustion, and Acupuncture Anesthesia 1986). Recent shifts in study design and analysis displayed at conferences in China and in newer publications suggest that the trend towards improved research design observed by Delis in the west might be at work in the east as well.

Acknowledgments

As is apparent from the text, this presentation owes a heavy debt to the work of Paul Unschuld and Nigel Wiseman. The scholarship and enterprise of these two individuals is reflected in their work and the help that they have provided to students of Chinese medicine such as myself. My wife and colleague Marnae Ergil contributed enormously by reviewing text, answering questions, and being willing to check technical points in Chinese language materials at any hour of the day or night. This project would not have been possible to complete without the deep institutional commitment to scholarship and the support provided of the Pacific College of Oriental Medicine.

References

Agren H. 1975. A new approach to Chinese traditional medicine. Am J Chin Med 3(3):207–212

Aloysio DD, Penacchioni P. 1992. Morning sickness control in early pregnancy by Neiguan point acupressure. Obstet Gyenecol 80(5, November):852–854

Auteroche B, Gervais G, Auteroche M, et al. 1992. Acupuncture and Moxibustion: A Guide to Clinical Practice. Churchill Livingstone. Edinburgh

Bannerman RH. 1979. The World Health Organization viewpoint on acupuncture. World Health, December, 24–29

Barlow J, Richardson C. 1979. China Doctor of John Day. Binford and Mort. Portland

Becker RO. 1985. The Body Electric: Electromagnetism and the Foundation of Life. Quill William Morrow. New York

Bensky D, Barolet R. 1990. Chinese Herbal Medicine: Formulas and Strategies. Eastland Press Inc. Seattle

Bensky D, Gamble A. 1986. Chinese Herbal Medicine: Materia Medica (Revised Edition). Eastland Press Inc. Seattle

Birch S. 1994. A historical study of radial pulse six position Diagnosis: naming the unnameable. J Acupun Soc NY 1(3&4):19–32

Birch S. 1995. A biophysical basis for acupuncture. In Birch S (ed). Proceedings of the Second Symposium of the Society for Acupuncture Research. Society for Acupuncture Research. Boston, pp. 274–294

Bowers JZ. 1970. Western Medical Pioneers in Feudal Japan. Johns Hopkins Press. Baltimore

Broffman M, McCulloch M. 1986. Instrument-assisted pulse evaluation in the acupuncture practice. Am J Acupuncture 14(3, July–September):255–259

Burton Goldberg Group. 1993. Acupuncture. In Alternative Medicine: The Definitive Guide. Strohecker J (ed). Future Medicine Publishing, Inc. Puyallup. p. 37–46

Chang HM. 1986. Pharmacology and Applications of Chinese Materia Medica. Hson-Mou Chang HM, Pui-Hay But P (eds). Yao S-C, Wang L-L, Chang-Shing Yeung S (trans). World Scientific Publishing Co. Singapore. p. 1–773

Chen KK. 1977. Half a century of ephedrine. In Kao FF, and Kao JJ. (eds). Chinese Medicine—New Medicine. Neale Watson Academic Publications, Inc. New York. pp. 21–27

Christensen BV, Iuhl IU, Vilbe KH, et al. 1992. Acupuncture treatment of severe knee osteoarthritis. Acta Anaesthesiol Scand (36):519–525

Chuang Y. 1982. The Historical Development of Acupuncture. Oriental Healing Arts Institute. Los Angeles

Coan R, Wong GT, Ku S-L, et al. 1980. The acupuncture treatment of low back pain: a randomized controlled study. Am J Chin Med 8(2):181–189

Delis K, Morris M. 1993. Clinical Trials in Acupuncture. In Birch S (ed). Proceedings of the First Symposium of the Society of Acupuncture Research. Society for Acupuncture Research. Boston. p. 68–71

Dundee JW, Ghaly RG, Fitzpatrick KTJ, et al. 1989. Acupuncture prophylaxis of cancer chemotherapy induced sickness. J R Soc Med 82:268–271

Ellis A, Wiseman N, Boss K. 1991. Fundamentals of Chinese Acupuncture. Paradigm. Brookline

Ergil KV. 1995. Chinese specific condition review: urinary tract infections. Protocol J Botan Med 1(1, Summer): 130–133

Ergil KV. 1995. Where tradition matters: identifying epistemological and terminological issues in research design. Proc 2nd Sym Soc Acupunc Res 59–69

Ergil MC. 1994. Medical education in China. CCAOM News 1(1, Spring):3–5

Farquhar J. 1987. Problems of knowledge in contemporary Chinese medical discourse. Soc Sci Med 24(12): 1013–1021

Foreman J. 1995. What the research shows. The Boston Globe, 22/5, 25, 27

Ghaly RG, Fitzpatrick KTJ, Dundee JW. 1987. Anaesthesia 42:1108–1110

Haller JS. 1973. Acupuncture in nineteenth century western medicine. NYS J Med

Hao LZ. 1983. An attempt to understand the substance of kidney and its disorders. Cheung CS (trans). J Am Coll Tradit Chin Med 1983(3):82–97

Helms JM. 1987. Acupuncture for the management of primary dysmenorrhea. Obstet Gynecol 69(1):51–56

Hirsch RC. 1985. Korean constitutional nutrition. J Am Coll Tradit Chin Med 1985(1):24–37

Hsu E. 1989. Outline of the history of acupuncture in Europe. J Chin Med (29, January):28–32

Hsu H, Peacher W. 1977. Chen's History of Chinese Medical Science. Modern Drug Publishers. Taipei

Huang B, Di F, Li X, et al. 1993. Syndromes of Traditional Chinese Medicine. Huang B (ed). Ma D, Guo'en W, Sun S, Cao H (trans). Heilongjiang Education Press. Heilongjiang

Huard P, Wong M. 1968. Chinese Medicine. McGraw Hill, World University Library. New York

Jobst K. 1995. A critical analysis of acupuncture in pulmonary disease: efficacy and safety of the acupuncture needle. J Altern Comple Med (1, January):57–86

Kaptchuk TJ. 1983. The Web That Has No Weaver: Understanding Chinese Medicine. Congdon and Weed. New York

Kiresuk TJ, Culliton PD. 1994. Overview of Substance Abuse Acupuncture Treatment Research. Workshop on Acupuncture. p. 1–17, 21/4

Kleinman A. 1986. Social Origins of Distress and Disease: Depression, Neurasthenia, and Pain in Modern China. Yale University Press. New Haven

Lee JK, Bae SKB. 1981. Korean Acupuncture Ko Mun Sa

Lin Y. 1942. Laotse, the Book of Tao. In Lin Y (ed). The Wisdom of China and India. The Modern Library. New York. p. 578–624

Lock M. 1980. East Asian Medicine in Urban Japan. Comparative Studies of Health Systems, vol. 4. University of California Press. Berkeley

Maciocia G. 1989. The Foundations of Chinese Medicine. Churchill Livingstone. Edinburgh

Manaka Y, Itaya K. 1994. Acupuncture as intervention in the biological information system. J Acupunct S NY 1(3 & 4):19–32

Muench C. 1984. One Hundred Years of Medicine: The Ah-Fong Physicians of Idaho. In Schwarz HG (ed). Chinese Medicine on the Golden Mountain: An Interpretive Guide. Washington Commission for the Humanities. Seattle. p. 51–80

Naeser MA, Michael PA, Stiassny-Eder D, et al. 1992. Real versus sham acupuncture in the treatment of paralysis in acute stroke patients: A CT Scan Lesion Study. J Neurol Rehab (6):163–173

Oschman J. 1993. A Biophysical Basis for Acupuncture. In Birch S (ed). Proceedings of the First Symposium of the Society for Acupuncture Research. Society for Acupuncture Research. Boston. p. 141–220

Osler W. 1913. The Principles and Practice of Medicine. D. Appleton and Co. New York

Patel M, Gutzwiller F, Paccand F, Marazzi A. 1989. A meta-analysis of acupuncture for chronic pain. Int J Epidemiol 18(4):900–906

Payer L. 1988. Medicine and Culture: Varieties of Treatment in the United States, England, West Germany, and France. Henry Holt and Company. New York

Peacher W. 1975. Adverse reactions, contraindications and complications of acupuncture and moxibustion. Am J Chin Med 3(1):35–46

Pomeranz B. 1988. Scientific Basis of Acupuncture. In Stox G (ed). The Basics of Acupuncture. Springer-Verlag. New York. p. 4–37

Qiu. 1993. Chinese Acupuncture and Moxibustion. Churchill Livingstone. New York

Reichmanis M, Marino AA, Becker RO. 1975. Electrical correlates of acupuncture points. IEEE Trans Bio Engineer November, 533–535

Seto A, Kusaka S, Nakazatio W, et al. 1992. Detection of extraordinary large bio-magnetic field strength from human hand. Intern J Acupunct Electrother 17:75–94

Shanghai College of Traditional Chinese Medicine. 1981. Acupuncture: A Comprehensive Text. O'Connor J, Bensky D (trans). Eastland. Seattle

Sivin N. 1987. Traditional Medicine in Contemporary China. Science, Medicine and Technology in East Asia, vol. 2. Center for Chinese Studies The University of Michigan. Ann Arbor

Takashima M. 1995. Pulse Research. Personal Communication

ter Riet G, Kleijnen J, Knipschild P. 1990. Acupuncture and chronic pain: a criteria-based meta-analysis. J Clin Epidemiol 43:1191–1199

Unschuld P. 1979. Medical Ethics in Imperial China: A Study in Historical Anthropology. University of California, Berkeley, California

Unschuld P. 1985. Medicine in China: A History of Ideas. University of California. Berkeley

Veith I. 1972. The Yellow Emperors's Classic of Internal Medicine. Veith I (trans). University of California Press. Berkeley

Vincent CA. 1989. A controlled trial of the treatment of migraine by acupuncture. Clin J Pain 5:305–312

Vincent CA. 1993. Acupuncture as a treatment for chronic pain. In Lewith GT, Aldridge D (eds). Clinical Research Methodology for Complementary Therapies. Hodder and Stoughton. London. p. 289–308

Wang G, Fan Y, Guan Z. 1990. Chinese Massage. In Zhang E (ed). WenPing Y (trans). A Practical English-Chinese Library of Traditional Chinese Medicine. Publishing House of Shanghai. College of Traditional Chinese Medicine. Shanghai

Wang X. 1986. Research on the Origin and Development of Chinese Acupuncture and Moxibustion. In Xiangtong Z (ed). Research on Acupuncture, Moxibustion and Acupuncture Anesthesia. Springer-Verlag. New York. p. 783–799

Wilhelm R. 1967. The I Ching. Third. Baynes CF (trans). Princeton University Press. Princeton

Wiseman N. 1993. A List of Chinese Formulas. unpublished paper, Taiwan

Wiseman N, Boss K. 1990. Glossary of Chinese Medical Terms and Acupuncture Points. Paradigm Publications. Brookline

Wiseman N, Ellis A, Zmiewski P, Li C. 1985. Fundamentals of Chinese Medicine. In Zmiewski P (ed). Wiseman N, Ellis A (trans). Paradigm. Brookline

Wiseman N, Ellis A, Zmiewski P, Li C. 1993. Fundamentals of Chinese Medicine. SMC Publishing Inc. Taipei

Wiseman N, Ellis A, Zmiewski P, Li C. 1995. In Wiseman N, Ellis A (trans). Fundamentals of Chinese Medicine. Paradigm. Brookline (in press)

Wong CK, Wu TL. 1985. History of Chinese Medicine: Being a Chronicle of Medical Happenings in China from Ancient Times to the Present Period. Southern Materials Center, Inc. Taipei

Xianytong Z. 1986. Research on Acupuncture, Moxibustion, and Acupuncture Anesthesia. Springer-Verlag. New York

Zhu B. 1991. Pulse Research in China. Personal Communication

Qigong in Traditional Chinese Medicine

Charles T. McGee
Kenneth Sancier
Effie Poy Yew Chow

Chinese Qigong is an ancient healing discipline that emerged from centuries of secrecy in the early 1980s. Because of its unusual nature, Qigong is rapidly attracting the interest of the public as well as scientists in China and elsewhere. In China, Qigong is referred to as the jewel of Traditional Chinese Medicine.

Qigong (pronounced chee goong and also spelled Chi Kung, Qi Gong, Chi Gong, Chi Gung, among others) is a discipline consisting of breathing and mental exercises. These are usually, but not always, combined with physical exercises. Qigong balances the subtle energy system in the body described in the theories of Traditional Chinese Medicine (TCM). As with many traditions in China, Qigong developed in many isolated locations over many years, leading to the development of literally thousands of variations.

History

For approximately 900 years, people in China gathered each morning to practice taiji (tai chi chuan), a martial art exercise that was developed from Qigong. Taiji is a useful discipline for maintaining health and energy levels, and for controlling some disease conditions such as high blood pressure. Most taiji practitioners have switched to Qigong, however, because Qigong exercises produce much stronger healing effects. Eighty million people in China now arise early every morning to practice Qigong in groups in parks. They continue this practice because of the improvements they experience in their own levels of energy and stamina. They also are aware of documented reports of miraculous healings that baffle western scientists. Improvements have been documented in a wide range of conditions including cases of complete recovery from paralysis caused by strokes and spinal cord injury, many forms of cancer, multiple sclerosis, and cerebral palsy (McGee et al 1994).

Widespread acceptance of Qigong in China occurred quickly because of two spectacular cases that were reported on national television. The first case was of a prominent 21-year-old athlete who developed lung cancer in the early 1980s. His physicians advised treatment with standard western approaches, but he rejected this recommendation. He tried to cure his condition using only the practice of Guo Lin Gong, a walking form of Qigong, which he practiced 10 to 14 hours every day. The method is named after a woman named Guo Lin who cured herself of widespread recurrent uterine cancer in the 1960s. The athlete's cancer slowly shrank and he achieved complete cure. Pretreatment chest radiographs showed a large tumor in the left upper chest that disappeared totally by the end of 10 months. Currently, one million cancer patients practice this form of Qigong daily in China.

The second highly publicized case was a 36-year-old man who was injured in a factory accident in 1987, suffering a depressed skull fracture, compression fracture of L2 vertebra with a spinal cord injury, and paraplegia. Seven months later, he still was unable to move his legs. At that time, a famous Qigong master (and doctor of TCM) treated him for 6 consecutive hours (from 10 miles away). The man walked with crutches immediately. Two months later, he walked up the Great Wall with only a slight limp, accompanied by the Qigong master and 11 other patients who had been cured miraculously. Qigong quickly became a household word in China.

Written records on Qigong go back 4000 years and document the input of energy concepts from India, Tibet, and China. For almost all of that time, the most effective forms of Qigong were secrets available only to elite classes in China such as dynasty family members, medical practitioners, monks in Buddhist monasteries, and intellectuals. In the late 1970s, the Chinese government became aware of an increase in Qigong activities, which had been banned during the Cultural Revolution. Officials expressed serious doubts about Qigong because it resembled religious and superstitious practices, which were banned routinely. The government commissioned and funded several scientific studies. When a scientific basis was established for Qigong, the government allowed it to be added to the list of treatment methods offered in the nationwide system of TCM hospitals (Personal communication). Shuyu Kong, PhD, President, Sino-Foreign Health Technology Exchange Center, Beijing.

The word Qigong is derived from two words, qi and gong. Qi is the modern pinyin Mandarin term for the vital energy and life force in our bodies, as well as breath. Gong can be translated as work or discipline. Qigong has been defined in many ways, including "air energy," "breath work," and "energy work."

For most people, Qigong is a do-it-yourself discipline that can improve health and prevent disease. Most practitioners spend about 30 minutes a day doing Qigong exercises, plus another 30 minutes in meditation. With serious practice, some become Qigong masters, defined as people who have developed the ability to emit healing energy from the body, and who have achieved proven success in healing with qi (energy). In addition, small numbers of people have been identified who have natural healing abilities yet never practiced Qigong, referred to as people with "natural abilities." It is common knowledge in China that top officials in the government and the Communist Party receive daily energy balancing treatments from their own personal Qigong masters.

Theory

According to the theories of TCM, a vital energy system exists in the body through which flows qi, the life force. The pathways of this system are called meridians or channels. They do not correspond to any identifiable anatomic structures such as nerves, veins, arteries, or lymphatics. Energy points along the pathways can be treated in a variety of ways to alter levels of energy. Treatment includes needles (acupuncture), heat, electric current, Qigong energy emission, laser, and pressure.

The existence of this energy system has been verified scientifically. Energy points themselves can be identified easily with electronic instruments because skin resistance over these points is markedly lower than that of surrounding skin. They can be seen with Kirlian high voltage photography techniques (Personal communication). Energy channels and the direction of energy flow through them have been verified in French and Chinese studies using radioisotopes. When injected into an energy point, a radioisotope will migrate up or down an energy channel in the precise direction and path described in 2000-year-old texts (Tiberiu 1981, Darras 1989, deVernejoul et al 1992).

According to TCM theories, when energy is flowing through this system at normal levels, in balance, the body stays healthy, resistant to disease, and can activate its own healing efforts. When imbalances or blockages occur, physiology is affected, followed eventually by pathologic changes.

Therefore, if a person is healthy, various modalities of TCM can be combined and practiced to maintain good health and prevent disease. If a person is ill, the person can regain health by re-establishing a normal balance in the energy system. All of the treatment modalities in TCM are designed to achieve this harmony, and Qigong is its most powerful method.

Research

Most clinical and experimental research on Qigong has been carried out in China during the past 15 years. With few exceptions, English descriptions of these research studies are contained in abstracts printed in the proceedings of nine international Qigong conferences dating back to 1986.* The abstracts number more than 800 and range in length from a few lines to short papers of several pages, making Qigong an intensively studied healing method in alternative and complementary medicine.

These abstracts often contain detailed information on research protocols including controlled experiments, results, statistical analysis, and conclusions. While the research may not always meet strict scientific standards, the immense scope of research on Qigong and the favorable results reported provide confidence in Qigong's potential for improving health care in the west. The body of scientific research performed in China on medical applications of Qigong is too large and significant to be ignored.

One of the most intriguing aspects of Qigong is the subject of emitted qi. Emitted qi is defined as energy that is emitted from the body of a Qigong master—generally, but not necessarily, from the hand—when the master is in the "Qigong state." In most cases, the master holds his or her hand above an object or person and concentrates on emitting energy to the object.

The effects of emitted qi have been demonstrated in many ways. Its application in human studies has been followed by improvement in many medical conditions, including the function of the immune system. In animal studies, emitted qi has altered heart rates and slowed the growth rate of induced cancers. In clinical laboratory experiments, emitted qi has been shown to kill bacteria and viruses progressively as the time of exposure to emitted qi increases. In agricultural studies, the germination rate of rice and wheat seeds has increased or decreased according to the intent of the Qigong master. In the physics laboratory, emitted qi has been reported to alter the physical properties of matter (McGee et al 1994).

The Qigong Institute, East West Academy of Healing Arts, has reviewed selected scientific studies of the medical applications of Qigong (Sancier 1991). Sancier has studied the effects of Qigong on the body (Sancier 1989, Sancier 1994) and has led an effort to systematize the information published on Qigong by developing a computerized Qigong database in English.

When first hearing of Qigong, it is natural for scientists and medical practitioners to seek evidence of Qigong's measurable effects on the body. A partial list of these is presented below: from the Qigong database. Most research studies used the self-practice of Qigong exercises but in a few cases, emitted qi was used as therapy. Research illustrates that Qigong can affect many functions of the body and can alleviate many different diseases and medical conditions. This list is far from complete. Furthermore, this information was developed in reference to studies of given diseases and medical conditions; it is reasonable to expect that Qigong can affect many different body functions. This suggests that western health care could benefit by incorporating Qigong into its treatment protocols (McGee et al 1994). Qigong's effects may be considered global, as it affects many different parts and functions of the body.

Diseases and Medical Conditions Studied in Which Beneficial Effects of Qigong Have Been Reported

- Aging
- Allergy
- Asthma
- Bone fractures
- Cancer
- Cardiovascular disorders
- Cervical spondylosis
- Circulation
- Deafness

(Continues)

---

* Proceedings of these conferences are available from the East West Academy of Healing Arts, 450 Sutter Street, Suite 2104, San Francisco, California 94108.

- Diabetes
- Digestion disorders
- Gallstones
- Gastrointestinal disorders
- Headache
- Hepatitis
- Hormone balance
- Hypertension
- Immunodeficiencies
- Impotency
- Inflammation
- Injuries
- Joint diseases
- Kidney disorders
- Liver disorders
- Lung disorders
- Mental health
- Myopia
- Paralysis
- Personality
- Stroke
- Tumors

The following section outlines the results of a small number of controlled studies conducted in academic institutions and hospitals throughout China.

Aging

Although aging is accepted as a natural phenomenon, research has shown that Qigong exercise confers beneficial effects on strength, health, and longevity. One double-blind, clinical study determined the effects of Qigong on blood levels of superoxide dismutase (SOD), which scavenges harmful superoxide radicals and promotes immunologic function (Hefen 1993). For this study, 100 male and 100 female retirees, aged 52 to 76 years, were divided into a Qigong exercise group and a control group. Each group consisted of 50 men and 50 women.

The Qigong exercise selected incorporated relaxation, breathing exercises with massage, a relaxation breathing exercise, and a walking exercise. Exercises were practiced for a minimum of 30 minutes per day for 1 year. Progress was evaluated by clinical observations and by determining SOD activity.

Analysis showed SOD levels were greater in sub-jects who practiced Qigong. In female subjects, the SOD level in blood erythrocytes was 2718.15 ± 593.6 u/g hemoglobin for the Qigong group and 1704.3 ± 572.84 u/g hemoglobin for the control group ($p < 0.001$). In male subjects, the SOD level was 2740.85 ± 602.16 u/g hemoglobin in the Qigong group and 1678.18 ± 484.14 u/g hemoglobin in the control group ($p < 0.001$). The results indicate that Qigong exercise can elevate blood levels of SOD. This may be one way in which Qigong promotes longevity while maintaining energy and good health in older people.

Cancer

One study involved 123 people with advanced cancer of several different types, who were treated simultaneously with drugs and Qigong (Quizhi 1988). Patients were divided into a Qigong group (N = 97) and a control group (N = 30). All patients received drug therapy, and in addition, the Qigong group did Qigong exercises for more than 2 hours a day for 3 to 6 months. Symptoms, signs, body weight, and immunologic indices were recorded before and after the study.

The Qigong group showed much greater improvements than the control group in symptoms and signs such as strength, appetite, bowel function, weight gain of 3 kg or greater, and phagocytic rate. The authors concluded that Qigong therapy is helpful to some extent in ameliorating symptoms, improving appetite, strengthening the constitution, and hence increasing the ability for self-cure. Furthermore, Qigong is simple, easy to learn, and has no side effects. This study suggests that a combination therapy of Qigong and drugs is superior to drug therapy alone.

In a study performed at the China Immunology Research Center, human stomach cancer cells in tissue culture were treated with emitted qi for 1 hour. In 41 separate trials, an average of 25 percent of qi-treated cells were either killed or inactivated, whereas cells in control specimens remained unaffected (Lida 1988).

In the same report, human uterine cervix cancer cells in tissue culture were treated with emitted qi for 20 minutes. In 20 separate trials the combined killing and inactivation rates were between 13 and 36 percent. In control samples, all cancer cells remained unaffected.

Paralysis

In one study, 43 patients with paralysis practiced Qigong themselves and also were treated with emitted qi. Before the study 6 patients walked without assistance, and 7 could manage daily necessities, these numbers rose to 20 and 34, respectively, following Qigong. After treatment, some patients who used wheelchairs could walk with crutches, and those who originally needed two crutches could walk with one crutch (Huang 1988).

Patients were evaluated by commonly used indices of rehabilitation. The treatment was judged to be excellent in 23 percent, good in 47 percent, fair in 23 percent, and ineffective in 7 percent. The total effectiveness rate was 93 percent.

In another study, 18 small pigs were divided into a treatment group (N = 12) and a control group (N = 6). All of the pigs were given a spinal cord injury by Allen's method, which stretches the spinal cord, producing a paraplegia. Twelve of the pigs were treated with Ba Gua Induction Qigong (emitted qi) two to three times a day. The six control pigs were not treated. After 89 consecutive days of treatment, 11 of 12 pigs treated with Qigong could walk using their previously paralyzed hind legs. None of the six control pigs regained the ability to walk (Jing 1993A).

Diabetes

A clinical study was carried out to determine the effect of Qigong on 31 subjects with type II diabetes (Jing et al 1993B). A group of 31 middle-aged to elderly subjects practiced Qigong exercises (hui-chungong exercises), and several observations were made. There was no effect on body weight. Fasting blood sugar reduced from an average of 10.19 ± 3.29 mmol/L to 6.93 ± 1.98 mmol/L ($p < 0.001$). Cholesterol levels fell from 6.75 ± 1.32 mmol/L to 5.51 ± 1.16 mmol/L ($p < 0.001$). Triglyceride levels fell from 2.80 ± 1.01 mmol/L to 1.34 ± 0.71 mmol/L ($p < 0.001$). Serum insulin levels (by IRI) fell from 16.604 ± 6.005 MCU/L to 12.62 ± 14.85 MCU/L ($p < 0.05$). Severe obstruction of nail-microcirculation was relieved greatly.

These results showed that one year of Qigong exercise had a comprehensive beneficial effect on type II diabetic patients. Properly conducted Qigong exercises may allow people with type II diabetes to manage their disease without drugs.

Clinical Setting

Many studies have been conducted to measure the types and quantities of energies being emitted from the hands of Qigong masters. Of 839 abstracts in the Qigong database, 166 refer to the measured effects of emitted qi in their titles. The Raman spectra and ultraviolet absorption spectra of some materials were altered. In addition, infrasonic emission in 1 to 12 hertz range, microwave emissions, magnetic field generation, and electrostatic field generation at abnormally high levels were detected coming from the hands of Qigong masters. In most cases, the amount of energy being emitted was several times greater than that measured from control individuals, or from the same Qigong masters when not in the "Qigong state."

In some studies, effects of emitted qi have been documented from distances as far as 1200 miles with responses similar to those carried out at close range. This type of response violates the currently accepted laws of physics.

Not all research has been conducted in China. A 1985 study in a Seattle nursing home tested the effectiveness of an integrated healing system that combined Qigong with many other health supporting practices (Chow 1985). Fifteen patients were selected for the study, all of whom had medical conditions considered to be untreatable.

Each patient was treated by a Qigong master for 1 hour once a month for 6 months. The staff provided specific supportive measures between these visits. Progress was verified by videotapes of each patient made by staff members during these hands-on treatments by the Qigong master. The majority of improvements seen in these patients occurred during these 1-hour Qigong treatment sessions.

All 15 patients in the study improved to some degree, many dramatically. One man with Parkinson's disease had been in the nursing home for 2 years and was unable to walk unassisted. At the beginning of the first session, he was sitting in a wheel chair, head leaning to the left, drooling, with a blank stare on his face and flat affect. When pulled to a vertical position, with difficulty, he walked with full assistance and on the outer side of his right foot.

By the third session, this patient was able to walk to the treatment room pushing his own wheelchair in front of him. By the end of that session, he was dancing with nurses, a favorite activity before his illness. At the end of the fourth session, he jogged around the room, with his head up and with excellent coordination. Once again, he danced with the nurses and even with the female Qigong master. At that point, he was able to move out of the nursing home, a most unusual event. His drug regimen had not changed throughout these months, to avoid interference with the study.

Several patients who were paralyzed and wheelchair-bound regained the ability to walk. One elderly woman with hemiplegia and severely atrophied leg muscles from a stroke regained the ability to walk, even though she was not in the study and was never treated with emitted qi. She learned how to practice Qigong secondhand from her sister (and roommate) who was in the study.

Future

Results seen from the practice of Qigong challenge our understanding of what might be possible in the healing process. It remains unknown how breathing and mental and physical exercises can produce dramatic healing responses in situations that western medicine considers to be hopeless and untreatable. These results cannot be explained by our current understanding of biomedicine.

Qigong is a fertile field for research and, undoubtedly, more studies will be done by western medicine in the future. Until then, Qigong remains available as a discipline that is compatible with other forms of treatment, incurs costs only in time and effort, and can pay off in better levels of health, energy, and stamina.

References

Chow EPY. 1985. Integrated Healing System, its Effects in Rehabilitation at the Lutheran Home for Aging. The East West Academy of Healing Arts, San Francisco

Darras JC. 1989. Energy Fields in Medicine. John E. Fetzer Foundation, Kalamazoo, Michigan

Feng L, Juqing Q, Shugine C. 1988. A study on the effect of the emitted qi of Qigong on human carcinoma cells. China Immunology Research Center, Beijing. Presented at the First World Conference for Academic Exchange of Medical Qigong, Beijing (Abstract)

Hefen X, Huining X, Meiguang B, et al. 1993. Clinical study of the anti-aging effect of Qigong, Jiangsu Provincial Institute of TCM, Nanjing, China. Presented at the Second World Conference on Academic Exchange of Medical Qigong, Beijing (Abstract)

Huang M. 1988. A study of the effect of the emitted qi combined with self-practice of Qigong in treating paralysis, The General Hospital of PLA, Beijing, China, presented at the First World Conference for the Academic Exchange of Medical Qigong, Beijing (Abstract)

Jing Y, Li X, Wang Z, et al. 1993A. Observations on the effects of emitted qi in treatment of spinal cord injury, Qigong Institute, Beijing Military Region and Hebei Langfarg People's Hospital, Beijing Agricultural University. Reported at the Second World Conference for Academic Exchange of Medical Qigong, Beijing (Abstract)

Jing Y, Li X, Wang Z, et al. 1993B. Observations on effects of 31 cases of diabetes treated by huichungong, Shandong Institute of TCM, Shandong Province, Jinan 250014, China. Presented at the Second World Conference for Academic Exchange of Medical Qigong, Beijing (Abstract)

McGee CT, Chow EPY. 1994. Miracle Healing From China . . . Qigong, Medipress, Coeur d'Alene, Idaho

Moss T. Personal communication.

Quizhi S, Li Z. 1988. A clinical observation of Qigong as a therapeutic aid for advanced cancer patients. Kuangan Men Hospital, China Academy of Traditional Chinese Medicine, Beijing. Presented at the First World Conference for Academic Exchange of Medical Qigong, Beijing (Abstract)

Sancier KM, Chow EPY. 1989. Healing with Qigong and quantitative effects of Qigong measured by a muscle test. J Am Coll Trad Chin Med 7(3):13.

Sancier KM, Hu B. 1991. Medical applications of Qigong and emitted qi on humans, animals, cell cultures, and plants: Review of selected scientific studies. Am J Acup 19:376

Sancier KM. 1994. Effect of Qigong on therapeutic balancing measured by electroacupuncture according to Vol 1, Acu Electrother Res 19:119

Tiberiu R. 1981. Radioactive trace study of the bladder meridian. Am J Acup 9(3):251.

14
Ayurveda

Traditional Ayurveda

Kenneth G. Zysk

As the health care professions look seriously at complementary and alternative modalities of medicine, a growing interest in traditional Indian medicine is emerging simultaneously. As with any popular development, aspects of the Indian medical system and its cures have sometimes been appropriated by individuals not wholly familiar with the basics of Ayurveda or the Science of Longevity. Over the past decade, however, a group of dedicated scholars has undertaken serious study of this ancient healing tradition. In this textbook, it is appropriate to present the fundamental principles and practices of traditional Ayurveda, as they may be understood from classical Sanskrit sources and traditional Indian practitioners.

History

Based on available literary sources, the history of Indian medicine occurred in four main phases. The first, or Vedic phase dates from about 1200 to 800 BCE. Information about medicine during this period is obtained from numerous curative incantations and references to healing that are found in the *Atharvaveda* and the *Rigveda,* two religious scriptures that reveal a "magico-religious" approach to healing. The second, or classical phase is marked by the advent of the first Sanskrit medical treatises, the *Caraka* and *Sushruta Samhitas,* which probably date from a few centuries before to several centuries after the start of the common era. This period includes all subsequent medical treatises dating from before the Muslim invasions of India at the beginning of the eleventh century, for these works tend to follow the earlier classical compilations closely and provide the basis of traditional Ayurveda. The third, or syncretic

phase is marked by clear influences on the classical paradigm from Islamic or Unani, South Indian Siddha, and other nonclassical medical systems. Bhavamishra's sixteenth century *Bhavaprakasha* is one text that reveals the results of these influences, which included diagnosis by examination of pulse or urine. This phase extends from the Muslim incursions to the present era. I would term the final phase as "New Age Ayurveda," wherein the classical paradigm is being adapted to the world of modern science and technology, including quantum physics, mind-body science, and advanced biomedical science. This recent manifestation of Ayurveda is most visible in the Western world, although there are indications that it is filtering back to India. These four phases of Indian medical history provide a chronologic grid necessary to understanding the development of this ancient system of medicine.

Theoretical Foundations

From its beginnings during the Vedic era, Indian medicine always has adhered closely to the principle of a fundamental connection between the microcosm and macrocosm. Human beings are minute representations of the universe, and contain within them everything that makes up the surrounding world. Comprehending the world is crucial to comprehending the human and, conversely, understanding the world is necessary to understanding the human.

The Human Body

According to Ayurveda, the cosmos is composed of five basic elements: earth, air, fire, water, and space. Certain forces cause these to interact, giving rise to all that exists. In human beings, these five elements occur as the three *doshas*, forces that, along with the seven *dhatus* (tissues) and three *malas* (waste products), make up the human body.

The Three Doshas

When in equilibrium, the three doshas maintain health; but when an imbalance occurs among them, they defile the normal functioning of the body, leading to the manifestation of disease. An imbalance indicates an increase or decrease in one, two, or all three of the doshas. The three doshas are *vata, pitta,* and *kapha.*

Vata or *Vayu* meaning wind, is composed of the elements air and space. It is the principle of kinetic energy, and is responsible for all bodily movement and nervous functions. It is located below the navel, in the bladder, large intestines, nervous system, pelvic region, thighs, bone marrow, and legs; its principal seat is the colon. When disrupted, its primary manifestation is gas and muscular or nervous energy, leading to pain.

Pitta, or bile, is composed of the elements fire and water. It governs enzymes and hormones, and is responsible for digestion, pigmentation, body temperature, hunger, thirst, sight, courage, and mental activity. It is located between the navel and the chest, the stomach, small intestines, liver, spleen, skin, and blood; its principal seat is the stomach. When disrupted, its primary manifestation is acid and bile, leading to inflammation.

Kapha or *Shleshman,* meaning phlegm, is composed of the elements of earth and water. It connotes the principle of cohesion and stability. It regulates Vata and Pitta, is responsible for keeping the body lubricated and maintaining its solid nature, tissues, sexual power, and strength. It also controls patience. Its normal locations are the upper part of the body, the thorax, head, neck, upper portion of the stomach, pleural cavity, fat tissues, and areas between joints; its principal seat is the lungs. When it is disrupted, its primary manifestation is liquid and mucus, leading to swelling, with or without discharge.

The attributes of each dosha helps to determine the individual's basic bodily and mental makeup and to isolate which dosha(s) is responsible for a disease. The qualities of *Vata* are dryness, cold, light, irregu-

larity, mobility, roughness, and abundance. Dryness occurs when Vata is disturbed, and is a side effect of motion. Too much dryness produces irregularity in the body and mind. *Pitta* is hot, light, intense, fluid, liquid, putrid, pungent, and sour. Heat appears when Pitta is disturbed, resulting from change caused by Pitta. The intensity of excessive heat produces irritability in the body and mind. *Kapha* is heavy, unctuous, cold, stable, dense, soft, and smooth. Heaviness occurs when Kapha is disturbed, and results from firmness caused by Kapha. The viscosity of excessive heaviness and stability produces slowness in body and mind.

The Seven Dhatus

The seven dhatus or tissues are responsible for sustaining the body. Each dhatu is responsible for the one that comes next in the following order.

1. Rasa, meaning sap or juice, includes the tissue fluids, chyle, lymph, and plasma, and functions as nourishment. It comes from digested food.
2. Blood includes the red blood cells, and functions to invigorate the body.
3. Flesh includes muscle tissue, and functions as stabilization.
4. Fat includes adipose tissue, and functions as lubrication.
5. Bone includes bone and cartilage, and functions as support.
6. Marrow includes red and yellow bone marrow, and functions as filling for the bones.
7. Shukra includes male and female sexual fluids, and functions in reproduction and immunity.

The Three Malas

These are the waste products of digested and processed food and drink. Ayurveda delineates three principal malas, urine, feces, and sweat. A fourth category of other waste products includes fatty excretions from the skin and intestines, ear wax, mucus of the nose, saliva, tears, hair, and nails. According to Ayurveda, an individual should evacuate the bowels once a day, and eliminate urine six times a day.

Ayurveda considers digestion to be the most important function that takes place in the human body. It provides all that is required to sustain the organism and is the principal cause for all maladies from which an individual suffers. The process of digestion and assimilation of nutrients will be discussed under the topics of the Agnis (enzymes), Ama (improperly digested food and drink), and the Srotas (channels of circulation).

The Thirteen Agnis

The Agnis, or enzymes, assist in the digestion and assimilation of food, and are divided into three types.

Jatharagni is active in the mouth, stomach, and gastrointestinal tract, and helps to break down food. The waste product of feces results from this activity.

Bhutagnis are five enzymes located in the liver. They adapt the broken down food into a homologous chyle according to the five elements, and assist the chyle to assimilate with the corresponding five elements in the body. The homologous chyle circulates in the blood channels as rasa, nourishing the body and supplying the seven dhatus.

Dhatvagnis are seven enzymes which synthesize the seven dhatus from the assimilated chyle homologized with the five elements. The remaining waste products result from this activity.

Ama

Ama, the chief cause of disease, is formed when there is a decrease in enzyme activity. A product of improperly digested food and drink, it takes the form of a liquid sludge that travels through the same channels as the chyle. Because of its density, however, it lodges in different parts of the body, blocking the channels. It frequently mixes with the doshas that circulate through the same pathways and it gravitates to a weak or stressed organ, or to a site of a disease manifestation. Since all diseases invariably come from Ama, the word *Amaya,* meaning "coming from Ama," is a synonym for disease. Internal diseases begin with Ama, and external diseases produce Ama. In general, Ama can be detected by a coating on the tongue; turbid urine with foul odor; and feces that is passed with undigested food, an offensive odor, and abundant gas. The principal course of treatment in Ayurveda involves the elimination of Ama and the restoration of the balance of the doshas.

The Thirteen Kinds of Srotas

The srotas are the vessels or channels of the body through which all substances circulate. They are either large, such as the large and small intestines, uterus, arteries, and veins, or small, such as the capillaries. A healthy body has open and free-flowing channels. Blockage of the channels, usually by Ama, results in disease.

1. Pranavahasrotas convey vitality and vital breath (*prana*) and originate in the heart and alimentary tract.
2. Udakavahasrotas convey water and fluids and originate in the palate and pancreas.
3. Annavahasrotas convey food from the outside and originate in the stomach.
4. Rasavahasrotas convey chyle, lymph, and plasma, and originate in the heart and in the ten vessels connected with the heart. Ama primarily accumulates within them.
5. Raktavahasrotas convey red blood cells and originate in the liver and spleen.
6. Mamsavahasrotas convey ingredients for muscle tissue and originate in the tendons, ligaments, and skin.
7. Medovahasrotas convey ingredients for fat tissue and originate in the kidneys and fat tissues of the abdomen.
8. Asthavahasrotas convey ingredients for bone tissue and originate in hip bone.
9. Majjavahasrotas convey ingredients for marrow and originate in the bones and joints.
10. Shukravahasrotas convey ingredients for the male and female reproductive tissues and originate in the testicles and ovary.
11. Mutravahasrotas convey urine and originate in the kidney and bladder.
12. Purishavahasrotas convey feces and originate in the colon and rectum.
13. Svedavahasrotas convey sweat and originate in the fat tissues and hair follicles.

This broad outline exhibits that Ayurveda understands that the human body's anatomical parts are composed of the five basic elements, which have undergone a process of metabolism and assimilation in the body. Human beings differ, depending upon their normal bodily constitution (*prakriti*), which is determined at the moment of conception and remains until death. The four factors that influence constitutional type include the father, the mother (particularly her food intake), the womb, and the season of the year. A large imbalance of the doshas in the mother will affect the growth of the embryo and fetus, and a moderate excess of one or two of the doshas will affect the constitution of the child.

Prakriti

There are seven normal body constitutions based on the three doshas: *vata, pitta, kapha, vata-pitta, pitta-kapha, vata-kapha,* and *sama.* The latter is balanced, which is best, but extremely rare. Most people are a combination of doshas, in which one dosha predominates. In general, Vata-type people tend to be anxious and fearful, exhibit light and "airy" characteristics, and are prone to vata-diseases. Pitta-type people are aggressive and impatient, exhibit fiery and hotheaded characteristics, and are prone to pitta-diseases. Kapha-type people are stable and entrenched, exhibit heavy, wet, and earthy characteristics, and are prone to kapha-diseases.

These are the principal factors that help the Ayurvedic physician determine the correct course of treatment to be administered to a patient for a particular ailment.

Three Mental States

In addition to physical constitution, Ayurveda understands that an individual is influenced by three mental states, based on the three qualities (*gunas*) of balance (*sattva*), energy (*rajas*), and inertia (*tamas*). In the state of balance, the mind is in equilibrium and can discriminate correctly. In the state of energy, the mind is excessively active, causing weakness in discrimination. In the state of inertia, the mind is excessively inactive, also creating weak discrimination.

Ayurveda always has recognized that the body and the mind interact to create a healthy, normal (*prakriti*) or unhealthy, abnormal (*vikriti*) condition. A good Ayurvedic physician will determine both the mental and physical condition of the patient before proceeding with any form of diagnosis and treatment.

Disease

Aspects of the Ayurvedic understanding of disease have been mentioned in the previous section. Here I shall focus specifically on the Ayurvedic classification of disease, the naming of disease, and the manifestations of disease.

Classification of Disease

Ayurveda identifies three broad categories of disease, based on causative factors.

Adhyatmika diseases originate within the body, and may be subdivided into hereditary diseases, congenital disease, and diseases caused by one or a combination of the doshas.

Adhibhautika diseases originate outside the body, and include injuries from accidents or mishaps, and in the terminology of the modern era, from germs, viruses, and bacteria.

Adhidaivika diseases originate from supernatural sources, including diseases that are otherwise inexplicable, such as maladies stemming from providential causes, planetary influences, curses, and seasonal changes.

Disease Names

In Ayurveda, diseases receive their names in one of six ways. A disease is named for the misery it produces (fever, or *Jvara*); its chief symptom (diarrhea, or *Atisara*); its chief physical sign (jaundice, or *Pandu*); its principal nature (piles, or *Arshas*); the chief dosha(s) involved (wind-disease, or *Vata-roga*); or the chief organ involved (disease of the duodenum, or *Grahani*). Regardless of its given name, most diseases will involve one or more of the doshas.

Manifestation of Disease

During the course of a disease, an Ayurvedic physician seeks to identify its site of origin, its path of transportation, and its site of manifestation. The site of manifestation of a disease usually differs from its site of origin. Recognizing this distinction enables the physician to determine the correct course of treatment.

Ayurveda describes the manifestation of all diseases in the same fundamental way. Causative factors (such as food, drink, regimen, season, and mental state) suppress enzyme activity in the body, leading to the formation of Ama. The circulating Ama blocks the channels. The site of the disease's origin is where the blockage occurs. The circulating Ama, often combining with one or more of the doshas, then takes a divergent course, referred to as the path of transportation. Finally, the dosha(s) and Ama mixture comes to rest in and afflicts a certain body part, which is known as the site of disease manifestation. Treatment entails correction of all the steps in the process resulting in disease manifestation, thus restoring the entire person to his or her particular, balanced state.

Therapeutics

In Ayurveda, restoring a person to health is not viewed simply as the eradication of disease. It entails a complete process of diagnosis and therapeutics that takes into account both mental and physical components integrated with the social and physical worlds in which the patient lives. I shall therefore briefly explain Ayurvedic diagnosis, examination of the disease, and types of therapeutics.

Ayurvedic Diagnosis

Ayurveda established a detailed system of diagnosis, involving examination of pulse, urine, and physical features.

After a preliminary examination by means of visual observation, touch, and interrogation, the Ayurvedic physician undertakes an eightfold method of detailed examination to determine the patient's type of physical constitution and mental status and to get an indication of any abnormality.

Pulse Examination

Pulse examination is first mentioned in a medical treatise from the late 13th or early 14th century of the common era. It is a highly specialized art. Not every Ayurvedic physician uses pulse examination. The diagnostic process involves evenly placing the index, middle, and ring fingers of the right hand on the radial artery of the right hand of men and the left hand of women, just at the base of the thumb. A pulse resembling the movement of a snake at the index finger indicates a predominance of Vata; a pulse resembling the movement of a frog at the middle finger indicates a predominance of Pitta; a pulse resembling the movement of a swan or peacock at the ring finger indicates a predominance of Kapha; and a pulse resembling the movement of a woodpecker indicates a predominance of all three doshas. To get an accurate reading, the physician must keep in mind the times when each of the doshas are normally excited, and should take the pulse at least three times early in the morning when the stomach is empty, or three hours after eating in the afternoon, making sure to wash his or her hands after each reading.

Urine Examination

Like pulse examination, urine examination probably was formalized in the syncretic phase. After collecting the morning's midstream evacuation in a clear glass container, the physician submits the urine to two kinds of examination after sunrise. First, he studies it in the container to determine its color and degree of transparency. Pale-yellow and unctuous urine indicates Vata; intense yellow, reddish, or blue urine indicates Pitta; white, foamy, and muddy urine indicates Kapha; urine with a blackish tinge indicates a combination of doshas; and urine resembling lime juice or vinegar indicates Ama. The physician also puts a few drops of sesame oil in the urine and examines it in sunlight. The shape, movement, and diffusion of the oil in the urine indicate the prognosis of the disease. The shape of the drops also reveals which dosha(s) is involved. Snake-like shape indicates Vata; umbrella shape, Pitta; and pearl shape, Kapha.

Examination of Bodily Parts

The physician concludes his diagnostic examination with careful scrutiny of the tongue, skin, nails, and physical features to determine which dosha(s) is affected. Using the basic characteristics of each of the doshas, he will examine the different parts of the body. Coldness, dryness, roughness, and cracking indicate Vata; hotness and redness indicate Pitta; and wetness, whiteness, and coldness indicate Kapha.

Having completed this phase of the diagnosis, the Ayurvedic physician proceeds to examine any malady present.

Examination of the Disease

A detailed examination of the disease involves a five-step process, leading to a complete understanding of the abnormality.

Etiology

A disease results from one or several of the following factors: mental imbalances resulting from the effects of past actions (*karma*); unbalanced contact between the senses and the objects of the senses affecting the body and the mind; effects of the seasons on the mental and doshic balance; and the immediate causes of diet, regimen, and microorganism; doshas and Ama; and the combination of interaction of individual components such as doshas and tissues, or doshas and microorganisms.

Early Signs and Symptoms

Early signs and symptoms that appear before the onset of disease provide clues to the diagnosis. Proper diet and administration of medicine can avert disease if it is recognized early enough.

Manifest Signs and Symptoms

The most crucial step in the diagnostic process is manifest signs and symptoms. It involves determining the site of origin and of manifestation, and of the path of transportation of the Ama and dosha(s). Most signs and symptoms are associated with the site of disease manifestation, from which the physician must work his way back to the site of the origin of disease to effect a complete cure. Although symptomatic treatment was largely absent in traditional Ayurveda, modern medicine in India has introduced Ayurvedic physicians to techniques of symptomatic treatment in cases of acute disease.

Exploratory Therapy

Exploratory therapy involves 18 different experiments that use drugs, diet, and regimens to determine the precise nature of the malady and suitable therapy by allopathic and homeopathic means.

Pathogenesis

Pathogenesis is a six-step process that determines the manner by which a dosha becomes aggravated and moves through the different channels to produce disease. An accumulation of a dosha leads to its aggravation, which causes it to spread through the channels until it lodges in a particular organ of the body, bringing about a manifestation of disease. Once a general form of the disease appears, it progressively splits into specific varieties. As in systems of medicine the world over, many patients consult the Ayurvedic physician only after the disease appears.

Ayurveda delineates seven basic varieties of disease, based on the doshas: diseases involving a single dosha; diseases involving two doshas; and diseases involving all three doshas together.

Prognosis is the final step in the Ayurvedic diagnostic process. Since Ayurvedic physicians traditionally did not treat persons with incurable diseases, it was important for the physician to know precisely the patient's chances of full recovery. Therefore, disease is one of three types. It is easily curable, palliative, or incurable or difficult to cure. In general, if the disease type (Vata, Pitta, Kapha) is different from the person's normal physical constitution, the disease is easy to cure. If the disease and constitution are the same, the disease is difficult to cure. If the disease, constitution, and season correspond to doshic type, the disease is nearly impossible to cure.

Having determined the patient's normal constitution, diagnosed his illness, and established his prognosis for recovery, the Ayurvedic physician can begin a proper course of treatment.

Ayurvedic Treatment

Ayurveda recognizes two courses of treatment, based on the condition of the patient. The first is prophylaxis, for the healthy person who wants to maintain a normal condition based on his or her physical constitution, and to prevent disease. The second is therapy, for an ill person who requires health to be restored. Once healthy, Ayurveda recommends continuous prophylaxis based on diet, regimen, medicines, and regular therapeutic purification procedures.

When a person is diagnosed with a doshic imbalance, either purification therapy, alleviation therapy, or a combination of these is prescribed.

Purification Therapy

Purification therapy involves the fundamental *Pañchakarma*, or Five Action treatment. The fivefold process varies slightly in different traditions and regions of India, but a standard regimen generally is followed. All five procedures can be performed, or a selection of procedures can be chosen, based on different factors such as the physical constitution of the patient, his or her condition, the season, and the nature of the disease. Before any action is taken, the patient is given oil internally and externally (with massage), and is sweated to loosen and soften the dosha(s) and Ama. An appropriate diet of food and drink is prescribed. Following this twofold preparatory treatment, called *Purvakarma*, the five therapies are administered in sequence over the period of about a week. Because of the profound effects on the mind and body, the patient is advised to set aside time for treatment. First the patient might be given an emetic, and vomits until bilious matter is produced thus removing Kapha. Second, a purgative is given until mucus material appears, thus removing Pitta. Third, an enema, either of oil or decocted medicines, is administered to remove excess Vata. Fourth, head purgahon is given in the form of smoke inhalation or nasal drops to eradicate the dosha(s) that have accumulated in the head and sinuses. Fifth, leeches may be applied and bloodletting performed to purify the blood. Some physicians do not consider bloodletting in the five therapies of *Pañchakarma*, instead counting oily and dry (decoated medicine) enemas as two separate forms.

Alleviation Therapy

Alleviation therapy uses the basic condiments honey, butter or ghee, and sesame oil or castor oil to eliminate Kapha, Pitta, and Vata, respectively. This therapy and Pañchakarma often are used in conjunction with one another.

Pharmaceutics

Ayurveda prescribes a rich store of natural medicines that have been collected, tested, and recorded in medical treatises from ancient times. The tradition of collecting and preserving information about medicines in recipe-books called *Nighantus* continues to the present day. The most traditional sources of Ayurvedic medicine is the kitchen. It is likely that, at an early stage of its development, Indian medical and culinary traditions worked hand-in-hand with each other.

Because of the close association between food and medicine, Ayurveda classifies foods and drugs (usually vegetal) by the tongue, potency, and taste after digestion.

Rasa, taste by the tongue, is categorized into six separate tastes, with their individual elemental composition and doshic effect as follows:

1. Sweet, composed of earth and water, increases Kapha and decreases Pitta and Vata.
2. Sour, composed of earth and fire, increases Kapha and Pitta and decreases Vata.
3. Saline, composed of water and fire, increases Kapha and Pitta and decreases Vata.
4. Pungent, composed of wind and fire, increases Pitta and Vata and decreases Kapha.
5. Bitter, composed of wind and space, increases Vata and decreases Pitta and Kapha.
6. Astringent, composed of wind and earth, increases Vata and decreases Pitta and Kapha.

Virya, potency comprises eight types that are divided into four pairs: hot-cold, unctuous-dry, heavy-light, and dull-sharp.

Vipaka, postdigestive taste, identifies three kinds of after-taste: sweet, sour, and pungent.

Contrary foods and drugs are to be avoided always. For instance, clarified butter and honey should not be taken in equal quantities; alkalies and salt must not be taken for a long period of time; milk and fish should not be consumed together; and honey should not be put in hot drinks.

Four important criteria are considered when compounding plant substances and other ingredients into medical recipes. The substances that make up the recipe should have many attributes that enable it to cure several diseases; they should be usable in many pharmaceutical preparations; they should be suitable for the recipe and not cause unwanted side-effects; and they should be culturally appropriate to the patients and their customs. Every medicine should be able to treat the disease's site of origin, site of manifestation, and its spread, simultaneously.

A brief survey of the different kinds of medical preparations indicates the depth and content of Ayurvedic pharmaceuticals. The botanically-based medicines derive largely from the Ayurvedic medical tradition, while the mineral and inorganic-based drugs derive from the Indian Alchemical traditions, called *Rasashastra*.

1. Juices are cold-presses and extractions made from plants.
2. Powders are prepared from parts of plants that have been dried in the shade, and other dried ingredients.
3. Infusions are parts of plants and herbs that have been steeped in water and strained.
4. Cold infusions are parts of plants and herbs that were soaked in water overnight and filtered the next morning.
5. Decoctions are vegetal products boiled in a quantity of water proportionate to the hardness of the plant part and then reduced by a fourth. It is then filtered and often used with butter, honey, or oils.
6. Medicated pastes and oils. Often the plant and herbal extracts are combined with other ingredients and formed into pastes, plasters, and oils. Used externally, pastes and plasters are applied for joint, muscular, and skin conditions, and oil is used for hair and head problems. Medicate oils also are used for massages and enemas.
7. Large and small pills and suppositories. Plant and herbal extracts are also formed into pills and suppositories to be used internally.
8. Alcoholic preparations are made via fermentation or distillation. Two preparations are delineated: One requires the drug to be boiled before it is fermented or distilled, and in the other, the drug is simply added to the preparation. Fifteen percent is the maximum allowable amount of alcohol content in a drug.

   Several Ayurvedic medicines are prepared from minerals and metals, and are derived ultimately from ancient traditions.
9. Sublimates. These are prepared by an elaborate method leading to the sublimation of sulphur in a glass container. They are found in recipes (*Rasayanas*) used in rejuvenation therapies.
10. *Bhasmas* are ash residues produced from the calcination of metals, gems, plants, and animal products. Most are metals and minerals that are first detoxified and then purified. An important bhasma is prepared from mercury, which undergoes an 18-stage detoxification and purification process. Ayurveda maintains that bhasmas are quickly absorbed in the blood and increase the red blood cells.
11. *Pishtis* are fine powders made by trituration of gems with juices and extracts.
12. Collyrium is made from antimony powder, lead oxide, or the soot from lamps burned with castor oil. Collyrium is used especially to improve vision.

Space does not allow a discussion of the individual plants used in Ayurvedic recipes. It is safe to say, however, that of the hundreds of plants mentioned in various Ayurvedic treatises, only a small portion are commonly employed by most Ayurvedic physicians.

Ayurvedic Clinical Approach

An example of a specific disease will illustrate the traditional Ayurvedic clinical approach. In Sanskrit terminology, the malady *Amavata* refers approximately to arthritic and rheumatic conditions.

Amavata

As the word itself indicates, Amavata involves Ama and the dosha Vata (wind). Traditional Ayurveda does not distinguish types of arthritis. This disease is caused by all factors that lead to the formation of Ama: unwholesome foods and regimens, bad digestive power, insufficient exercise, and excessive intake of unctuous foods and meat. The site of origin is principally the colon, but the entire alimentary canal is involved. Contrary foods and mental disturbance aggravate Vata and lead to the formation of Ama in the colon. Ama, propelled by Vata, leaves the site of origin and affects the enzymes, causing Ama to form at every level. Ama then becomes lodged in the joints and the heart, the sites of manifestation. The path of transport is the *Rasavahasrotas*, the vessels transporting chyle, lymph, and plasma.

Vata is the principal dosha affected. With the aggravation of Vata, symptoms include severe pain in the joints, rough skin, distension of the stomach, and indigestion. If Pitta is involved, a burning sensation spreads all over the body, especially in the joints. If Kapha is involved, the patient gradually becomes crippled. Little pain is experienced in the early morning because Ama is just beginning to move. The Ayurvedic treatment of Amavata involves actions, medicines, and procedures to reduce Ama and alleviate Vata. The first course of action is to put the patient on a mild fast and to administer medicines that have a bitter taste, hot potency, and pungent postdigestive taste, all of which help to reestablish the digestive powers. Sweating might be recommended to aid the digestive process.

The second step of the treatment involves the purification therapy of Pañchakarma. The two preparatory actions, oleation and sweating, are administered first to dislodge and soften the Ama. The remaining five procedures are performed over the period of a week, during which time the patient maintains a strict diet. These will eradicate the dislodged Ama from the system, and restore the balance of the doshas, especially Vata. One of two types of enema will be used, depending upon the amount of Ama present. If Ama persists, an enema with decoctions is administered until Ama is removed when an oily enema is given.

After the Pañchakarma therapy, the patient should assume a regimen that includes avoiding sleep during the day and after meals, as well as heavy foods that hinder digestion. Effective treatment of arthritic conditions, especially in children, has included wet massage therapy in conjunction with the enemas of Pañchakarma. The affected areas are patted with a cloth bag filled with rice that has been cooked with milk and herbs. Massages with oils also are routinely prescribed.

Conclusions

Traditional Ayurveda is a sophisticated system of medicine that has been practiced in India for over 2,500 years. Like other forms of alternative and complementary medicine, it focuses on the whole organism and its relation to the external world, in order to reestablish and maintain the harmonious balance that exists within the body and between the body

and its environment. Only a glimpse of this ancient form of medicine has been offered; there is much to be learned from a deeper exploration of Ayurveda. Studies of Ayurveda and related traditions in Tibetan medicine are being undertaken in India, Europe, and North America. The recently established Indo-Tibetan Medical Project at Columbia University, New York, is devoted to scientific and scholarly investigation and public education.

Very few reliable sources for traditional Ayurveda are available in English. Most of the sound works are by and for specialists and are virtually inaccessible to the reader without knowledge of Sanskrit. In order to provide information on Ayurveda, the University of California Press has undertaken the publication of a series of books devoted to Indian and Tibetan Medicine, specifically aimed at informing the general public, health care professionals, and scholars about these medical traditions. A selective list of trustworthy and available books in English on traditional Ayurveda follows.

Suggested Readings

Bhishagratna KK (trans). 1983. An English Translation of the Sushruta Samhita Based on Original Sanskrit Text. 3. Vols. 1907-16, Reprint. The Chowkhamba Sanskrit Series Office. Varanasi

Dash B. 1980. Fundamentals of Ayurvedic Medicine. Bansal & Co. Delhi

Dash B, Kashyap L. 1980. Basic Principles of Ayurveda Based on Ayurveda Saukhyam of Todarananda. Concept Publishing Company. New Delhi

Jolly J. 1977. Indian Medicine. Kashikar GC (trans). Munshiram Manoharlal. New Delhi

Lad V. 1990. Ayurveda. The Science of Self-Healing. Lotus Press. Wilmot, Wisconsin

Meulenbeld GJ. 1974. The Madhavanidana and Its Chief Commentary. EJ Brill. Leiden

Nadkarni AK. 1908. Dr. K. M. Nadkarni's Indian Materia Medica. 3rd Ed. Reprint. Popular Prakashan. Bombay

Sen Gupta KN. 1984. The Ayurvedic System of Medicine. 1906, Reprint. Logos Press. New Delhi

Sharma PV (trans). 1981-1994. Caraka-Samhita. Agnivesha's Treatise Refined and Annotated by Caraka and Redacted by Dridhabala. 4 Vols. Chaukhambha Orientalia. Varanasi

Singh RH. 1992. Pañchakarma Therapy. Chowkhamba Sanskrit Series Office. Varanasi

Singhal GD, et al (trans). 1972–1993. Ancient Indian Surgery. [Sushruta Samhita]. 10 Vols. Singhal Publications. Varanasi

Srikanta Murthy KR (trans). 1984. Sharngadharasamhita of Shrangadhara. Chaukhambha Orientalia. Varanasi

Svoboda RE. 1984. Prakruti. Your Ayurvedic Constitution. Geocom. Albuquerque

Upadhyay SD. 1986. Nadivijana (Ancient Pulse Science). Chaukhamba Sanskrit Pratisthan. Delhi

Zysk KG. 1991. Asceticism and Healing in Ancient India. Medicine in the Buddhist Monastery. Oxford University Press. New York

Zysk KG. 1993. Religious Medicine. The History and Evolution of Indian Medicine. Transaction Publishers. New Brunswick, New Jersey

Maharishi Ayurveda

Hari M. Sharma

History

Ayurveda is a holistic system of natural health care that originated in the ancient Vedic civilization of India. During the centuries of foreign rule in India, which began in the 15th century, Ayurvedic institutions declined or were suppressed, and much of the Ayurvedic knowledge was fragmented, misunderstood, and not used in its totality. Recently, Ayurveda has been revived in its completeness in accordance with the classical texts by Maharishi Mahesh Yogi, and in collaboration with leading Ayurvedic scholars and physicians, known as vaidyas. This specific reformulation of Ayurveda is known as Maharishi Ayurveda (MAV).

The Sanskrit name "Ayurveda" is a compound of two words: *Ayus,* which means "life" or "lifespan," and *Veda,* which means "knowledge," with a connotation of completeness or wholeness of knowledge. The element of "wholeness" in Ayurvedic knowledge has profound clinical significance: the Maharishi Ayurveda clinician uses more than 20 treatment approaches that deal with the full range of the patient's life—the body, mind, behavior, environment, and most importantly, the patient's consciousness, his or her "innermost life." MAV considers consciousness to be of primary importance in maintaining optimal health, and emphasizes meditation techniques to develop integrated holistic functioning of the nervous system.

MAV includes a sophisticated theoretical framework that provides clinical insight into the functioning of both mind and body. Understanding of the patient's mind/body type is essential to diagnosis and treatment, and special emphasis is placed on the therapeutic effects of diet and healthy digestion, as well as techniques to balance behavior and emotions.

An extensive materia medica describes the therapeutic use of medicinal plants, and there is a detailed understanding of biologic rhythms, which form the basis for daily and seasonal behavioral routines to strengthen the immune system and homeostatic mechanisms.

Ancient Ayurvedic texts* typically begin with a thorough description of strategies of prevention before discussing modalities for treatment. In addition to preventive techniques, MAV offers a holistic theory of prevention. Western medical attempts to develop preventive medical strategies, although laudable, conspicuously lack such a theory. As for the fields of diagnosis and treatment, Maharishi Ayurveda offers a large body of procedures and protocols, including a set of noninvasive diagnostic techniques, and addresses certain deficiencies of Western allopathic medicine. For example, functional diseases, such as irritable bowel syndrome and poor digestion, account for approximately one-third of patient visits to family practitioners: Western medicine, however, lacks well-developed theories or methods of treatment for these disorders.

Another example is iatrogenic (physician-caused)

---

* These include three major texts (*Brihat Trayi*), the *Charaka Samhita, Sushruta Samhita* and *Ashtanga Hridaya* of Vagbhata, and three minor texts (*Laghu Trayi*), the *Sarngadhara Samhita, Bhavaprakash Samhita,* and *Madhava Nidanam.* Most of these texts have been translated into English (Vagbhata, 1982; Madhavakava, 1986; Sarngadhara, 1984; Charaka Samhita, 1977; and Sushruta Samhita, 1963). These texts address eight main sections of Ayur-Veda: *Shalya,* surgery in general; *Shalakya,* surgery for supraclavicular diseases; *Kaya chikitsa,* treatment, diagnosis and internal medicine; *Kaumarya Birtya,* pediatrics, obstetrics, and gynecology; *Agad Tantra,* toxicology and medical jurisprudence; *Bhut Vidya,* psychosomatic medicine; *Rasayana,* materia medica to promote vitality, stamina, resistance to disease, and longevity; and *Vajikarana,* fertility and potency.

243

diseases, which studies have found to afflict more than one-third of hospitalized patients (Steel et al 1981). For instance, Western approaches to cancer treatment have severe side effects, and some anti-tumor drugs even contribute to development of new cancers. MAV modalities have been effective in reducing the side effects of several of these treatments (Misra et al 1994, Sharma et al 1994A), and laboratory research has shown that some MAV herbal preparations reduce cancer growth directly (Sharma et al 1990, Arnold et al 1991, Sharma et al 1991A, Patel et al 1992, Prasad et al 1992).

MAV is being practiced in clinics worldwide, in India, Europe, Japan, Africa, Russia, Australia, and South and North America, by specially-trained physicians, many of whom also practice privately. In various ways, MAV directs its objectives not only to individual patients but to the life of society as a whole.

Theoretical Basis: A "Consciousness Model" of Medicine

Maharishi Ayurveda's contribution to patient care and clinical practice results from the model of health and disease on which it is based. Whereas Western medicine bases its model for understanding health and disease on the *material* of the body, Maharishi Ayurveda is based on the body's *non*material substrate, which is conceived as a field of pure intelligence. Western medicine's paradigm may seem to be seen as more scientific, but in certain respects, Ayurveda's may be seen to presaged today's advanced theories of physics.

From the time of Newton until the early twentieth century, the field of physics was based on a materialist approach to the natural world (see Chapter 1). The allopathic medical paradigm, developed in the 19th century, is based on this theory of materialism; it views the body as a complex machine. However, discoveries by twentieth-century physicists have undermined this materialist worldview, and uncovered a fundamental role for consciousness in the physical world. Because the nature and importance of consciousness are not commonly considered in allopathic medicine, twentieth-century physics provides a useful background for understanding Maharishi Ayurveda.

According to the materialist theory that dominated physics until the 1900s, the universe is composed of solid, discrete bits of matter. These particles affect each other only through direct interactions. Four basic principles support this "common sense" view of reality:

1. Solid matter: The world is composed fundamentally of solid material objects, the building blocks of nature.
2. Strict causality: Change in motion of one object can be caused only by direct interaction with another object.
3. Locality: Interactions between particles can occur only through collisions or through influences radiated through the electromagnetic or gravitational fields at the speed of light, or less. No nonlocal interaction can occur.
4. Reductionism: Large systems in nature—including, in principle, the human body and even the entire universe—can be understood completely by understanding the properties and local, causal interactions of their smallest discrete components.

In the materialist theory, the consciousness of the scientist is considered to be separate from the material objects being studied. The knower (consciousness) and the known (object) are thought to exist in completely distinct domains. This separation is thought to be the basis of "objective" science. Throughout the history of science, however, the separation of consciousness from the apparently material world has led to theoretical difficulties. For one thing, if consciousness is completely separate from matter, it is difficult to explain how consciousness could arise from the purely mechanical interactions of solid matter within the brain.

In the twentieth century, the terms of this discussion have been changed by the fundamental discoveries of quantum physics. Experiments performed in the first quarter of this century indicated that subatomic particles, the supposed building blocks of nature, did not appear to be composed of solid matter. In some of these experiments, particles behaved as if they were waves. In others, electrons took instantaneous, discontinuous quantum jumps from one atomic orbit to another, with no intervening time and no journey through space—an impossible act for a classical particle. It also was shown that an individual subatomic particle cannot have both a precise position and a precise momentum simultaneously (the "uncertainty" principle), another situation that would not apply to a solid material particle. Finally, it was found that electrons can, with predictable regularity, tunnel through a solid barrier that, classically, would be impenetrable.

Based on these findings, the basic principles of quantum mechanics (often known as the Copenhagen interpretation) challenge the materialist worldview.

1. No solid matter: This interpretation accepted the scientific findings (wave/particle, quantum jumps, uncertainty, tunneling) that contradict the notion of solid matter.
2. No strict causality: Precise predictions for individual subatomic particles are impossible. Quantum mechanics thus loses the ability to trace causal relations among individual particles.
3. No locality: Quantum mechanical equations indicate that two particles, once they have interacted, are instantaneously connected, even across astronomical distances. This defies the strictly local connections allowed in classical materialism.
4. No reductionism: If apparently separate particles actually are connected nonlocally, a reductionist view based on isolated particles is untenable.

The Copenhagen interpretation was not put to experimental test for decades, leaving some physicists unconvinced that solidity, causality, locality, and reductionism had to be abandoned. In the 1980s, however, a number of different experiments produced results that consistently contradicted the theories of materialism (often called local realism), and consistently confirmed the predictions of quantum mechanics (Aspect et al 1981, Rarity & Tapster 1990). These studies found that once two particles have interacted, they are instantaneously correlated nonlo-

cally, over arbitrarily vast distances—an impossibility in materialism.

These results do not invalidate materialism altogether. In the everyday world of "large" objects, the mechanistic causation of Newtonian physics is approximately correct, which is why much of medicine has been able to rely on it without apparently ill consequences. But at the fundamental, subatomic level, materialism conflicts both with theory and with frequently replicated experimental evidence. This gives rise to a fundamentally different worldview. Many physicists now argue that nature is composed of *probability waves* that are a function of *intelligence alone,* not of discrete physical particles. The equations of quantum mechanics thus describe a world made of abstract patterns of intelligence.

> In view of these uniformly idea-like characteristics of the quantum-physical world, the proper answer to our question, "What sort of world do we live in?" would seem to be this: "We live in an idea-like world, not a matter-like world." There is, in fact, in the quantum universe no natural place for matter. This conclusion, curiously, is the exact reverse of the circumstance that in the classical physical universe there was not a natural place for mind (Stapp 1994).

Quantum field theory, the most accurate version of quantum mechanics, can be related to the core tenet of Maharishi Ayurveda's paradigm. In quantum field theory, the probability wave for a particle is described as a fluctuation in an underlying, nonmaterial field (known as a force field or matter field). Furthermore, in the most recent superunified theories, physicists have described all the force and matter fields that comprise the universe as modes of vibration of one underlying, unified field, sometimes called the superfield or superstring field. All the order and intelligence of the laws of nature arise from this one fundamental, nonmaterial field, as does all matter. Not only are particles really just waves; those waves ultimately are made of an underlying field, as ocean waves are made of ocean water. This field is one of pure intelligence, having the attributes that we associate with consciousness. This lends support to the statement of the quantum mechanical pioneer Max Planck, who said, "I regard consciousness as primary. I regard matter as derivative from consciousness," and to Sir Arthur Eddington, the physicist who first provided evidence in support of Einstein's general theory of relativity, who said, "The stuff of the world is mind-stuff" (Eddington 1974).

Unified field theory may seem worlds away from the concerns of a clinician. Today's allopathic approach assumes that the body can be explained by material reductionism, analogous to machinery. Maharishi Ayurveda, by contrast, has viewed it as an abstract pattern of intelligence. Since this latter view appears to be consistent with fundamental science, it is not unreasonable to consider that it might contribute to the clinician's capacity to promote health. Let us examine how Maharishi Ayurveda's "consciousness model" is applied in clinical practice.

Applying the Consciousness Model in Maharishi Ayurveda

Transcendental Meditation

To understand the most basic application of the consciousness model, we must briefly touch on physics again. Vedic thought discusses a unified field of pure, nonmaterial intelligence and consciousness whose modes of vibration manifest as the material universe. These modes of vibration are called *Veda*.* The Vedic description is strikingly similar to that of physics, but emphasizes an idea less often discussed in physics—that the unified field is the field of pure consciousness. The differentiation between consciousness and matter, between knower and known, loses its significance at the level of the unified field.

In Maharishi Ayurveda, the ultimate basis of disease is losing one's connection to (or, to use a central Vedic description, one's memory of) the unified field, which is the innermost core of one's own being

and experience. This loss is known technically as *pragya-aparadh*. The ultimate basis of prevention and cure is restoring one's conscious connection to (or, memory of) this innermost core of one's being and experience. This reconnection is the basis of an integrated approach to health care; integration of the different layers of life begins with reconnecting one's life to the substrate upon which all its layers are based. The innermost core of one's experience is considered identical to the home of all the laws of nature that operate throughout the universe. The body contains, at its basis, the total potential of natural law, and all of Maharishi Ayurveda's modalities aim to enable the full expression of the body's inner intelligence.

The foremost means for accomplishing this are the Vedic techniques for developing consciousness, the most important of which is Transcendental Meditation (TM). The term "transcendental" indicates that the mind *transcends* even the subtlest impulses of thought and settles down to the simplest state of awareness (in MAV terms, identical to the unified field). This state of awareness is known technically as transcendental consciousness (TC).

Interestingly, a large body of published research has demonstrated that, during the subjective experience of TC, the body's metabolism and EEG (electroencephalogram), take on a unique pattern of profound physiological rest and balance, with a metabolic reduction significantly deeper than that experienced during sleep or eyes-closed rest (Wallace 1970, Gallois 1984). Periods of clear experience of TC have been characterized by suspension of respiration without oxygen deprivation (Farrow & Hebert 1982, Badawi et al 1984); stabilization of the autonomic nervous system (Orme-Johnson 1973); and a decrease in plasma lactate, a chemical marker of metabolic activity (Jevning et al 1983) and cortisol levels (Jevning et al 1978). Simultaneous with this metabolic rest, the brain displays "restful alertness," characterized by greatly increased coherence between the EEG patterns of different areas of the brain (that is, stable phase relations between two EEG signals, as measured by Fourier analyses that attain correlations of over 0.95) (Levine 1976, Badawi et al 1984). Also, blood flow to the brain increases markedly (Jevning et al 1978).

The state of transcendental consciousness can thus be defined physiologically and experientially. This

---

* These various modes of vibration known as Veda are described and written down in the voluminous Vedic literature. Recently, the different aspects of Vedic literature have been found to correspond with different areas of the human physiology (Nader 1993).

corroborates Maharishi Ayurveda's view of TC as the fourth major state of human consciousness, in the sense that the three common states of waking, sleeping, and dreaming can be defined physiologically as well. MAV also discusses three higher states of consciousness (as yet untested in the laboratory) in which the full potential of consciousness progressively unfolds.

Maharishi Ayurveda views unfolding consciousness as the single most important strategy of both prevention and cure. Consistent with this theory, data suggest that regular experience of TC has significant health benefits. Such research supports the MAV concept that "remembering" the unified field enlivens the orderly patterns that prevail in a healthy body. For example, a Harvard study of elderly nursing home residents compared TM with two other types of meditation and relaxation techniques over three years; the TM group had the greatest reductions in stress and blood pressure, and by far the lowest mortality rate (Alexander et al 1989). A meta-analysis of research on meditation and trait anxiety conducted at the Stanford Research Institute found that TM is approximately twice as effective as other meditation techniques at reducing trait anxiety (Eppley et al 1989). Schneider et al, in press found TM to be approximately twice as effective as progressive muscle relaxation in reducing hypertension in older African Americans. Similar studies and meta-analyses have found TM to be more effective than other techniques in bringing improvement on several other variables (Alexander et al 1991, Alexander et al in press, Alexander et al 1994), which raises the question of why these techniques differ. An explanation suggested by the MAV viewpoint is that the crucial factor is not meditation per se, but experiencing the fourth state of consciousness, TC, an experience TM is known to produce.

Regular practice of TM also has been found to significantly reduce health care costs, as measured by insurance statistics; TM practitioners needed hospitalization for illness or surgery 80 percent less often than a matched control group (Orme-Johnson 1987A). A more recent study found reduced government payments for Canadian health insurance plan enrollees who learned TM (Herron et al in press). TM also has been found in several studies to retard biological aging (Wallace et al 1982, Glaser et al 1992). TM has been found to significantly reduce

high blood pressure (Cooper & Aygen 1978, Alexander et al 1989, Schneider et al 1992, Wallace et al 1982) and cholesterol (Cooper & Aygen 1978, 1979).

More than 500 studies have been conducted on TM in over 220 universities and research institutions in 27 countries. They have documented a wide range of benefits in such areas as rehabilitation and intellectual development (Chalmers et al 1989, Wallace et al 1989, Orme-Johnson & Farrow 1977).

Prevention, Pathogenesis, and Balance

Seeing the body as a pattern of intelligence is the basis of a central tenet of MAV: For optimal health, it is necessary to maintain the body's natural state of internal balance. This tenet has applications for strengthening immunity, as well as for prevention, diagnosis, and treatment. The natural state of balance is understood in terms of another important Ayurvedic concept—three principles known as *doshas,* which govern the functioning of the body. The three doshas are called, Vata, Pitta, and Kapha; each has specific qualities and governs certain physiological activities. The doshas are not thought of as specifically physiological, but as subtle principles that emerge early in the manifestation of the unified field. Therefore, they are understood to operate throughout nature.*

In terms of the body, Vata—which governs flow and motion—is said to be at the basis of the activity of the locomotor system. It controls functions such as blood circulation and the expansion and contraction of the lungs and heart; intestinal peristalsis and elimination; activities of the nervous system; the contractile process in muscle; ionic transport across membranes (such as the sodium pump); cell division; and unwinding of DNA during the process of transcription or replication. Vata is of prime importance in all homeostatic mechanisms and controls the other two principles, Pitta and Kapha.

---

* The doshas are considered to derive from combinations of still subtler expressions, the five mahabhutas, or "great elements." The physicist John Hagelin, a major contributor to grand unification theory, has pointed out that physics too now identifies five basic "elements," known as "spin types." All the force and particle fields of physics belong to one of these five categories, and the characteristics of the five spin types correspond closely to those of the five mahabhutas.

Pitta governs bodily functions concerned with heat and metabolism, and directs all biochemical reactions and the process of energy exchange. For example, it regulates digestion, functions of the exocrine glands and endocrine hormones, and intracellular metabolic pathways such as glycolysis, the tricarboxylic acid cycle, and the respiratory chain.

Kapha governs the structure and cohesion of the organism. It is responsible for biological strength, natural tissue resistance, and proper body structure. Microscopically, it is related to anatomical connections in the cell, such as the intracellular matrix, cell membrane, membranes of organelles, and synapses.

On a biochemical level, it structures receptors and the various forms of chemical binding.

When the doshas are balanced in their natural states and bodily locations, they produce health; when aggravated or imbalanced, they produce disease. A balanced Pitta dosha, for example, ensures healthy digestion, but an aggravated Pitta can cause ulcers and acid indigestion. MAV holds that all disease results from disruption of the natural balance of the doshas, and immune strength results from maintaining balance of the doshas. As Table 14-1 shows, the natural dosha balance can be thrown off by a wide variety of factors, such as unhealthy diet,

Table 14-1. The Three Doshas

Dosha	Effect of Balanced Dosha	Effect of Imbalanced Dosha	Factors Aggravating Dosha
Vata	Exhilaration Clear and alert mind Perfect functioning of bowels and urinary tract Proper formation of all bodily tissues Sound sleep Excellent vitality and immunity	Rough skin Weight loss Anxiety, worry Restlessness Constipation Decreased strength Arthritis Hypertension Rheumatic disorder Cardiac arrhythmia Insomnia	Excessive exercise Wakefulness Falling Bone fractures Tuberculosis Suppression of natural urges Cold Fear or grief Agitation or anger Fasting Pungent, astringent, and bitter foods Late autumn and winter (November–February)
Pitta	Lustrous complexion Contentment Perfect digestion Softness of body Perfectly balanced heat and thirst mechanisms Balanced intellect	Yellowish complexion Excessive body heat Insufficient sleep Weak digestion Inflammation Inflammatory bowel diseases Skin diseases Heartburn Peptic ulcer	Anger Strong sunshine Burning sensations Fasting Sesame products Linseed Yogurt Wine, vinegar Pungent, sour, or salty foods Midsummer and early autumn (July–October)
Kapha	Strength Normal joints Stability of mind Dignity Affectionate, forgiving nature Strong and properly proportioned body Courage Vitality	Pale complexion Coldness Lethargy Excessive sleep Sinusitis Respiratory diseases Asthma Excessive weight gain Loose joints Depression	Sleeping during daytime Heavy food Sweet, sour, or salty food Milk products Sugar Spring and early summer (March–June)

poor digestion, unnatural daily routine, pollutants, and certain behaviors. The balance is restored by a variety of dietary and behavioral modalities, as well as other modalities discussed in this chapter, such as TM and herbal mixtures.

Each dosha has five subdivisions that govern different aspects of the body. For example, one subdivision of Pitta, *Bhrajaka* Pitta, relates to the skin. When balanced, it gives luster to the skin; when aggravated, Bhrajaka Pitta results in acne, boils, and rashes.

The concept of doshas—underlying metabolic principles—simplifies the practitioner's tasks and increases his or her effectiveness. The tri-dosha concept can help in clarifying the possible side effects of any treatment, customizing treatments for a specific patient, predicting risk factors and tendencies toward specific diseases, and noticing clusters of apparently unrelated syndromes that may have a similar underlying cause.

Some of these aspects result from the doshas' ability to provide the basis for a more precise description of the individual's natural state of balance. An individual may have a natural predominance of one or more doshas. These doshas need not be present in equal proportion to ensure physiologic balance, but they need to be functioning in harmony with each other. This state is called *prakriti*. When the doshas are out of balance, they create *vikriti*, resulting in disorder and disease. Table 14-2 describes the classic characteristics of Vata, Pitta, and Kapha prakritis. More common than these are mixed prakritis, which involve various combinations of the three classic types, such as Vata/Pitta, or Pitta/Kapha, also describing the normal state of balance for individuals who possess them. Treatment in MAV is tailored to the individual patient through careful evaluation of both prakriti and vikriti.

Since Maharishi Ayurveda views disease as resulting from disruption of the natural balance of the doshas, it follows that the doshas play a key role in MAV's approach to understanding pathogenesis. In Western medicine, a disease is detected as a result of its symptoms. The emergence of symptoms, however, must be preceded by earlier stages of imbalance. MAV locates six stages of pathogenesis, the first three of which have highly subtle symptoms with

Table 14-2. Classic Characteristics of Vata, Pitta, and Kapha Prakritis

Vata prakriti
- Light, thin build
- Performs activity quickly
- Tendency to dry skin
- Aversion to cold weather
- Irregular hunger and digestion
- Quick to grasp new information, also quick to forget
- Tendency toward worry
- Tendency toward constipation
- Tendency toward light and interrupted sleep

Pitta prakriti
- Moderate build
- Performs activity with medium speed
- Aversion to hot weather
- Sharp hunger and digestion
- Medium time to grasp new information
- Medium memory
- Tendency toward irritability and temper
- Enterprising and sharp in character
- Prefers cold food and drink
- Cannot skip meals
- Good speakers
- Tendency toward reddish complexion and hair, moles, and freckles

Kapha prakriti
- Solid heavier build
- Greater strength and endurance
- Slow, methodical in activity
- Oily, smooth skin
- Tranquil, steady personality
- Slow to grasp new information, slow to forget
- Slow to become excited or irritated
- Sleep is heavy and for long periods of time
- Hair is plentiful, tends to be dark color
- Slow digestion, mild hunger

which allopathic medicine is not familiar. These first three stages involve aggravation of the normal functioning of the doshas. A skilled MAV diagnostician can detect these early pathogenic stages before overt symptoms emerge, using the techniques discussed in the next section.

Diagnosis

Maharishi Ayurveda adds a number of diagnostic techniques to the clinician's repertoire. All of them are noninvasive and reveal much information both about specific illnesses and about underlying imbalances. Chief among these techniques is *nadi vigyan* (pulse diagnosis), which allows one to retrieve detailed information about the internal functioning of the body and its organs through signals present in the radial pulse. This information involves not only the cardiovascular system, but other bodily systems as well. From the pulse, the diagnostician gains information about the functioning of the bodily tissues, the state of the doshas, and much more. Pulse diagnosis reveals early stages of imbalance that precede full-blown symptoms. In this and other MAV diagnostic modalities, perceiving the body as a pattern of intelligence enables physicians to retrieve enormous amounts of information in a noninvasive manner.

Pharmacology

This paradigm in which the body is understood in terms of patterns of intelligence also is demonstrated in Maharishi Ayurveda's approach to pharmacology, which makes sophisticated use of thousands of herbs and other plants.

Western pharmacology—applying the mechanistic model of the body—isolates and then synthesizes single active ingredients from herbs and plants. For example, the Ayurvedic remedy willow bark was the source of acetylsalicylic acid, and the Ayurvedic remedy rauwolfia was the source of reserpine. The active-ingredient model reflects a weakness of the scientific method—its inability to deal with complex systems, and its requirement that the researcher radically simplify a process in order to evaluate it (Sharma, in press A). By contrast, Ayurvedic pharmacology, called *dravyaguna*, utilizes the synergistic cooperation of substances as they *co*-exist in natural sources. It uses either single plants, or more often, mixtures of plants whose effects are complementary. Such synergistic effects are gaining consideration in Western medical research, which is finding, for example, that *combinations* of antioxidants may stop oxidation damage and cancer cell growth more effectively than these substances acting alone. In terms of MAV's consciousness model, the effectiveness of herbal mixtures relative to active ingredients can be explained by the idea that plants, especially herbs, are concentrated repositories of nature's intelligence which, when used properly, can increase the expression of that intelligence in the body. Research and experience with Maharishi Ayurveda herbal mixtures, known as *rasayanas,* shows that synergism enhances the free radical-scavenging properties of herbs and mitigates the harmful side effects that often accompany Western drugs.

According to Maharishi Ayurveda, rasayanas promote longevity, stamina, immunity, and overall well-being (Sharma 1993). Research has shown several of them to have significant antioxidant properties (Fields et al 1990, Niwa 1991, Tomlinson & Wallace 1991, Dwivedi et al 1991, Engineer et al 1992, Sharma et al 1992, Hanna et al 1994, Sharma et al 1995). The rasayana known as Maharishi Amrit Kalash (MAK) is approximately 1000 times more effective at scavenging free radicals than such active ingredients as vitamins C and E, and a commonly used pharmaceutical antioxidant (Sharma et al 1992). Research also has found these herbal mixtures to be effective in clinical use. For example, in angina patients using MAK, the angina frequency and systolic blood pressure were reduced significantly, and exercise tolerance was improved (Dogra et al 1994). MAK also increased resistance of low-density lipoprotein to oxidation in hyperlipidemic patients, which is important for the prevention of atherosclerosis (Sundaram et al 1995). As aforementioned, MAK also is effective in protecting against the side effects of chemotherapy (Misra et al 1994). MAK has been found to improve age-related visual discrimination, which also might involve attentional capacity and alertness (Gelderloos et al 1990). Another MAV herbal mixture known as Student Rasayana improved the performance of children on a test of nonverbal intelligence (Nidich et al 1993).

MAK was found in laboratory research to have anticancer and anticarcinogenic properties (Sharma et al 1990, Sharma et al 1991A, Arnold et al 1991, Prasad et al 1992, Patel et al 1992, Dileepan et al 1993); to prevent atherosclerosis and human platelet aggregation (Lee 1995, Sharma et al 1989); to improve immunity (Dileepan et al 1990, 1993); and to protect against the toxic effects of toluene, an industrial chemical that can cause brain damage (Bondy et al 1994, Sharma et al 1995).

Diet and Digestion

Western medical research is accumulating more and more evidence that diet plays a critical role in the development of heart disease and cancer. For example, researchers now suspect that diet plays a role in at least 35% of cancer deaths. Ayurveda has long considered problems of diet and digestion to be among the central causes of all disease, and has considered improvement of diet and digestion to be crucial to almost any therapeutic regimen. Ayurveda views faulty diet as not only contributing to specific degenerative diseases, but also to throwing off the body's natural balance, thus weakening immunity.

MAV's approach to diet rests on the "consciousness model;" food is viewed as not only providing matter and energy to the body, but also intelligence, order, and balance. This brings to mind the observations of the Nobel Laureate physicist Erwin Schrödinger that food helps the body to resist the Second Law of Thermodynamics, which normally leads any complex system into chaos (Schrödinger 1967). By this view, when we eat, we are eating not only nutrients, but also orderliness. MAV dietetics considers not only the nutritional value and caloric content of food, but also the food's impact on the body's underlying state of balance; food affects the doshas, and diet must be suited to the individual vikriti and prakriti. It also must reflect the climate and season, as well as specific health conditions.

The influence of food on the doshas is specific to the food, but usually can be determined by knowing in which generic categories of tastes and qualities the food belongs. According to MAV, the six categories of taste are: sweet, sour, salty, pungent, astringent, and bitter. The six major categories of quality are: heavy, light, cold, warm, oily, and dry. Table 14-3 summarizes how taste and food qualities affect the doshas, and Table 14-4 gives examples of foods that possess these various qualities and tastes.

To give an example of how this information would be applied clinically, a patient with Kapha syndromes (such as sinusitis or certain types of obesity) would be told to minimize eating cold, oily, and heavy foods, as well as foods with sweet, sour, and salty tastes. The patient would be advised instead to give predominance to foods exhibiting the remaining qualities and tastes.

Maharishi Ayurveda recommends a lacto-vegetarian diet for optimal health. Meat is more difficult to digest and has been linked to numerous diseases, including heart disease and cancer. MAV also recommends the use of fresh produce. These emphases

Table 14-3. Taste and Food Quality Effects on the Doshas

Tastes	
Decrease Vata	Increase Vata
Sweet	Pungent
Sour	Bitter
Salty	Astringent
Decrease Pitta	Increase Pitta
Sweet	Pungent
Bitter	Sour
Astringent	Salty
Decrease Kapha	Increase Kapha
Pungent	Sweet
Bitter	Sour
Astringent	Salty
Major Food Qualities	
Decrease Vata	Increase Vata
Heavy	Light
Oily	Dry
Hot	Cold
Decrease Pitta	Increase Pitta
Cold	Hot
Heavy	Light
Oily	Dry
Decrease Kapha	Increase Kapha
Light	Heavy
Dry	Oily
Hot	Cold

Table 14-4. Common Examples of the Six Tastes and the Major Food Qualities

The Six Tastes and Some Common Examples

Sweet: Sugar, milk, butter, rice, breads, honey

Sour: Yogurt, lemon, cheese

Salty: Salt

Pungent: Spicy foods, peppers, ginger, cumin

Bitter: Spinach, other green leafy vegetables

Astringent: Beans

The Six Major Food Qualities and Some Common Examples

Heavy: Cheese, yogurt, wheat products

Light: Barley, corn, spinach, apples

Oily: Dairy products, fatty foods, oils

Dry: Barley, corn, potato, beans

Hot: Hot (temperature) food and drink

Cold: Cold food and drink

map well with emerging Western findings on diet, which have shown significant health benefits from a meatless diet and from increasing consumption of plant-based foods.

Maharishi Ayurveda focuses not only on what one eats, but also on how one digests it. The emphasis on digestion contrasts with Western allopathic medicine, which deals with digestion only when it is significantly disrupted. In MAV, excellent digestion is critical to robust health. MAV contains a number of techniques for improving digestion and treating digestive disorders. They center around the concept of *agni*, which literally means "fire," and refers to metabolic and digestive activities that convert foodstuff into bodily substances. Ayurveda describes 13 types of agni in the body. Their importance in Ayurvedic health care is suggested by the fact that one of the eight branches of Ayurveda, *Kaya Chikitsa* (internal medicine), focuses on the strength or weakness of the agnis.

This becomes clearer when we consider the end product of poor digestion, which Ayurveda calls *ama*. Ama plays a key role in pathogenesis, interacting with aggravated doshas, and causing them to "stick" to areas where they do not belong. Healthy digestion reduces the amount of ama produced.

To rid the body of accumulated ama, pollutants, and other pathogenic impurities that disrupt or block the natural expression of the body's inner intelligence, Maharishi Ayurveda emphasizes the importance of purification therapies that rid the body of these substances. Foremost among these purification therapies is *panchakarma*, which literally means "five activities," because it includes five main treatment modalities:

1. Whole-body massage with herbalized oil (*abhyanga*)
2. Continuous flow of warm herbalized oil on the forehead (*shirodhara*)
3. Fomentation of the body with herbalized heat (*swedana*)
4. Special herbalized oil head massage and nasal administration of herbs (*nasya*)
5. Sesame oil retention or herbalized eliminative enemas (*basti*).

Daily treatments, administered for two to fourteen days or longer, are recommended with each change of the seasons. Certain aspects of panchakarma can fit easily into a patient's daily preventive regime. Preliminary research has shown that regular panchakarma reduces several cardiovascular risk factors, including cholesterol (Sharma et al 1993A, Waldschutz 1994). Sesame oil, which is used topically and for colonic irrigation in panchakarma, has been shown to inhibit *in vitro* malignant melanoma growth (Smith & Salerno 1992) and human colon adenocarcinoma cell line growth (Salerno & Smith 1991).

The central role of food and digestion is demonstrated particularly well by consideration of another central MAV concept—the importance of a substance called *ojas*. Ojas is said to be the finest manifestation of the unified field, which serves as a sort of glue to link consciousness and matter. Ojas maintains the integrity of the seven bodily tissues (*dhatus*): plasma (*rasa*), blood (*rakta*), muscle (*mamsa*), fat (*meda*), bone (*asthi*), bone marrow and nervous system (*majja*), and sperm/ovum (*sukra*). The majority of MAV therapies and behavioral advice are designed to maximize the presence of ojas, and almost all MAV proscriptions are designed to minimize the depletion of ojas. The end product of truly healthy diet and digestion is said to contain significant amounts of ojas. According to an MAV expression, "like a bee which gets honey from the flowers, we get ojas from our food." MAV also asserts that positive, loving emotions increase the abundance of ojas; food should be eaten in a warm, congenial, and uplifting atmosphere. Arguing, or any other negativity at meals interferes with digestion, producing a harmful end product instead of ojas.

Behavior, Emotions, and the Senses

The recommendation for a positive emotional tone during meals reflects a general concept of MAV regarding behavior, speech, and emotions, and their effect on health. This concept springs naturally from the model that places consciousness at the basis of the body. Emotions can be understood as fine fluctuations of consciousness (or the unified field); as such, their impact on the more expressed physical levels of the body are immense. Recently, Western medicine has begun to investigate the effect of emotions on health, with interesting findings; Ayurveda has discussed this field for millennia. Ayurvedic texts include detailed discussions of lifestyle and behavior, and their impact on health. Interestingly, traditional virtues—such as respect for elders, teachers, loved ones, and family members, pardoning those who wrong you, practicing nonviolence, and not speaking ill of others—are understood to promote health for the individual's mind and body, as well as for the community and society.

In addition to emotion, sensory input is understood to have an impact on health. This idea is applied clinically, not only in terms of behavioral advice, but also in the form of sensory therapies, such as aromatherapy and sound therapy involving both music (called *Gandharva-Veda*) and primordial sounds that are used for their healing qualities. A study on Maharishi Ayurveda primordial sound therapy (specifically, Vedic sounds known as *Sama Veda*) found it to reduce in vitro human tumor cell growth significantly, whereas hard rock music tended to increase the growth significantly (Sharma et al, in press).

Biological Rhythms

In Maharishi Ayurveda, attuning the patient's lifestyle to natural biorhythms is considered a crucial element of prevention and treatment. MAV gives a detailed analysis of circadian (daily) and circannual (seasonal) rhythms, with recommendations for daily and seasonal routines. These include such advice as rising and retiring early and eating one's main meal at lunchtime, when the digestive "fires" are strongest. This advice must be suited to the individual. Emerging Western data on biorhythms correlates well with Ayurvedic knowledge. Again, the idea of a connection between patterns of order in nature and in the human body was obvious to Ayurveda millennia ago.

The three-dosha concept plays a key role in understanding these connections. Different times of the day are associated with different doshas, as are different seasons and the different stages of the human life cycle. For example, the summer is dominated by Pitta (the dosha that governs heat and metabolism), while the spring is dominated by Kapha (which has qualities of coolness and moisture). Childhood is dominated by Kapha (which governs structure, substance, and growth), old age by Vata. In fact, physicians see a preponderance of Kapha-based disorders in children, such as colds and respiratory illnesses, and an ever-increasing number of Vata disorders in

elderly patients, such as constipation and lighter, shorter, and more frequently interrupted sleep. They also see more Kapha-type disorders in spring and Pitta disorders in summer. Understanding the concept of doshas is helpful in treating these ailments.

The Seasons and Times of Day Classified According to the Doshas

- Kapha season: Spring-early summer (approximately March to June)
- Kapha time: Approximately 6 AM (sunrise) to 10 AM and 6 PM to 10 PM
- Kapha period in life cycle: Childhood
- Pitta season: Midsummer-early autumn (approximately July to October)
- Pitta time: Approximately 10 AM to 2 PM and 10 PM to 2 AM
- Pitta period in life-cycle: Adulthood
- Vata season: Late autumn-winter (approximately November to February)
- Vata time: Approximately 2 AM to 6 AM (sunrise) and 2 PM to 6 PM
- Vata period in life cycle: Old age

Collective Health and the Environment

Maharishi Ayurveda holds great promise in several areas of collective health. In terms of infectious disease and epidemics, the Western approach of using antibiotics has an inherent limitation and risk, caused by the process of natural selection that produces new resistant strains of microbes. As a result, overreliance on antibiotics can foster the growth of serious new infectious diseases. MAV's focus on strengthening immunity, and its techniques for dealing directly with epidemics offers a more effective and safer means of ensuring collective health.

In terms of chronic disease, Western medicine has long recognized that preventing and treating these disorders requires changes in lifestyle, diet, and behavior. However, allopathic medicine has been at a loss as to how to effect these changes in patients for a prolonged period of time. Research has shown that those who practice TM are better able to give up harmful habits such as cigarette smoking, alcohol consumption, and illegal drug use, and incorporate healthy dietary and lifestyle changes (Monahan 1977, Gelderloos et al 1991, Alexander et al 1994). MAV also offers other time-tested modalities that benefit individual patients, such as daily routine and purification procedures, which could be useful in large-scale applications. Finally, MAV offers an overall theory of prevention, involving such elements as the three-dosha concept, that could have value for future research on preventive medicine.

The most significant public health approach of Maharishi Ayurveda deals with larger social disorders and the dangers they pose. War, crime, and violence rarely are considered subjects of public health policy, but their implications for health are obvious. As with individual disease, Maharishi Ayurveda understands these as originating not in material factors but ultimately in consciousness—in this case, both individual and collective consciousness. Just as an abstract field of consciousness underlies the individual's mind and body, so such a field underlies societal trends. Society reflects the influence of its members not only in a linear, additive way—in the sense that a green forest is made of green trees—but also through a field effect—in the sense that a gravitational field's influences are not localized. If the individual consciousness of a sufficient number of members of a society is coherent, harmonious, and life-supporting, those influences spread through the "field" of the collective consciousness of the society, influencing the whole society.

This idea has been tested by a number of studies. One study found that when a sufficiently large group of practitioners of the TM and advanced TM-Sidhi techniques meditated together as a group in Israel, war deaths in Lebanon were significantly reduced, compared to casualty rates on days when the number of practitioners meditating together decreased below a certain threshold (Orme-Johnson et al 1987B). Similar findings have emerged in studies of other localities, usually involving reductions in the rate of violent crime (Orme-Johnson & Gelderloos 1988, Dillbeck et al 1981, Dillbeck et al 1988). For example, a 1993 study in Washington, DC showed that when a large group of practitioners of the TM and TM-Sidhi programs assembled to meditate during the summer, it produced an 18 percent reduction in violent crime compared to levels that had been predicted based on the previous years' crime and weather trends (Hagelin et al 1994). There has been much discussion and debate regarding these observations and the validity of what has been called the Maharishi effect.

Future Directions

Many central elements of Ayurveda—such as the ideas that diet and emotions play a crucial role in disease and in prevention—were not taken seriously by Western medicine a generation ago, but are now major themes of research. Other concerns of MAV might prove to be of value both in clinical work and in research. Already, Maharishi Ayurveda's Transcendental Meditation technique and herbal preparations have produced bodies of significant research findings whose implications have yet to be fully explored. Other areas, such as prakriti and vikriti, will likely prove equally interesting to researchers.

The clinical use of Maharishi Ayurveda has appeared to be most dramatic when applied to diseases that Western medicine finds difficult to treat, such as poor digestion, cancer, and chronic disease (Orme-Johnson 1987A, Janssen 1989). Its clinical value extends to other areas not discussed above, such as pediatrics, where it has been found to significantly reduce the incidence of childhood ailments such as frequent colds, or gynecology, where it has been able to reduce the severity of menstrual and pre-menstrual problems.

Hundreds of physicians worldwide have been trained in Maharishi Ayurveda and have incorporated its principles into their practice. Maharishi Ayurveda schools, institutions, and universities are being opened in each state of the United States, to train physicians, technicians, and nurses, and to teach the general public various areas of health-care management. Several medical institutions have incorporated this teaching into their curriculums. Maharishi Ayurveda continues to make significant contributions to the health care profession in the United States and around the world.

REFERENCES

Alexander CN, Langer EJ, Davies JL, et al. 1989. Transcendental Meditation, mindfulness and longevity: an experimental study with the elderly. J Pers Soc Psychol 57:950–964

Alexander CN, Rainforth MV, Gelderloos P. 1991. Transcendental Meditation, self-actualization, and psychological health: A conceptual overview and statistical meta-analysis. J Soc Behav Pers 6:189–247

Alexander CN, Robinson P, Orme-Johnson DW, et al. In press. The effects of Transcendental Meditation compared to other methods of relaxation and meditation in reducing risk factors, morbidity and mortality. Homeostasis

Alexander CN, Robinson P, Rainforth M. 1994. Treating alcohol, nicotine, and drug abuse through Transcendental Meditation: A review and statistical meta-analysis. Alcohol Treat Q 11:13–87

Arnold JT, Wilkinson BP, Korytynski EA, Steel VE. 1991. Chemopreventive activity of Maharishi Amrit Kalash and related agents in rat tracheal epithelial and human tumor cells. Proc Am Assoc Cancer Res 32:128(abstract)

Aspect A, Grangier P, Roger G. 1981. Experimental tests of realistic local theories via Bell's theorem. Physical Rev Let 47:460

Badawi K, Wallace RK, Orme-Johnson DW, Rouzere AM. 1984. Electrophysiologic characteristics of respiratory suspension periods occurring during the practice of the Transcendental Meditation program. Psychosom Med 46:267–276

Bondy SC, Hernandez TM, Mattia C. 1994. Antioxidant properties of two Ayurvedic herbal preparations. Biochem Arch 10:25–31

Carr T. 1991. Medicine at the mind-body interface: The approach of Maharishi Ayur-Ved. Intl Clin Nutr Rev 11(4):190–220

Chalmers RA, Clements G, Schenkluhn H, Weinless M (eds). 1989. Scientific Research on Maharishi's Transcendental Meditation and TM-Sidhi Program: Collected Papers, Vols. 2, 3, 4. MVU Press, Vlodrop, The Netherlands

Charaka S. 1977. Sharma RK, Dash B, (trans.) Chowkhamba Sanskrit Series Office, Varanasi, India

Cooper MJ, Aygen MM. 1978. Effect of Transcendental Meditation on serum cholesterol and blood pressure. Harefuah 95(1):1–2

Cooper MJ, Aygen MM. 1979. A relaxation technique in the management of hypercholesterolemia. J Hum Stress 5:24–27

Dileepan KN, Patel V, Sharma HM, Stechschulte DJ. 1990. Priming of splenic lymphocytes after ingestion of an Ayurvedic herbal food supplement: evidence for an immunomodulatory effect. Biochem Arch 6:267–274

Dileepan KN, Varghese ST, Page JC, Stechschulte DJ. 1993. Enhanced lymphoproliferative response, macrophage mediated tumor cell killing and nitric oxide production after ingestion of an Ayurvedic drug. Biochem Arch 9:365–374

Dillbeck MC, Banus CB, Polanzi C, Landrith III G. 1988. Text of a field model of consciousness and social change: the transcendental meditation and TM-Sidhi program and decreased urban crime. Mind Behav 9(4):457–486

Dillbeck MC, Landrith III G, Orme-Johnson DW. 1981. The Transcendental Meditation program and crime rate change in a sample of 48 cities. J Crime Justice 4:24–45

Dogra J, Grover N, Kumar P, Aneja N. 1994. Indigenous free radical scavenger MAK 4 and 5 in angina pectoris: Is it only a placebo? J Assoc Physicians India 42(6):466–467

Dwivedi C, Sharma HM, Dobrowki S, Engineer F. 1991. Inhibitory effects of Maharishi Amrit Kalash (M-4) and Maharishi Amrit Kalash (M-5) on microsomal lipid peroxidation. Pharmacol Biochem Behav 39:649–652

Eddington A. 1974. The Nature of the Physical World. University of Michigan Press, Ann Arbor, p. 276

Engineer FN, Sharma HM, Dwivedi C. 1992. Protective effects of M-4 and M-5 on Adriamycin-induced microsomal lipid peroxidation and mortality. Biochem Arch 8:267–272

Eppley KR, Abrams A, Shear J. 1989. Differential effects of relaxation techniques on trait anxiety: a meta-analysis. J Clin Psychol 45:957–974

Farrow JT, Hebert JR. 1982. Breath suspension during the transcendental meditation technique. Psychosom Med 44(2):133–153

Fields J, Rawal P, Hagen J, et al. 1990. Oxygen free radical (OFR) scavenging effects of an anti-carcinogenic natural product, Maharishi Amrit Kalash (MAK). Pharmacologist 32:A155(abstract)

Gallois P. 1984. Modifications neurophysiologiques et respiratoires lors de la practique des techniques de relaxation. L'encephale 10:139–144

Gelderloos P, Ahlstrom HHB, Orme-Johnson DW, et al. 1990. Influence of a Maharishi Ayur-Vedic herbal preparation on age-related visual discrimination. Int J Psychosom 37:25–29

Gelderloos P, Walton KG, Orme-Johnson DW, Alexander CN. 1991. Effectiveness of the Transcendental Meditation program in preventing and treating substance misuse: A review. Int J Addic 26:293–325

Glaser J, Brind J, Vogelman J, et al. 1992. Elevated serum dehydroepiandrosterone sulfate levels in practitioners of the Transcendental Meditation (TM) and TM Sidhi programs. J Behav Med 15(4):327–341

Hagelin JS, Orme-Johnson DW, Rainforth M, et al. 1994. Results of the national demonstration project to reduce violent crime and improve governmental effectiveness in Washington, D.C. Institute of Science, Technology, and Public Policy Technical Report ITR-94:1

Hanna AN, Sharma HM, Kauffman EM, Newman HAI. 1994. In vitro and in vivo inhibition of microsomal lipid peroxidation by MA-631. Pharmacol Biochem Behav 48:505–510

Herron R, Hills S, Mandarino J, et al. Reducing medical costs: the impact of transcendental meditation on government payments to physicians in Quebec. Am J Health Promotion. (in press)

Janssen GWHM. 1989. The application of Maharishi Ayur-Ved in the treatment of ten chronic diseases: a pilot study. Ned Tijdschr Geneeskd 5:586–94

Jevning JR, Wilson AF, Davison JM. 1978. Adrenocortical activity during meditation. Horm Behav 10:54–60

Jevning JR, Wilson AF, O'Halloran JP, Walsh RN. 1983. Forearm blood flow and metabolism during stylized and unstylized states of decreased activation. Am J Physiol 245(Regul Integr Comp Physiol 14):R100–R116

Lee JY. 1995. The antioxidant and antiatherogenic effects of MAK-4 in WHHL rabbits. Ph.D. dissertation, The Ohio State University, Columbus, Ohio

Levine JP. 1976. The Coherence Spectral Array (COSPAR) and its application to the study of spatial ordering in the EEG. Proc San Diego Biomed Symp 15:237–247

Lonsdorf N, Butler V, Brown M. 1993. A Woman's Best Medicine: Health, Happiness and Long Life Through Ayur-Veda. Jeremy P. Tarcher/Putnam. New York

Madhavakava. 1986. Madhava Nidanam. Srikanta Murthy KR (trans). Chaukambha Orientalia. Delhi, India

Misra NC, Sharma HM, Chaturvedi A, et al. 1994. Antioxidant adjuvant therapy using a natural herbal mixture MAK during intensive chemotherapy: reduction in toxicity—A prospective study of 62 patients. In: Rao RS, Deo MG, Sanghvi LD (eds). Proceedings of the Sixteenth International Cancer Congress, Monduzzi Editore, Bologna, Italy, pp. 3099–3102

Monahan RJ. 1977. Secondary prevention of drug dependence through the transcendental meditation program in metropolitan Philadelphia. Int J Addict 12:729–754

Nader T. 1993. Human Physiology: Expression of Veda and the Vedic Literature. MVU Press. Vlodrop, The Netherlands

Nidich SI, Morehead P, Nidich RJ, et al. 1993. The effect of the Maharishi Student Rasayana food supplement on non-verbal intelligence. Person Individ Diff 15:599–602

Niwa Y. 1991. Effect of Maharishi-4 and Maharishi-5 on inflammatory mediators—with special reference to their free radical scavenging effect. Indian J Clin Prac 1:23–27

Orme-Johnson DW. 1973. Autonomic stability and transcendental meditation. Psychosom Med 35:341–349

Orme-Johnson DW. 1987A. Medical care utilization and the transcendental meditation program. Psychosom Med 49:493–507

Orme-Johnson DW, Alexander CN, Davies JL, et al. 1987B. International peace project in the Middle East: The effects of the Maharishi Technology of the Unified Field. J Conflict Resolution 32(4):776–812

Orme-Johnson DW, Farrow JT (eds). 1977. Scientific Research on the Transcendental Meditation Program: Collected Papers, Vol. 1. MERU Press. Rheinweiler, Germany

Orme-Johnson DW, Gelderloos P. 1988. The long term effects of the Maharishi Technology of the Unified Field on the quality of life in the United States (1960–1983). Soc Sci Per J 2(4):127–146

Patel VK, Wang J, Shen RN, et al. 1992. Reduction of metastases of Lewis Lung Carcinoma by an Ayurvedic food supplement in mice. Nutr Res 12:667–676

Prasad KN, Edwards-Prasad J, Kentroti S, et al. 1992. Ayurvedic (science of life) agents induce differentiation in murine neuroblastoma cells in culture. Neuropharmacology 31:599–607

Rarity JG, Tapster PR. 1990. Experimental violation of Bell's inequality based on phase and momentum. Physical Rev Lett 64:2495

Salerno JW, Smith DE. 1991. The use of sesame oil and other vegetable oils in the inhibition of human colon cancer growth in vitro. Anticancer Res 11:209–216

Sarngadhara. 1984. Sarngadhara Samhita. Srikanta Murthy KR (trans). Chaukhambha Orientalia. Delhi, India

Schneider RH, Alexander CN, Wallace RK. 1992. In search of an optimal behavioral treatment for hypertension: a review and focus on transcendental meditation. In Johnson EH, Gentry WD, Julius S (eds). Personality, Elevated Blood Pressure, and Essential Hypertension. Hemisphere. Washington, DC, pp. 123–131

Schneider RH, Staggers F, Alexander CN, et al. A randomized controlled trial of stress reduction for the treatment of hypertension in older African Americans. Hypertension (in press)

Schrödinger E. 1967. What is Life? Cambridge University Press. Cambridge

Sharma H. 1993. Freedom from Disease: How to Control Free Radicals, a Major Cause of Aging and Disease. Veda Publishing. Toronto

Sharma HM. The fallacy of the active ingredient. In Alternative Perspectives on Health: An Ecological Approach. Chesworth J (ed). Sage Publications. Thousand Oaks, California (in press)

Sharma HM, Dwivedi C, Satter BC, Abou-Issa H. 1991A. Antineoplastic properties of Maharishi Amrit Kalash, an Ayurvedic food supplement, against 7, 12-dimethylbenz(a)anthracene-induced mammary tumors in rats. J Res Educ Indian Med 10(3):1–8

Sharma HM, Dwivedi C, Satter BC, et al. 1990. Antineoplastic properties of Maharishi-4 against DMBA-induced mammary tumors in rats. Pharmacol Biochem Behav 35:767–773

Sharma HM, Feng Y, Panganamala RV. 1989. Maharishi Amrit Kalash (MAK) prevents human platelet aggregation. Clin Ter Cardiovasc 8:227–230

Sharma H, Guenther J, Abu-Ghazaleh A, Dwivedi C. 1994A. Effects of Ayurvedic food supplement M-4 on cisplatin-induced changes in glutathione and glutathione-S-transferase activity. In Rao RS, Deo MG, Sanghvi LD, (eds). Proceedings of the Sixteenth International

Cancer Congress, Vol. 1. Monduzzi Editore, Bologna, Italy pp. 589–592

Sharma HM, Hanna AN, Kauffman EM, Newman HAI. 1992. Inhibition of human LDL oxidation in vitro by Maharishi Ayur-Veda herbal mixtures. Pharmacol Biochem Behav 43:1175–1182

Sharma HM, Hanna AN, Kauffman EM, Newman HAI. 1995. Effect of herbal mixture Student Rasayana on lipoxygenase activity and lipid peroxidation. Free Radic Biol Med 18:687–697

Sharma HM, Kauffman EM, Dudek A, Stephens RE. Effect of different sounds on growth of human cancer cell lines in vitro. J Res Educ Indian Med (in press)

Sharma HM, Nidich SI, Sands D, Smith DE. 1993A. Improvement in cardiovascular risk factors through Panchakarma purification procedures. J Res Educ Indian Med 12(4):2–13

Smith DE, Salerno JW. 1992. Selective growth inhibition of a human malignant melanoma cell line by sesame oil in vitro. Prostaglandins Leuko Essen Fatty Acids 46: 145–150

Stapp HP. 1994. Mind, Matter and Quantum Mechanics. Springer-Verlag. New York, pp. 220–221

Steel K, Gertman PM, Crescenzi C, Anderson J. 1981. Iatrogenic illness on a general medical service at a university hospital. N Engl J Med 304:638–642

Sundaram V, Hanna AN, Lubow G, et al. 1995. Increased resistance of human LDL to oxidation in hyperlipidemic patients supplemented with oral herbal mixture MAK-4. FASEB J 9(3):A141(abstract)

Sushruta S. 1963. Ghisagrantne KL (trans). Chowkhamba Sanskrit Series Office. Varanasi, India

Tomlinson PF, Wallace RK. 1991. Superoxide scavenging of two natural products, Maharishi-4 (M-4) and Maharishi-5 (M-5). FASEB J 5(5):A1284(abstract)

Vagbhata. 1982. Ashtanga Hridayam. Upaohyaya VY (ed). Chaukambha Sanskrit Sansthan. Varanasi, India

Waldschütz R. 1994. Influence of Maharishi Ayur-Veda purification treatment on physiological and psychological health. Translation; original German version appeared in 1988, Erfahrungsheilkunde-Acta medica empirica 11:720–729

Wallace RK. 1970. Physiological effects of transcendental meditation. Science 167:1751–1754

Wallace RK. 1993. The Physiology of Consciousness. MIU Press, Fairfield, Iowa

Wallace RK, Dillbeck MC, Jacobe E, Harrington B. 1982. The effects of the transcendental meditation and TM-Sidhi program on the aging process. Int J Neurosci 16: 53–58

Wallace RK, Orme-Johnson DW, Dillbeck MC (eds). 1989. Scientific Research on Maharishi's Transcendental Meditation and TM-Sidhi Program: Collected Papers, Vol. 5. MIU Press, Fairfield, Iowa

15
Curanderismo

Robert T. Trotter II

History

Curanderismo, from the Spanish verb *curar* (to heal), is a healing tradition found in Mexican American communities throughout the United States. Its historic roots are common with traditional healing practices in Puerto Rican and Cuban American communities, as well as traditional practices found throughout Latin America. At the same time, it has a history and a set of traditional medical practices that are unique to Mexican cultural history and to the Mexican American experience in the United States.

There are seven historic roots embedded in modern curanderismo. Its theoretical beliefs partly trace their origins to Greek humoral medicine, especially the emphasis on balance, and the influence of hot and cold properties of food and medicines on the body. Many of the rituals that provide both a framework and a meaningful cultural healing experience in curanderismo date to healing practices contemporary to the beginning of the Christian tradition, and even into earlier Judeo-Christian writings. Other healing practices derive from the European Middle Ages, including the use of traditional medicinal plants and magical healing practices.

The Moorish conquest of Southern Europe is visible in the cultural expression of curanderismo. Some common Mexican-American folk illnesses originated in the Near East and then were transmitted throughout the Mediterranean, such as belief in *mal de ojo*, or the evil eye (the magical influence of staring at someone). Homeopathic remedies for common health conditions such as earaches, constipation, anemia, cuts and bruises, or burns were brought from Europe to the New World, to be passed down to the present time within curanderismo. There also is significant sharing of beliefs with Aztec and other Native American cultural traditions in Mexico. Some of the folk illnesses treated in pre-Columbian times, such as a fallen fontanelle (caida de la mollera) and perhaps the blockage of the intestines (*empacho*) are parts of this tradition. The pharmacopeia of the New World also is important in curanderismo (and added significantly to the plants available for treatment of diseases in Europe from the 1600s to the present). Some healers (*curanderos*) keep track of developments in parapsychology and New Age spirituality, as well as acupuncture and Eastern healing traditions, and have incorporated these global perspectives into their own practices.

Finally, curanderismo is a traditional healing system, but it exists within the modern world. Biomedical beliefs, treatments, and practices are very much a part of curanderismo, and are supported by curanderos. On the border between the United States and Mexico, it is not unusual for healers to recommend the use of prescription medications (which can often be purchased in Mexico across the counter) for infections and other illnesses. These healers also use information obtained from television and other sources to provide the best advice on preventive efforts such as nutrition and exercise, and on explanations for biomedical illnesses. Individual healers vary greatly in their knowledge of the practices that stem from each of these seven historical sources. The overall system of curanderismo is complex and not only maintains its cultural link to the past, but evolves toward accommodation with the future as well.

Cultural Context

This article is based partly on research that was conducted in the Lower Rio Grande Valley of Texas for more than 15 years. That information is enhanced by data from other regions near the border between America and Mexico, and from Mexican American communities in Colorado, Nebraska, Chicago, and Florida. A multiplicity of research environments, both rural and urban, has affected the practice of curanderismo. Alger (1974) has described one possible outcome of urbanized curanderismo, in which the folk healing system mimics the modern medical system. Yet this mimicry does not exist to any significant extent in South Texas, where both curanderos and their clients have extensive knowledge of the medical system in urban and rural areas. However, unlike attitudes reported in earlier studies of the area (Madsen 1961, Rubel 1966), curanderos and their patients accept the utility of modern medicine. These multiple environments of curanderismo practice create a complex healing system with core elements that are common to each place, and modifications that respond to local cultural, political, and legal circumstances.

The earliest systematic research was done on curanderismo in the late 1950s; when modern medicine was inaccessible, or only recently available to significant segments of the Mexican American population. Since that time, the efficacy of modern medicine has been demonstrated empirically numerous times, so it is an integrated part of the cultural system, although many access barriers still exist to prevent its full utilization by everyone. These barriers reflect the same reasons that the holistic health movement and the charismatic healing movements are becoming increasingly popular. Although traditional healers in Mexican American communities believe that modern medicine is as capable in certain types of healing, their experience shows that their own practices are not recognized in hospitals and clinics, and that they can accomplish those same tasks better than modern medicine. Thus, curanderismo and modern medicine often assume complementary roles in the minds of the curanderos and their patients, although not necessarily in the minds of the medical professionals of the area.

Intellectual Tradition

Traditional Mexican American healers perceive health and illness to contain a duality of "natural" and "supernatural" illnesses. This duality forms the theoretical base upon which curanderismo is constructed. The natural source of illness is essentially a biomedical model of illness that includes lay interpretations of some diseases inspired by Mexican American culture. Biomedical aspects such as the germ theory of disease, genetic disorders, psychological conditions, and dietary causes for medical conditions are accepted. These natural illnesses are treated by physicians using herbal remedies. A parallel supernatural source of illness also is recognized by this healing tradition. These illnesses are not considered amenable to treatment by the medical establishment. They can be repaired only by the supernatural manipulations of curanderos. The curanderos fault the scientific medical system for its failure to recognize the existence of magic or of supernatural causation. One curandero commented that as many as ten percent of patients in mental institutions were really *embrujados* (hexed or bewitched), and because doctors could not recognize this condition, it went untreated.

Supernaturally induced illnesses are most commonly said to be initiated by either evil spirits (*espiritos malos*) or by *brujos* (individuals practicing antisocial magic). They form a significant part of the curanderos' work; these healers explain that any particular illness experienced by a patient could be caused theoretically by either natural or supernatural processes. For example, that there is a natural form of diabetes, and a form that is caused by a supernatural agent, such as a *brujo*. The same is true for alcoholism, cancer, and other diseases. Identifying the nature of the causal agent for a particular illness is a key problem for the curandero. Some identify more supernatural causes for illnesses, and others take a more biomedically balanced approach. In either case, there is far less dichotomizing of physical and social problems within curanderismo than within the medical care system (Kiev 1968, Holland 1963).

Curanderos routinely deal with problems of a social, psychological, and spiritual nature, as well as physical ailments. Many cases overlap into two or more categories. Bad luck in business is a common problem presented to curanderos. Other problems encountered were marital disruptions, alcoholism or alcohol abuse, infidelity, supernatural manifestations, cancer, diabetes, and infertility. One healer distinguishes between the problems presented by females and males. The central focus of the problems brought by women is the husband—the husband drinks too much, does not work, does not give them money, or is seeing other women. Men bring problems of a more physical nature, such as stomach pain, headaches, weakness, and bladder dysfunction. Men also bring problems that deal directly with work; they need to find a job, cannot get along with people at work, or are having trouble setting up a business. The wife rarely is the focal point of their problems. The total list of problems presented to curanderos includes nearly every situation that can be thought of as an uncomfortable human condition. Curanderismo seems to play an important, culturally appropriate psychotherapeutic role in Mexican American communities (Galvin 1961, Klineman 1969, Torrey 1972).

Another element of curanderismo that forms an important intellectual foundation for its practices is the concept that healers work by virtue of "a gift of healing" (*el don*) (Hudson 1951, Romano 1964, Rubel 1966, Madsen 1965). This inherent ability allows the healer to practice his or her work, especially in the supernatural area. In the past, this was believed to be a gift from God. However, a secular interpretation of the *don* is competing with the more traditional explanation. Many healers still refer to the *don* as a gift from God and support this premise with Biblical passages (Corinthians 12:7 and James 5:14), but other healers explain the *don* as an inborn trait that is present in all human beings, just like the ability to sing, run, or talk. Almost any human being can do these things, but some do them better than others, and a few people can do them extremely well. Curanderos, according to this theory, are the individuals with a better ability to heal than is normative

for the population as a whole. Healers refer to this concept as "developed abilities."

Another element common to Hispanic-based folk medicine is the hot-cold syndrome (Ingham 1940, Foster 1953, Currier 1966). This belief system is not common in South Texas (Madsen 1961), where the only indications of a hot-cold syndrome found amongst the patients were scattered folk beliefs such as not eating citrus during menses, not ironing barefoot on a cement floor, or taking a cold shower after prolonged exposure to the sun. None of these beliefs were organized in a systematic fashion, nor were they extensively shared within the Mexican American population. In other areas, there is extensive knowledge and use of this system of classifying foods, treatments, and elements of illnesses to provide the basis for deciding which remedies apply to specific illnesses.

Theoretic Basis

The community-based theoretic structure for curanderismo has three primary areas of concentration, called levels (*niveles*) by the healers—the material level (*nivel material*), the spiritual level (*nivel espiritual*), and the mental level (*nivel mental*). More *curanderos* have the *don* for working at the material level, which is organized around the use of physical objects to heal or to change the patient's environment. This theoretic area can be subdivided into physical and supernatural manipulations. Physical treatments are those that do not require supernatural intervention to assure a successful outcome. *Parteras* (midwives), *hueseros* (bone setters), *yerberos* (herbalists), and *sobadores* (people who treat sprains and tense muscles), are healers who work on the *nivel material* and effect cures without any need for supernatural knowledge or practices. All of the *remedios caseros* (home remedies) used in Mexican American communities are part of this healing tradition.

The supernatural aspect of this level is involved in cures for common folk illnesses found in Mexican American communities, such as *susto, empacho, caida de mollera, espanto,* and *mal de ojo.* These illnesses are unique to Hispanic cultural models of health and illness. This area of healing also includes the spells and incantations that are derived out of medieval European witchcraft and earlier forms of magic, such as the cabala, that have been maintained as supernatural healing elements of curanderismo. Supernatural manipulations involve prayers and incantations in conjunction with such objects as candles, ribbons, water, fire, crucifixes, tree branches, herbs, oils, eggs, and live animals. These treatments use a combination of common objects and rituals to cure health problems.

The spiritual level (*nivel espiritual*) is an area of healing that is parallel to the channeling found in New Age groups and in shamanistic healing rituals around the world (Macklin 1967, 1974a, 1974b, 1974c, Macklin & Crumrine 1973). Individuals enter an altered state of consciousness and, according to the curanderos, make contact with the spirit world by one or all of the following methods: opening their minds to spirit voices; sending their spirits out of the body to gain knowledge at a distance; or allowing spirits the use of the body to communicate with this world, or all three.

The mental level (*nivel mental*) is the least commonly encountered of the three levels. One healer described working with the mental level as the ability to transmit, channel, and focus mental vibrations (*vibraciones mentales*) in a way that would affect the patient's mental or physical condition directly. Both patients and healers are confident that the curanderos can effect a cure from a distance using this technique.

The three levels are discrete areas of knowledge and behavior, each necessitating the presence of a separate gift for healing. They involve different types of training, and different methods of dealing with both the natural and the supernatural world. The material level involves the manipulations of traditional magical forces found in literature on Western witchcraft. Spiritualism involves the manipulation of a complex spirit world that exists parallel to our own, and the manipulation of *corrientes espirituales*, spiritual currents that can both heal and provide information or diagnosis from a distance. The mental level necessitates the control and use of the previously mentioned *vibraciones mentales*. Thus, the levels are separate methods of diagnosing and treating human problems that are embedded into a single cultural tradition.

Not all problems can be successfully dealt with using each level. An example of this is serious alcohol abuse (Trotter & Chavira 1978, Trotter 1979). Alcohol abuse and alcoholism are treated by curanderos, using techniques of both the material and the mental level. The techniques of the spiritual level, however, were considered ineffective in dealing with alcohol-related problems. So if one has the *don* for working with the spiritual level alone, he or she is excluded from the process of curing alcohol problems.

One theme that is common to the practices of all three levels is the use of energy to change the health status of the client. On the material level, this energy often is discussed in relation to the major ritual of that level, known as the *barrida* or *limpia* (a sweeping, or cleansing). In that ritual, a person is "swept" from head to foot with an object that is thought to be able to either remove bad vibrations (*vibraciones malos*), or to give positive energy (*vibraciones positives*) to the patient. The type of object used (such as egg, lemon, garlic, crucifix, or broom) depends on the nature of the patient's problem and whether it is necessary to remove or to replace energy. On the spiritual level, the energy that is used for both diagnosis and healing is the previously mentioned *corrieiites espirituales*. The mental level is nearly totally oriented around generating and channeling *vibraciones mentales*. The following sections provide more detail on the actual practices of the curandero's work on each level.

The Material Level (nivel material)

The material level is the easiest of the three levels to describe; it is the most extensively practiced and the most widely reported. At this level, the curandero manipulates physical objects and performs rituals (or trabajas, spells). The combination of objects and rituals is widely recognized by Mexican-Americans as having curative powers. Practitioners of the material level employ common herbs, fruits, nuts, flowers, animals and animal products (chickens, doves, and eggs), and spices. Religious symbols are widely used, such as the crucifix, pictures of saints, incense, candles, holy water, oils, and sweet fragrances, and secular items as well, such as cards, alum, and ribbons. The curandero allows his patients to rely extensively on their own resources by prescribing items that either are familiar or have strong cultural significance; thus, a significant characteristic of the objects used at the material level is that they are common items used for daily activities such as cooking and worship.

Natural Illnesses and Herbal Cures

Curanderos recognize that illnesses can be brought about by natural causes, such as dysfunction of the body, carelessness or the inability of a person to take proper care of himself or herself, and infection. Curanderos at the material level utilized large amounts of medicinal herbs (*plantas medicinales*) to treat these natural ailments. Some traditional curanderos classify herbs as having the dichotomous properties considered essential for humoral medicine, based on a hot-cold classification system common throughout Latin America (Foster 1953). They use these dual properties to prescribe an herb or combination of herbs, depending on the characteristics of the illness. If a person's illness supposedly is caused by excessive "heat," an herb with "cold" properties is given. Conversely, if a person's illness is believed to be caused by excessive "coldness and dryness," a combination of herbs having "hot and wet" properties is administered.

Other curanderos recognize herbs for their chemical properties, such as poisons (*yerba del coyote, Karwinskia humboldtuna Roem. et Sch.*), hallucinogens (*peyote, Lophaphora williams Lem.*), sedatives (*flor de tila, Talia mexicana Schl.*), stimulants (*yerba del trueno*), and purgatives (*cascara sagrada*). These individuals refer to the beneficial chemical properties of the herbs that allow them to treat natural illnesses.

Curanderos prescribe herbs most frequently as teas, baths, or poultices. The teas act as a sort of formative chemotherapy. *Borraja* (borage: *Borajo officialis L.*), for example, is taken to cut a fever; *flor de tila*, a mild sedative, is taken for insomnia; *yerba de la golondrina* (*Euphorbia prostrate* Ait.) is used as a douche for vaginal discharges; and *peilos de elote* are used for kidney problems. Herbal baths usually are prescribed to deal with skin diseases; *fresno* (ash tree, *Fraxinus* Sp.) is used to treat scalp problems such as eczema, dandruff, and psoriasis; and *linaza* is prescribed for body sores. For specific sores such as boils, *malva* (probably a *Malvastrum*) leaves are boiled until soft and then applied to the sores as a poultice. Other herbs are used as decongestants. A handful of *oregano* (oregano: *Oregenum vulgare* L.) is placed in a humidifier to treat someone with a bad cold.

Some herbal lore is passed on as an oral tradition, and other information is available in Spanish language books for Mexico that are widely circulated among both curanderos and the public (Arias; Wagner). These works describe and classify numerous herbs. Herbal remedies are so important to Mexican-American folk medicine, that their use often is confused with the art of curanderismo itself by the mass culture. Indeed, some curanderos known as *yerberos* or *yerberas*, specialize in herbs, but their knowledge and skills go beyond the mere connection of one disease to one herbal formula. In order for a curandero to be genuine, even at the material level, an element of mysticism must be involved in their practice. Herbs are used commonly for their spiritual or supernatural properties. Spiritual cleansings (*barridas*) often are given with *ruda* (*Ruta graveolens L.*), *romero* (rosemary, *Rosmarinus officiates* L.), and *albacar* (sweet basil, *Ocimum basiticum L.*), among others. Herbs are used as amulets, *verbena* (verbena, *Verbena officinalis L.*), worn as an amulet, is used to help open a person's mind to learn and retain knowledge.

Some curanderos have successful practices on the material level without resorting to the use of herbs. Some nonherbal treatments are described below.

Supernaturally Caused Illnesses and Ritual Cures

Supernatural illnesses, which occur when supernatural negative forces damage a person's health, sometimes can be confused with natural illnesses. One healer stated that these supernatural illnesses may manifest as ulcers, tuberculosis, rheumatism, or migraine headaches, but in reality, they are believed to be hexes that have been placed on the person by an enemy. Supernatural influences also disrupt a person's mental health and his or her living environment. Physicians cannot cure a supernatural illness. The curandero commonly deals with social disruption, personality complexes, and sometimes with serious psychological disturbances. One healer gave the following description of a case that contained several of these elements:

> This patient worked for the street maintenance department of (a small city in south Texas). Every day after work a voice would lead him out into the brush and sometimes keep him there until 2:00 AM. This activity was wearing out the man and his family and he was going crazy. A bad spirit was following this man and would not leave him alone. The man was cured, but it took three people to cure him: myself, a friend, and a master (*maestro*) from Mexico. This man was given three *barridas* each day for seven days, one by each of us. The tools used were eggs, lemons, herbs, garlic, and black chickens. The man was also prescribed herbal baths and some teas to drink. He was also given a charm made from the *haba mijrina* designed to ward off any more negative influences which might be directed at him. This patient regained his sanity.

There also are a number of illnesses that are both supernaturally caused and of a supernatural nature, which can be treated on the material level. The following account is an example of such an illness and cure.

> My brother-in-law was working at a motel . . . in Weslaco. When he started working they laid off this other guy who had been working there for several years. This guy didn't like it, and he's been known to be messing around with black magic. I don't know what he did to my brother-in-law, but every other day he'd have to be taken home because he was sick. He started throwing up, had shaky knees, and weak joints. So my mother and I went over to see this lady in Reynosa, and she told my mother just what to do. My sister rubbed her husband with a lemon every night for three days. She also gave him some kind of tea . . . On the third day, a big black spot appeared on the lemon, so we threw it away, and he's been fine ever since.

Rituals and the Material Level

Curanderos use several types of rituals for supernatural cures. The *barrida* is one of the most frequent rituals. These cleansings are designed to remove the negative forces that are harming the patient, while simultaneously giving the patient the spiritual strength necessary to enhance recovery. Patients are always "swept" from head to toe, with the curandero makes sweeping or brushing motions with an egg, lemon, herb, or whatever object is deemed spiritually appropriate. Special emphasis is given to areas in pain. While sweeping the patient, the curandero recites specific prayers or invocations that appeal to God, saints, or other supernatural beings to restore health to the patient. The curandero may recite these prayers and invocations out loud or silently. Standard prayers include the Lord's Prayer, the Apostles' Creed, and *Las Doce Verdades de Mundo* (The Twelve Truths of the World).

The following description of a *barrida* illustrates how the material objects, the mystical power of these objects, the invocations, the curandero, and the patient come together to form a healing ritual designed for a specific patient and a specific illness: In this case, five eggs, four lemons, some branches of *albacar* (sweet basil), and oil were used. To begin the healing process, the lemons and eggs were washed with alcohol and water to cleanse them spiritually. Before beginning the ritual, the participants were instructed to take off their rings, watches, and other jewelry; high frequency spiritual and mental vibrations can produce electrical discharges on the metal, which might disturb the healing process. The sweeping itself is done by interchanging an egg and a lemon successively. Sweeping with the egg is intended to transfer the problem from the patient to the egg by means of conjures (*conjures*) and invocations (*rechasos*). The lemon is used to eliminate the *trabajo* (magical harm) that has been placed on the patient. The patient is swept once with *albacar* (sweet basil) that has been rinsed in *agua preparada* (prepared water). This sweeping purifies the patient, giving strength and comfort to his spiritual being. The ritual ends by making crosses with *aceite preparado* (specifically prepared oil) on the principal joints of the patients, such as the neck, under the knees, and above the elbow. This oil serves to cut the negative currents and vibrations that surround the patient, which have been placed there by whoever is provoking the harm. The crosses protect against the continued effect of these negative vibrations. *Agua preparada* is then rubbed on the patient's forehead and occiput (*cerebro*) to tranquilize and to give mental strength. All the objects used in the *barrida* are then burned, in order to destroy the negative influences or harm transferred from the patient.

Another common ritual is called a *sahumerio,* or incensing. The *sahumerio* is a purification rite, used primarily for treating businesses, households, farms, and other places of work or habitation. This ritual is executed by treating hot coals with an appropriate incense. The curandero may prepare his own incense, or he may prescribe some commercially prepared incense such as *el sahumerio maravilloso* (miraculous incense). A pan with the smoking incense is carried throughout the building, making sure that all corners, closets, and hidden spaces, such as under the beds, are properly filled with smoke. While "incensing," the healer or someone else recites an appropriate prayer. If the *sahumerio maravilioso* is used, the prayer often is one to Santa Marta, requesting that peace and harmony be restored to the household. After the *sahumerio,* the healer may sprinkle holy water on the floor of every room in the house and light a white candle that stays lit for seven days. The *sahumerio* is an example of the curandero treating the general social environment, seeking to change the conditions of the persons who live or work there. Incensing of a house removes negative influences such as bad luck (*salaciones*), marital disruptions, illness, or disharmony. For business and farms, incensing helps assure success and growth, and protects against jealous competitors. These rituals are designed to affect everyone in the environment that has been treated.

Another type of ritual, called a *sortilegio* (conjure) uses material objects such as ribbons to tie up the negative influences that harm the curandero's patients. These negative influences are frequently personal shortcomings such as excessive drinking, infidelity, rebellious children, unemployment, or any other problem believed to be imposed by antisocial magic (*un trabajo*). One *sortilegio* that the author observed required four ribbons in red, green, white, and black, each approximately one yard in length. The color of each ribbon represents a type of magic, which the curanderos can activate to deal with specific problems. Red magic involves domination, green deals with healing, white with general positive forces, and black with negative or debilitating forces.

When working with a specific area of magic, one uses material objects that are the appropriate color naturally or that have been made that color artificially. The color-based division of magic also is carried over into another type of ritual system used on the material level, *velacione,* or burning candles to produce supernatural results. The *velaciones* and the colored material objects used in the *sortilegios* tie into the energy theme that runs throughout curanderismo, because the colors and objects are believed to have specific vibratory power or energy that can affect the patient when activated by the incantations used in conjunction with the objects. For example, blue candles are burned for serenity or tranquility; red candles are burned for health, power, or domination; pink candles are burned for good will; green candles are burned to remove a harmful or negative influence; and purple candles are burned to repel and attack bad spirits (*espiritus obscuros*) or strong magic. Once the proper color of candle has been chosen to produce the proper mental atmosphere, the candles are arranged in the correct physical formation and activated by the *conjuros y rechasos.* If a patient asks for protection, the candles might be burned in a triangle, which is considered to be the strongest formation, one whose influence cannot be broken easily. If they want to dominate someone—a spouse, a lover, or an adversary—the candles might be burned in circles. Other formations include crosses, rectangles, and squares, depending on the results desired (Buckland 1970).

Another relatively common use of candles is to diagnose problems by studying the flame or the ridges that appear on the melted wax. A patient may be swept with a candle while the healer recites an invocation asking the spirit of the patient to allow its material being to be investigated for any physical or spiritual problems that may be affecting the person. This ritual also can be performed by burning objects used in a *barrida.* Lighting the candle or burning the object after the *barrida* helps the curandero to reveal the cause and extent of the patient's problems. Similarly, if a petitioner asks for candling, the wax of the candles burned for the velacion may be examined for figures or other messages that point to the source of a patient's problems.

One of the organizing principles of the material level of curanderismo is synchronicity with Christianity in general and the Catholic Church in particular. Special invocations often are directed at saints or spirits to bring about desired results. For example, San Martin de Porres is asked to relieve poverty; San Martin Caballero is asked to assure success in business; San Judas Tadeo is asked to help in impossible situations; and Santa Marta is asked to bring harmony to a household. Ritual materials used by the church, such as water, incense, oils, and candles, are extensively used by folk healers. The ways in which these religious objects are used and the theories for their efficacy closely mirror the concepts found within the healing ministry of the Church, which are not incompatible with European witchcraft, from which curanderismo partly derives.

The Spiritual Level (*Nivel Espiritual*)

Curanderos who have the *don* for working on the spiritual level (*nivel espiritual*) of curanderismo are less numerous than those who work on the material level. These practitioners also must go through a developmental period (*desarrollo*) that can be somewhat traumatic. Spiritual practices in communities revolve around a belief in spiritual beings who inhabit another plane of existence, but who are interested in making contact with the physical world periodically. Healers become a direct link between this plane of existence and that other world. In some cases, the curanderos claim to control these spirit beings, and in other cases, they merely act as a channel through which messages pass. Some of these practices are carried out by individual healers, while other activities occur in conjunction with spiritual centers (*centros espiritistas*) that are staffed by trance mediums and other individuals with occult abilities. These centers frequently work through two prominent folk saints: El Nino Fidencio from Northern Mexico and Don Pedrito Jaramillo from South Texas (Macklin 1974a, 1974b, 1974c). This trend in visiting spiritualist centers appears to be relatively recent, having not been reported during the 1950s and 1960s by those doing research on Mexican American folk medicine (Madsen 1964, Rubel 1960, 1966, Clark 1959).

The practice of spiritualism rests on "soul concept," a belief in the existence of spirit entities derived from once-living humans. The soul is thought to be the immortal component, the life and personality force of human beings—an entity that continues to exist after physical death on a plane of reality separate from the physical world. This concept is important not only to curanderismo but also to the religions and mystical beliefs found in all western cultures.

The soul is alternately described by curanderos as a force field, ectoplasm, concentrated vibrations, or as a group of electrical charges that exist separate from the physical body. It is thought to retain the personality, knowledge, and motivations of the individual even after the death of the body. Under proper conditions, the soul is ascribed the ability to contact and affect persons living in the physical world. Although souls occasionally can be seen as ghosts or apparitions by ordinary human beings, they exist more often in the spiritual realm mentioned above. Some people view this realm as having various divisions that have positive or negative connotations associated with them, for example, heaven, limbo, purgatory, or hell. Other people see the spiritual realm as parallel to the physical world. They state that the spiritual is a more pleasant plane on which to live, but few attempt any suicidal test of this belief. One healer commented that "spirit" [*espiritos*], "souls" [*almas*], are the same thing. These spirits' activities closely parallel their former activities in this world. Since the personality, knowledge, and motivation of the spirits are much the same as they were for the living being, there are both good and evil spirits, spirits who heal and spirits who harm, wise spirits and fools.

These spirits might communicate with or act upon the physical plane. Some have left tasks undone in their physical lives they wish to complete; others want to help or cause harm; many wish to communicate messages to friends and relatives, telling them of their happiness or discontent with their new existence. Curanderos with the ability to work on the spiritual realm, therefore, become the link between these two worlds. Some curanderos believe that there are multitudes of spirits who want to communicate with the physical world, and they tend to hover around those who have the *don* to become a medium, waiting for an opportunity to enter their bodies and possess them. This explains the cases of spirit possession in Western cultures. Individuals who become possessed are people with a strong potential to be trance mediums, who have not had the opportunity to learn how to control this condition.

The ability to become a medium is thought to be centered in the *cerebro,* that portion of the brain found at the posterior base of the skull. Those with the gift are said to have a more fully developed *cerebro,* while those who do not are said to have a weak cerebros (*un cerebro debil*). This weakness has no relationship either to the intelligence or to the moral nature of the individual, only to his or her ability to communicate with the spiritual realm. Weak cerebros represent a danger for anyone who wishes to become a medium. Only rare individuals demonstrate mediumistic potential spontaneously and can practice as mediums without further training. So, curanderos frequently test their clients and friends for this gift of healing, and those with the gift are encouraged to develop their ability. The development of this ability is called *desarrollo,* and is a fairly lengthy process that might last from two months to more than six initially, with periodic refresher encounters often available from the *maestro* (teacher). *Desarrollo* is a gradual process of increasing an apprentice's contact with the spirit world, giving him or her more and more experiences in controlled trances and possessions, as well as the knowledge necessary to develop and protect himself or herself as a spiritualist. The teacher also is responsible for giving the apprentice knowledge at a safe pace. The curandero does not always explain what each sensation means; each person, as he or she develops, becomes more sensitive to his or her environment. The apprentice must expect to encounter odd sensations such as bright light, noises, changes in pressure, and other sensations associated with developing powers. At the end of these *desarrollo* sessions, the conversation reverts to social chatting for some time before the apprentice takes his leave. This developmental process continues, with variations, until the apprentice is a fully developed medium.

Fully developed mediums control how, where, and when they work, and there are several options available to them. Some mediums work alone and only treat family problems; others might use their abilities only for their own knowledge and gratification. Some mediums work in groups with other mediums or with other persons whom they feel have complimentary spiritual or psychic powers. Some mediums

work in elaborate spiritual centers (*centros espiritistas*) that are formal churches, often dedicated to a particular spirit (such as Fidencio, Francisco Rojas, or Don Pedrito Jaramillo). The spiritual centers and the activities surrounding them take on the major aspects of a formalized religion.

Many curanderos able to work on the spiritual level prefer to work at home, alone. Their practices tend to be less uniform than the practices of mediums working at spiritual centers, because they do not have to conform to the calendric and ritual structure found in more formalized temples. However, there is enough commonality to their actions to provide an accurate description of a lone medium. This healer is described by a student in his early twenties who was one of her clients; she had been handling problems for him and his family for several years.

R: Can you describe how this *curandera* works, in as great detail as you can?

S: We drive up into the driveway of a fairly decent-looking place. She walks out and greets us, shakes our hands, asks how we are doing and how we have been. Then we go inside. She's got a small room perhaps eight by ten feet. She has an altar with saints and candles and flowers on it. She has a small vase shaped like a crystal ball sitting on a table. Sometimes it has water on it and sometimes turned upside down.

You walk in there and sit down and she's talking with you. She's not in her trance; it's just social talk. Then she sits and puts her hand on that crystal-deal. She taps it, closes her eyes, and she starts asking you what kind of problem you have or whatever you want to ask her.

R: Her voice changes?

S: Yes, it does. It's a lot lower. All of a sudden her voice becomes soft, sort of like whispering. Really mild.

R: Does she keep her hands on the glass all of this time?

(*Continues*)

S: No. Sometimes she grabs a folder with papers in it and starts writing down things on it, using her finger.

R: Can she read what she has written?

S: I'm pretty sure she can.

R: How does she cure people?

S: She does it in a number of ways. Some time ago my mother had pains on both of her heels. She went to the doctor and the doctor didn't find anything wrong. So she went over to this lady again who said it was something (a *trabajo* or hex) that [a woman across the alley from his house] had put in the yard. When my mother's out hanging up clothes she's barefooted and she stepped on it. And that's what was hurting her. So the *curandera* gave her a "shot" on her arm like a regular shot. And that cured her.

R: How did she give her the shot?

S: (Simulated the action of giving an injection without a syringe or hypodermic.)

R: Could your mother feel it?

S: She told me she didn't. But it cured her.

The informant went on to tell of several other cures this curandera had performed for his family. She had prescribed herbs, suggested the use of perfumes to ward off the *envidia* (envy) of their neighbors, and suggested that the mother perform a series of *barridas* on her son-in-law to remove a hex against him that was making him ill and keeping him from work. Each of these cures could just as easily have been suggested or performed by a curandero working on the material level of curanderismo, but this curandera did it from a trance state. Therefore, what sets this curandera apart from those working strictly on the material level is not the tools she uses or the rituals she suggests to her clients, but the source of her diagnosis and cure—her contact with a spirit world.

Sometimes a trance session is open to more than one person at the same time. This group session can be carried out by a lone curandero, but more often is found at spiritual centers. The process of the development of these centers is described elsewhere (Trotter & Chavira 1975a). Once a temple has been established, it may house from one to 20 mediums. The more mediums, the better; otherwise, a medium may have to let his or her body be used by too many different spirits, exhausting them and laying them open to supernatural harm. Larger temples might have four or five *videnntes* (clairvoyants), as well as the mediums, and might be putting several apprentices through *desarrollo* at the same time. Many of the accounts provided to these authors about spiritual healing were from individuals who had had experiences with spiritual temples in Mexico. Some temples were located in *Espinaso*, the home of El Niño Fidencio and a center of pilgrimage for mediums practicing in his name, and others were in urban centers such as Tampico and Mexico City. Large numbers of people make pilgrimages to these healing centers in Mexico, to deal with health care problems that they have not resolved in the United States.

One healing center is called Roca Blanca, after the spirit that speaks most often in that place. The owner, Lupita, founded it 25 years ago, after discovering her ability to cure. She was granted permission to practice by a spiritual association. This report is from a visitor to Lupita's healing center:

I went to this place simply because I was curious. I was swept with *albacar* and the medium was at my side. While I was being swept, the medium went into trance. The sister who was sweeping me asked the spirit who he wanted to talk to. He said, "with the one you are sweeping." Then, the sister finished sweeping me and directed me to talk with the person who was addressing me. When she (the medium in trance) talked to me, she sounded like a man. He asked me, "Do you know who I am?" I have a cousin who got killed in a place in Tampico. "You must be my cousin," I said. "Yes, exactly, I am your cousin." "Look," he said, "You have come here with your husband." On other occasions I really had been there with my husband, mother and different relatives. "You have come here with your husband because you think he is hexed and that is why he is sick.

But that's not true. He has a physical illness that the doctor can cure. Don't believe it's anything bad.''

He said, ''I'm going to prove who I am by coming to your house. Tell my cousin I'm going to see her.'' You see, I have a sister who's not nervous at all and who isn't afraid of anything. On Tuesday, as my sister was leaning by the window watching a television show, she felt someone embrace her. She turned and saw no one.

These spiritual centers vary according to their size, their owners and the spirits who are associated with them, yet there is considerable regularity in the services they perform. Sometimes mediums prescribe simple herbal remedies for physical problems. These recipes are virtually identical to the ones presented in the previous section on the material level although, occasionally, it is said that a spirit will recommend a new use for an herb. The mediums might suggest that the patient perform the already familiar rituals of curanderismo, such as the *barrida*. The spirits are thought to be able to influence people's lives directly, in addition to imparting knowledge about remedies. The curanderos state that spirits control spiritual currents (*Corrientes espirituales*) and mental vibrations (*vibraciones mentales*); they can manipulate the patient's health by directing positive or negative forces at them from the spiritual realm.

During spiritual sessions observed at a developing spiritual center in South Texas, a spirit repeatedly presented himself over the course of several weeks to treat several patients. One of these patients was a man suffering from lower back pain. One week the spirit told him to buy a bandage and bring it to the next session. The man did so, but then the spirit chided him for not following instructions correctly. The bandage was too narrow and not long enough. The man was instructed to buy a new bandage and place it on the window ledge to catch the morning dew, which is thought to have healing properties. He then was to place a glass of water under the head of his bed and a jar of alcohol at the side of the bed. He was to wrap himself in the bandage according to given instructions, and lie quietly on his bed for no

less than two hours, during which time the spirit promised to visit him and complete the cure. The man followed these instructions and stated that he did gain relief from his back pain. The same spirit treated a young college girl who periodically suffered asthma attacks. The girl's mother, a regular member of the group, brought her to the session. The spirit, in the person of the medium, stood and clasped the girl's head with one hand on her *cerebro* and the other on her forehead, sending *Corrientes espirituales* through her brain. The spirit then told her to take a sip of *agua preparada* and sit back down in the circle. The treatment was successful in overcoming this particular attack, and the mother mentioned after the session that these cures relieved her own asthma for several months.

Another patient requested a social and emotional treatment. Her husband recently had begun to practice witchcraft (*btujeria*), and she was worried that he or his friends might attack her or members of her family. A considerable amount of tension existed between the couple's families. She felt under continual stress and had gone to a doctor for help. The doctor prescribed a mild sedative, which she had taken for three weeks without relief. The medium's spirit probed her mind, and told her to take three sips of *agua preparada*, to break any spells that had been cast on her. The spirit promised to provide her with protection and help from the spiritual realm, to counteract anything that her husband might do. She appeared to be content with the spirit's activities on her behalf and was greatly relieved.

There are several aspects of the spiritual level that have not been covered in this brief description, but are described in more detail elsewhere (Trotter 1975). These include the actual techniques of testing for *el don*, the physical and supernatural dangers of trance mediumship, the acquisition of spiritual protectors to overcome those dangers, detailed descriptions of the trance state from the subjective perspective of the developing medium and the objective perspective of an observer, and finally, the existence and purpose of mediums' associations.

The Mental Level (*Nivel Mental*)

Conducting observational, descriptive, and experimental research on the practices of the mental level has proven to be the most difficult task in exploring all of the aspects of curanderismo. The mental level has the fewest rituals and the least outward complex behavior associated with it. And, to date, it has the fewest practitioners, which severely limits the number of people who could be approached for an opportunity to investigate the phenomenon. All of the cases the author observed followed a similar pattern. For example:

> After the curandero chatted with the patient and asked them about the basic problem, he asked the patient to state her complete name (*el nombre completo*). The curandero wrote the name on a piece of paper. Sitting behind the desk he used for consultations, he leaned his arms on the desk, bent forward slightly, closed his eyes, and concentrated on the piece of paper. After a few minutes, he opened his eyes, told the patient more about his or her problem, and stated that it was being resolved.
>
> The curandero stated that he had learned to use his mind as a transmitter through *desarrollo*. He could channel, focus, and direct *vibraciones mentales* at the patient. These mental vibrations worked in two ways—one physical, one behavioral. If he was working with a physical illness, such as cancer, he channeled the vibrations to the afflicted area, which he already had pinpointed, and used the vibrations to retard the growth of damaged cells and accelerate the growth of normal cells. In a case of desired behavioral changes, he sent the vibrations into the person's mind and manipulated them in a way that modified the person's behavior. The curandero gave an example of one such case in which a husband had begun drinking excessively, was seeing other women, was being a poor father to his children, and was in danger of losing his job. The curandero stated that he dominated the man's thought processes and shifted them so that the husband stopped drinking to excess, and became a model husband and father (Trotter 1981, p. 473).

There also are a number of syncretic beliefs, drawn from other alternative healing traditions—such as New Age practices, the "psychic sciences," and Eastern philosophy—that have been incorporated into this area of curanderismo. For example, some healers state that they are able to perceive "auras" around people, and that they can use these auras to diagnose problems that patients are encountering. They conduct the diagnosis based on the color or shape of the patient's aura. Some state that they learned these practices from other healers, while others indicate that they learned them from books on parapsychology.

The mental level is practiced most often by individual healers working with individual patients, rather than in groups. It appears to be a new addition to this healing system and does not have, as yet, a codified body of ritual associated with it. It therefore constitutes an area in which additional descriptive work will be necessary to unify healers' behavior.

Theoretical Unification

The three levels of curanderismo unify the theories of disease and illness found in the Mexican American folk medical model. They create a framework for determining the therapeutic approaches of curanderos in South Texas. The system emphasizes a holistic approach to treatment, and relies heavily on the intimate nature of the referral system and the extensive personal knowledge of the patient's social environment that is normally held by the curandero. Christian symbols and theology provide both tools (candles, incense, water) and organization models (rituals, prayers, animistic concepts) for the material and the spiritual levels, but not to a similar degree for the mental level. An energy concept is the central idea that integrates the three levels and forms a systematic interrelationship between them. This energy concept derives from belief in forces, vibration, and currents that center in the mind of those who have the gift for healing, and that can be transmitted to cause healing from a distance, by affecting the patient's social, physical, spiritual, or psychological environment.

All three levels of healing are still evolving. The variations in the practices of curanderismo can be explained partly by differences in the curanderos' personality; differences in their treatment preferences or abilities; and differences in their emphasis on theoretical or experiential approaches. There also are variations produced by individual interpretations of an underlying body of theory. A study of these variations would be useful, now that the underlying theoretical system provides a common starting point and common objectives.

Settings for Curanderismo Healing System

Curanderismo is a community-based healing system. It is complex and widespread. At one level, it may be practiced anywhere that there exist Mexican Americans who know about it. Part of this healing tradition is the information that is spread throughout the Mexican American culture on home treatments for common physical ailments (colds, flu, arthritis, asthma, or diabetes), and for common spiritual or "folk illnesses" (*susto, mal de ojo,* and *empacho*). This is analogous to the biomedical information that is spread throughout all European cultures, including the Mexican American culture, where the home is the first line of defense and diagnosis of illnesses that eventually might necessitate a doctor or a hospital. On the other hand, some aspects of curanderismo require the use of special locations, preparations, and tools. This is true especially of spiritual practices on the spiritual level, and for the effective treatment of supernatural harm on the material level.

The first setting where this knowledge is used is at home. When people become ill, they use their existing cultural model of health and illness to come up with solutions. One type of solution is home diagnosis and home treatment. Therefore, both biomedical concepts and folk medical concepts are applied immediately, and home treatments are attempted. In the case of curanderismo, this often results in the use of home remedies (*remedio caseros*) that have been part of the culture for generations, especially herbal cures. When the diagnosis identifies a magical or supernaturally caused illness, the illness results in a home-based ritual. These interventions are done by mothers, grandmothers, cousins, friends, or knowledgeable acquaintances.

Illnesses that appear to be too serious to handle at home, both natural and supernatural, are taken to professional healers who have a locally widespread reputation for being able to treat both biomedical and traditional health care problems. Most of these healers work in a silent, but positive, partnership with physicians, although the physicians often are unaware of the link. The curanderos interviewed in various studies of Mexican American folk medicine are consistent in their positive regard for modern medicine. They consistently refer patients to modern health care services, where they see the efficacy of that approach to be equal to or greater than their own. At the same time, they note significant differences in the models of health and illness between their own practices and modern medicine, especially in the areas of supernatural illnesses; in addressing social (marital, business, interpersonal) problems; and in dealing with psychological problems. In these cases, the treatments take place either in the patient's home or work environment, or in special workrooms established by the curanderos as part of their practices. The cure might call for working directly in the environment that is affected. In other cases, the venue of choice is the curandero's area because the cure depends on careful preparation and protection from outside influences. These work areas contain altars, medicinal plants, tools for supernatural rituals, and other items, and the atmosphere is considered to be most beneficial for the healing process, particularly in the case of supernatural problems and treatments (Trotter & Chavira 1981).

Research and Evaluations Approaches

The research that is available on curanderismo is broad in interest and historic depth. Unlike specific healing techniques, such as acupuncture, which can be studied in relation to specific illnesses with relative ease, curanderismo is a complex brew of both theoretical approaches to healing and an interrelated set of healing techniques. The techniques range from herbal cures, which must be approached from an ethnopharmacological perspective; to rituals, which can be studied symbolically as projective psychiatric techniques; to methods such as massages, natural birth, nutritional prescriptions, and dietary practices. Some studies have investigated the scientific efficacy of the practices of curanderismo, while others have approached it from a sociopolitical or symbolic viewpoint. Some practices have not been studied at all. Therefore, while the efficacy of some parts of the system are clearly defined, others remain to be explored.

Early research on curanderismo can be found in the classic anthropological works on Mexican-American folk medicine, published primarily in the 1960s (Clark 1959a, Currier 1966, Kiev 1968, Madsen 1961, 1964, Rubel 1960, 1964, 1966, Romano 1965). These authors produced descriptive baseline data on the prominent folk medical practices of Hispanic communities in the United States. They provide an initial view of curanderismo that is rich in descriptions of Mexican-American folk illnesses such as *susto, empacho, mal de ojo, caida de mollera, bilis,* and *espanto* (Nall 1967). These works generally treat traditional healing in Mexican American communities as a body of knowledge that is widely distributed throughout the culture, rather than as a theoretical healing system. Therefore, the works consider the consensual data on what is available to a significant segment of the existing Mexican American population, but spend less time describing the professional actions of curanderos, because these mass cultural phenomena are generally thought of as having themes or unifying elements, rather than a theoretical structure. This viewpoint is well represented in articles about curanderismo and its form and function within Mexican-American communities (Clark 1959b, Edgerton et al 1970, Foster 1953, Martinez & Martin 1966, Torrey 1969).

Later research maintains the strengths of this approach, but adds folk theoretical concepts. Early epidemiological approaches to folk illnesses give an idea of the geographical spread and variation in beliefs, illnesses, and healing rituals, while later studies identify or discuss the common denominators that unify curanderos—their underlying perception of illness. Traditional anthropological research techniques were used to gather the data for these studies, primarily participant observation and interviewing over prolonged periods of time. Most of the authors utilized personal networks to identify individuals who were known locally as healers. Emphasis often was placed on finding individuals who were full-time healers, rather than talking to those who treated only family members and neighbors. Therefore, a curandero can be defined as an individual who is recognized in his community as having the ability to heal, who sees an average of five or more patients a day, and who has knowledge of and utilizes the theoretical structure described in this paper. These people can be viewed as both specialists and professionals. Several areas of curanderismo have received a considerable amount of research attention.

Home Remedies

Herbal and chemical treatments for both natural and supernatural illnesses are very common in Mexican American communities. More than 800 *remedios caseros* have been identified on the U.S./Mexican border alone (Trotter 1981a, 1981b). Many of the remedies have been tested for biochemical and therapeutic activities (Etkin 1986, Trotter & Logan 1986, Trotter 1981, Trotter 1983). Overall, the remedies are not only biochemically active; more than 90 percent have demonstrated therapeutic actions that matched the folk medical model for their uses. At the same time, only a small proportion of the herbs have been tested. This lack of information is being overcome by an ongoing project to study the efficacy of the complete range of herbal cures available in Mexican American communities (Graham 1994), utilizing combined ethnographic and biomedical methodology (Browner et al 1988, Croom 1983, Trotter 1985, Ortiz de Montellano & Browner 1985).

The exceptions to the general rule of efficacy are the use of remedies for illnesses such as the common cold, where they relieve symptoms but do not directly treat the illness. The actions of these remedies, some of which are described above, include diuretics, treatments for constipation, abortifacient, analgesics, sedatives, stimulants, cough suppressants, antibacterial agents, coagulants and anticoagulants, vitamin and mineral supplements, and plants with antiparasitic actions. The majority have proven safe and effective, when used in the manner described and recommended by the curanderos. This area, and the therapeutic, culturally competent counseling practices of the healers are the most clearly acceptable and useful for articulation with modern medicine.

Additional Information on the Epidemiology of Folk Illnesses

Of all the complex areas of Mexican American traditional healing, the one that has received the most research attention has been the study of common folk illnesses that are experienced and treated in Mexican American communities. The most commonly reported are *susto*, an illness caused by a frightening event; *mal de ojo*, an illness that can be traced to the Near East, which involves a magically powerful glance taking away some of the vital essence of a susceptible person; *empacho*, a blockage of the intestines caused by eating the wrong type of food at the wrong time, or by being forced to eat unwanted food; and *caida de la mollera*, a condition of fallen fontanel in infants. A number of others also are well defined, if not as commonly studied, but these four take up most of the research attention.

The epidemiology and the cognitive models of these illnesses have been well documented (Rubel 1964, Trotter 1982, Trotter 1985, Weller et al 1993). They have been studied both singly and in combination with each other (Baer et al 1989, Rubel et al 1984, Weller et al 1991, Weller et al 1993, Logan & Morrill 1979), in terms of their cognitive structure within and between Hispanic cultural groups, their frequency of treatment, belief and mention in various communities, and their relationships to medical conditions and to the treatment of medical conditions (Trotter 1991, Trotter et al 1989, Collado-Ardon et al 1983). In the case of *susto*, there is clear evidence that it is linked directly to serious morbidity patterns in Latin American communities, and acts as an excellent indicator that biomedical personnel should investigate multiple conditions and problems among patients complaining of its symptoms. *Caida de la mollera*, upon investigation, is a folk medical label that corresponds to severe dehydration in infants, caused by gastrointestinal problems. It is life threatening and, when identified by parents, is an excellent indicator that the child should be brought in immediately for medical care. *Empacho* is a severe form of constipation, based on its description, and is treated with numerous remedies that cause diarrhea. Since it is thought to be a blockage of the intestines, the purgative effect of these remedies signals that treatment has been effective. To date, no studies have linked *mal de ojo* to any biomedical condition; however, since the symptoms include irritability, lethargy, and crying, it is possible that some connection will be made in the future.

Healing and Psychiatry

Another area of significant endeavor in curanderismo is the identification of parallels and areas of compatibility between the processes and rituals of curanderismo and the use of psychiatry in cross-cultural settings. The time period between 1969 and the mid-1970s saw the analysis and publication of several seminal works in this area (Kiev 1968, Klineman 1969, Torrey 1969, Trotter 1979, Velimirovic 1978). The parallels are clear, especially where healers concentrate on psychological conditions that they recognize from their knowledge of psychology and psychiatry. This is an area where a number of successful collaborations have been conducted between traditional healers and individuals from modern medical establishments in several states.

Unexpected Consequences

It is clear that Mexican American folk medicine contains a very high ratio of useful, insightful, and culturally competent healing strategies that work well in Hispanic communities. As seen above, these range from proven herbal cures, to therapeutic models, to culturally important labeling systems that can help physicians identify the cultural labels for certain types of biomedical problems. The complexity of curanderismo assures that these findings will increase.

At the same time, no health care system exists that does not have side effects and unexpected results. With allopathic medicine, these range from the birth defects of thalidomide, to dreadful side effects of chemotherapy, and the limited ability of psychology to deal with chronic mental health conditions such as alcohol and drug abuse. In curanderismo, conditions are not the bulk of the effects of its use, a few unexpected consequences have been discovered in treating *empacho* (Baer & Ackerman 1988, Baer 1989, Trotter 1983b). These occurrences are rare, but must be taken into account and understood within the overall cultural context of curanderismo, and within the context of the far more pervasive positive benefits that the communities derive from having these alternative health care practices available. With the complexity and the diversity of practices within this traditional healing system, there remains a great deal of useful and insightful research that can be conducted beneficially in relation to curanderismo.

Acknowledgments

The initial phase of the research findings reported for the author was supported by a grant from the Regional Medical Program of Texas (RMPT Grant No. 75-108G). Further efforts at data collection were supported by the Texas Commission on Alcoholism, Pan American University, and the authors themselves.

References

Alger N (ed). 1974. The Curandero-Supremo. In Many Answers. West Publishing Co. New York

Arias HyF, Costas: No date. Plantas Medicinales. Biblioteca Practica. Mexico

Baca J. (1969). Some health beliefs of the Spanish speaking. Am J Nurs 69:2171–2176

Baer R, Ackerman A. 1988. Toxic mexican folk remedies for the treatment of empacho: the case of azarcon, greta and albayalde. Ethnopharmacol 24:31–39

Baer R, Garcia de Alba DJ, Cueto LM, et al. 1989. Lead based remedies for empacho: patterns and consequences. Soc Sci Med 29(12):1373–1379

Bard CL. 1930. Medicine and surgery among the first Californians. Touring Topics

Bourke IH. 1894. Popular medicine customs and superstitions of the Rio Grande. J Am Folklore 7:119–146

Browner CH, Ortiz de Montellano BR, Rubel AJ. 1988. A new methodology for ethnomedicine. Curr Anthropol 29(5):681–701

Buckland R. 1970. Practical Candle Burning. Llewellyn Publications. Saint Paul, Minnesota

Capo N. Mis observaciones clinicas sobre el limon, el ajo, y la cebolla. Ediciones Natura

Cartou LSM. 1947. Healing herbs of the Upper Rio Grande. Laboratory of Anthropology. Santa Fe, New Mexico

Chavez LR. 1984. Doctors, curanderos and brujos: health care delivery and Mexican immigration in San Diego. Med Anthropol Q 15(2):31–6

Clark M. 1959a. Health in the Mexican American Culture. University of California Press, Berkeley

Clark M. 1959b. Social functions of Mexican-American medical beliefs. California's Health 16:153–55

Collado-Ardon R, Rubel AJ, O'Nell CW. 1983. A folk illness (susto) as indicator of real illness. Lancet 2:1362

Comas J. 1954. Influencia indigena en la Medicina Hipocratica, en la Nueva Espana del Sigio XVI. America Indigena XIV(4):327–361

Creson DL, McKinley C, Evans R. 1969. Folk medicine in Mexican American subculture. Dis Nervous Sys 30:264–266

Croom EM. 1983. Documenting and evaluating herbal remedies. Economic Botany 37(1):13–27

Currier RL. 1966. The hot-cold syndrome and symbolic balance in Mexican and Spanish American folk medicine. Ethnology 4:251–263

Davis J. 1979. Witchcraft and superstitions of Torrance County. NM Histor Rev 54:53–58

Dodson R. 1932. Folk curing among the Mexicans. In Toll the Bell Easy. Texas Folklore Society. Southern Methodist University Press

Edgerton RB, Karno M, Fernandez I. 1970. Curanderismo in the metropolis: the diminished role of folk psychiatry among Los Angeles Mexican-Americans. Am J Psychiatry 24:124–134

Esteyneffer J de SJ. 1711. Florilegio medicina vide todos las enfermedades, acadodevarios, y clasicos autores, para bien de los pobres y de los que tienen falia de medicos, en particular para las provincial remotas en donde administran los RRPP. Misioneros de la Compania de Jesus. Mexico

Esteyneffer J de SJ. 1887. Florilegio Medicinal o Oreve Epidomede las Medicinas y Cirujia. La primera obra sobre esta ciencia impresa en Mexico en 1713. Mexico

Etkin N (ed). 1986. Plants Used in Indigenous Medicine: Biocultural Approaches. Redgrave Publications. New York

Fabrega H Jr. 1970. On the specificity of folk illness. Southwest J Anthropol 26:305–315

Farfan A. 1944. Tractado breve de medicina. Obra impresa en Mexico por Pedro Orcharte en 1592 y ahora editada en facimil. Coleccion le Incinables Americanos, Vol. X. Ediciones Cultura Hispanica. Madrid

Foster GM. 1953. Relationships between Spanish and Spanish American folk medicine. J Am Folklore 66:201–247

Galvin JAV, Ludwig AM. 1961. A case of witchcraft. J Nerv Men Dis 161–168

Gillin J. 1977. Witch doctor? a hexing case of dermatitis. Cutis 19(1):103–105

Gobeil O. 1973. El susto: a descriptive analysis. Int J Soc Psychiatry 19:38–43

Graham JS. 1994. Mexican American herbal remedies: an evaluation. Herbalgram 31:34–35

Gudeman S. 1976. Saints, symbols and ceremonies. Am Ethnologist 3(4):709–730

Guerra F. 1961. Monardes. Diologo de Hierro. Compania

Fundido de Fierro y Acero de Monterrey, SA., Mexico. D. LosCronistas-Hispanoamericano.sdelaMate-riaMedicinaColonial.al Profesor Dr. Teofilo Hernando por sus amigos y in Homenaje O discipulos. Libreria y Casa Editorial Hernando. SA., Madrid

Hamburger S. 1978. Profile of Curanderos: a study of Mexican folk practitioners. Int J Soc Psychiatry 24: 19–25

Holland WR. 1963. Mexican-American medical beliefs: science or magic? Arizona Med 20:89–102

Hudson WM. 1951. The healer of Los Olmos and other Mexican lore. Texas Folklore Soc XXIV

Ingham IM. 1940. On Mexican folk medicine. Am Anthropol 42:76–87

Jaco EG. 1957. Social factors in mental disorders in Texas. Soc Probl 4(4):322–328

Jaco EG. 1959. Mental health of the Spanish-American in Texas. In Upler MK (ed). Culture and Mental Health. The Macmillan Co. New York

Johnson CA. 1964. Nursing and Mexican-American folk medicine. Nurs Forum 4:100–112

Karno M. 1965. The Enigma of Ethnicity in a Psychiatric Clinic. A paper presented at the Southwestern Anthropological Association Annual Meeting, UCLA. April 16, 1965

Karno M. 1969. Mental health roles of physicians in a Mexican-American community. Community Ment Health J 5(1)

Karno M, Edgerton RB. 1969. Perception of mental illness in a Mexican-American community. Arch Gen Psychiatry 20:233–238

Kay M. 1972. Health and illness in the Barrio: Women's Point of View. Dissertation for Ph.D. University of Arizona. Tucson, Arizona

Kay M. 1974a. The fusion of Utoaztecan and European ethnogynecology in the florilegio medicinal. Paper presented at Medical Anthropology Symposium, XLI International Congress of Americanists. Mexico City, Mexico. Proceedings XLI International Congress of Americanists (in press)

Kay M. 1974b. Florilegio Medicinal: Source of Southwestern Ethnomedicine. Paper presented to the Society for Applied Anthropology. Boston. 1978 Parallel, Alternative, or Collaborative: Curanderismo in Tucson, Arizona. In Modern Medicine and Medical Anthropology in the United States-Mexico Border Population. Boris Velimirovic (ed). Pan American Health Organization. Scientific Publication No. 359. Washington, DC

Kiev A. 1968. Curanderismo: Mexican American Folk Psychiatry. The Free Press, New York

Klein J. 1978. Susto: the anthropological study of diseases of adaptation. Soc Sci Med 12:23–28

Kleinman A. 1978. Culture, illness, and care: clinical lessons from anthropological cross-cultural research. Ann Intern Med 88:251–258

Klineman A. 1969. Some factors in the psychiatric treat-

ment of Spanish-Americans. Am J Psychiatry 124: 1674–1681

Kreisman JJ. 1975. Curandero's Apprentice: a therapeutic integration of folk and medical healing. Am J Psychol 132:81–83

Langner TS. 1965. Psychophysiological Symptoms and the Status of Women in Two Mexican Communities. Approaches to Cross-Cultural Psychiatry. Cornell University Press. pp. 360–392

Macklin J. 1965. Current Research Projects. Curanderismo Among Mexicans and Mexican-Americans. Connecticut College. New London, Connecticut

Macklin J. 1967. El Niño Fidencio: Un Estudio del Curanderismo en Nuevo Leon. Anuario Huminitas. Centro de Estudios Humanisticos, Universidad de Nuevo Leon

Macklin J. 1974a. Santos folk, curanderismo y cullos espiritistas en Mexico: eleccion divina y seleccion social. Anuario Indigenista 34:195–214

Macklin J. 1974b. Folk saints, healers and spirit cults in northern Mexico. Rev Interamericana 3(4):351–367

Macklin J. 1974c. Belief, ritual and healing: New England spiritualism and Mexican American spiritism compared. In Zaretsky IT, Leone MP (eds). Religious Movements in Contemporary America. Princeton University Press. Princeton, New Jersey

Macklin J, Crumrine NR. 1973. Three north Mexican folk saint movements. Comp Studies Soc History 15(1): 89–105

Madsen C. 1965. A study of change in Mexican folk medicine. Mid Am Res Inst 25:93–134

Madsen W. 1955. Shamanism in Mexico. Southwest J Anthropol 11:48–57

Madsen W. 1961. Society and Health in the Lower Rio Grande Valley. Hogg. Austin, Texas. Foundation for Mental Health

Madsen W. 1964a. The Mexican Americans of South Texas. Holt, Rinehart and Winston, Inc. New York

Madsen W. 1964b. Value conflicts and folk psychotherapy in South Texas. In Kiev A (ed). Magic, Faith and Healing. Free Press. New York, pp. 420–440

Madsen N. 1966. Anxiety and witchcraft in Mexican-American acculturation. Anthropol Q 110–127

Maduro R. 1983. Curanderismo and Latino views of disease and curing. West J Med 139:868–874

Marcos LR, Alpert M. 1976. Strategies and Risks in Psychotherapy with Bilingual Patients. Am J Psychiatry 113(11):1275–1278

Marin BV, Marin G, Padilla AM. 1983. Utilization of traditional and nontraditional sources of health care among Hispanics. Hispanic J Behav Sci 5(1):65–80

Martinez C, Martin HW. 1966. Folk diseases among urban Mexican-Americans JAMA 196:161–164

Martinez C Jr, Alegria D, Guerra E. El Hospital Invisible: A Study of Curanderos. Mimeograph. Department of Psychiatry, University of Texas Health Science Center at San Antonio. San Antonio, Texas

Montiel M. 1970. The social science myth of the Mexican-

American family. El Grito 3:4 Morales A. 1970. Mental health and public health issues: the case of the Mexican Americans in Los Angeles. El Grito 111(2)

Moustafa A, Weiss G. 1968. Health Status and Practices of Mexican-Americans. University of California Graduate School of Business

Moya B. 1940. Superstitions and Beliefs among the Spanish Speaking People of New Mexico. Masters Thesis. University of Mexico

Nall FC, Speilberg J. 1967. Social and cultural factors in the responses of Mexican-Americans to medical treatment. J Health Soc Behav 7(1):299–308

Ortiz de Montellano BR, Browner CH. 1985. Chemical basis for medicinal plant use in Oaxaca, Mexico. J Ethnopharmacol 13:57–88

Padilla AM. 1973. Latino Mental Health: Bibliography and Abstracts. United States Government Printing Office

Paredes A. 1968. Folk Medicine and the Intercultural Jest in Spanish-Speaking People in the U.S. University of Washington Press. pp. 104–119

Pattison M. 1973. Faith healing: A study of personality and function. J Nerv Ment Dis 157:397–409

Press I. 1971. The urban Curandero. Am Anthropol 73:741–756

Press I. 1978. Urban folk medicine. Am Anthropol 78(1):71–84

Romano O. 1960. Donship in a Mexican-American community in Texas. Am Anthropol 62:966–976

Romano O. 1964. Don Pedrito Jaramillo: The emergence of a Mexican-American folk saint. PhD Dissertation, University of California. Berkeley, California

Romano O. 1965. Charismatic medicine, folk-healing, and folk sainthood. Am Anthropol 67:1151–1173

Romano O. 1969. The anthropology and sociology of the Mexican-American history. El Grito 2

Rubel AJ. 1990. Ethnomedicine. In Johnson TM, Sargent CF (eds). Medical Anthropology: Contemporary Theory and Methods. Praeger. New York. pp. 120–122

Rubel AJ. 1960. Concepts of disease in a Mexican-American community in Texas. Am Anthropol 62:795–814

Rubel AJ. 1964. The epidemiology of a folk illness: Susto in Hispanic America. Ethnology 3:268–283

Rubel A. 1966. Across the Tracks: Mexican-Americans in a Texas City. University of Texas Press. Austin, Texas

Rubel AJ, O'Neil CW. 1978. Difficulties of presenting complaints to physicians: Susto illness as an example. In Velimirovic B (ed). Modern Medicine and Medical Anthropology in the United States-Mexico Border Population. Washington, D.C.: Pan American Health Organization. Scientific Publication No. 359

Ruiz P, Langrod J. 1976. Psychiatry and folk healing: a dichotomy? Am J Psychiatry 133:95–97

Samora J. 1961. Conceptions of disease among Spanish Americans. Am Cath Soc Rev 22:314–323

Sanchez A. 1971. The defined and the definers: A mental health issue. El Sol

Sanchez A. 1954. Cultural Differences and Medical Care: The Case of the Spanish-Speaking People of the Southwest. Russell Sage Foundation. New York

Saunders L, Hewes GW. 1953. Folk medicine and medical practice. J Med Educ 28:43–46

Smithers WD. 1961. Nature's Pharmacy and the Curanderos. Sul Ross State College Bulletin. Alpine, Texas

Snow LF. 1974. Folk medical beliefs and their implications for care of patients. Ann Intern Med 81:82–96

Speilberg J. 1959. Social and Cultural Configurations and Medical Cure: A Study of 'Mexican-American's Response to Proposed Hospitalization for the Treatment of Tuberculosis. Masters Dissertation. University of Texas

Torrey FE. 1969. The case for the indigenous therapist. Arch Gen Psychiatry 20(3):365–373

Torrey FE. 1972. The Mind Game: Witch Doctors and Psychiatrists. Bantam Books, Emerson Hall Pub. New York

Trotter RT II. 1991. A survey of four illnesses and their relationship to intracultural variation in a Mexican American community. Am Anthropol 93:115–125

Trotter RT II. 1990. The cultural parameters of lead poisoning: a medical anthropologist's view of intervention in environmental lead exposure. Environ Health Perspect 89:79–84

Trotter RT II. 1988. Caida de mollera: A newborn and early infancy health risk. Migrant Health Newsline

Trotter RT II. 1986. Folk medicines and drug interactions. Migrant Health Newsline. 3(7):3–5

Trotter RT II. 1986. Folk medicine in the Southwest: myths and medical facts. Postgrad Med 78(8):167–179

Trotter RT II. 1985. Greta and Azarcon: a survey of episodic lead poisoning from a folk remedy. Health Care Hum Organization. 44(1):64–71

Trotter RT II. 1983. Greta and Azarcon. Unusual sources of lead poisoning from Mexican American folk medicine. Tex Rural Health J May–June:1–5

Trotter RT II. 1983. Azarcon and Greta: ethnomedical solution to an epidemiological mystery. Med Anthropol Q 14(3):3–18

Trotter RT II. 1983d. Letter to the editor: Greta and Azarcon: two sources of lead poisoning on the United States-Mexico border. J Ethnopharmac 8(1):105–106

Trotter RT II. 1983. Ethnography and bioassay: combined methods for a preliminary screen of home remedies for potential pharmacologic activity. J Ethnopharmac 8(1):113–119

Trotter RT II. 1983. Community morbidity patterns and Mexican American folk illness: a comparative approach. Med Anthropol 7(1)33–44

Trotter RT II. 1982. Susto: within the context of community morbidity patterns. Ethnology 21:215–226

Trotter RT II. 1982b. Contrasting models of the healer's role: South Texas case examples. Hispanic J Behav Sci 4(3):315–327

Trotter RT II. 1981a. Don Pedrito Jaramillo. Slide series/

filmstrip. Institute of Texas Cultures. San Antonio, Texas

Trotter RT II. 1981b. Remedios caseros: Mexican American home remedies and community health problems. Soc Sci Med 15B:107–114

Trotter RT II. 1981. Folk remedies as indicators of common illnesses. J Ethnopharmac 4(2):207–221

Trotter RT II. 1979. Evidence of an ethnomedical form of aversion therapy on the United States-Mexico border. J Ethnopharmac 1(3):279–284

Trotter RT II. 1979. Las Yerbas de Mi Abuela (Grandmother's Tea), slide series/filmstrip. Institute of Texas Cultures. San Antonio, Texas

Trotter RT II. 1978. Discovering New Models for Alcohol Counseling in Minority Groups. In Velimirovic B (ed). Modern Medicine and Medical Anthropology in the United States-Mexico Border Population. Scientific Publication No. 359. Pan American Health Organization. Washington, DC. pp. 164–171

Trotter RT II. 1978. A case of lead poisoning from folk remedies in Mexican American communities. In Fiske S, Wulff R (eds). Anthropological Praxis. Westview Press. Boulder, Colorado

Trotter RT II, Chavira JA. 1980. Curanderismo: an emic theoretical perspective of Mexican American folk medicine. Med Anthropol 4(4):423–487

Trotter RT II, Chavira JA. 1981. Curanderismo: Mexican American Folk Healing System. University of Georgia Press. Athens, Georgia

Trotter RT II, Chavira JA. 1975a. The Gift of Healing. A monograph on Mexican American Folk Healing. Pan American University. Edinburg, Texas

Trotter RT II, Chavira JA. 1975b. Los Que Curan. A 43-minute color 16 mm film of South Texas Curanderismo

Trotter RT II, Logan M. 1986. Informant consensus: a new approach for identifying potentially effective medicinal plants. In Etkin N (ed). Plants Used in Indigenous Medicine: Biocultural Approaches. Redgrave Publications pp. 91–112

Trotter RT II, Ortiz de Montellano B, Logan M. 1989. Fallen fontanelle in the American Southwest: its origin, epidemiology, and possible organic causes. Med Anthropol 10(4):201–217

Unknown. 1951. Rudo Ensayo. By an unknown Jesuit. Tucson: Arizona Silhouettes Publication. Original 1763 by Johann Nentuig

Uzzell D. 1974. Susto Revisited: illness as a strategic role. Am Ethnol 1(2):369–378

Velimirovic B (ed). 1978. Modern Medicine and Medical Anthropology in the United States Mexico Border Population. Pan American Health Organization. Washington, DC. Scientific Publication No. 359

Wagner F. Remedios Caseros con Plantas Medicinales. D.F. Medicina, Mexico. Hermanos, S.A.

Weclew RV. 1975. The nature, prevalence and levels of awareness of "Curanderismo" and some of its implications for community mental health. Comm Ment Health J 11:145–154

Weller SC, Pachter LM, Trotter RT II, Baer RM. 1993. Empacho in four latino groups: a study of intra- and inter-cultural variation in beliefs. Med Anthropol 15(2): 109–136

16
Global Health Traditions*

Gerard C. Bodeker

*A*t the basis of the global concern about the ever-increasing cost of health care lies the issue of sustainability. Developing countries recognize that their health care systems are based on expensive, imported medicines and technologies, and that continued reliance on these systems will result in health care costs consuming national finances and stifling national economic growth.

Basic questions are now being asked about priorities in health expenditures and national economic development: How can countries address the health needs of their people without continuing to rely on expensive, imported medicines? Furthermore, how can local, existing systems of health care be utilized to provide basic health services to rural and poor communities? Increased attention is being paid to the potential of locally available medicinal plants and inexpensive herbal medicines in providing effective primary health care. This in turn has raised concerns about the sustainable use of wild sources of medicinal plants, the conservation of biodiversity, appropriate forms of local cultivation and production, the safety and effectiveness of natural medicines, and the regulatory environment that should accompany the incorporation of traditional systems of health into national health care.

In this article, some of these recent trends will be discussed and illustrated with experiences from countries and communities in Africa, the Americas, and Asia. We will consider economic, cultural, environmental, and other factors that have led to the resurgence of interest in traditional systems of health. We will conclude with a review of several myths about traditional systems of health care, and a discussion of policy options for incorporating traditional ecological and medicinal knowledge into national and international environmental, health, and economic policy and planning.

Background

The terms *traditional medicine* or *traditional systems of health*, refer to the long-standing indigenous systems of health care found in developing countries and among the indigenous populations of industrialized countries. The paradigms of these traditional medical systems view humanity as being linked intimately with the wider dimensions of nature. Long relegated to marginal status in the health care plans of developing countries, traditional medicine—or more appropriately, traditional systems of health care, since they provide comprehensive approaches to prevention and treatment that are beyond the scope of medicine alone—have undergone a major renewal in the past decade or more.

The World Health Organization (WHO) has referred to these systems as *holistic*, meaning, "that of viewing man in his totality within a wide ecological spectrum, and of emphasizing the view that ill health

* This article was published originally as "Traditional health knowledge and public policy," in Nature & Resources, 30, (2), UNESCO, 1994. Reprinted by permission.

or disease is brought about by an imbalance, or disequilibrium, of man in his total ecological system and not only by the causative agent and pathogenic evolution" (WHO 1978). Traditional medicine has been described as "one of the surest means to achieve total health care coverage of the world population, using acceptable, safe, and economically feasible methods."

The treatment strategies utilized by traditional systems of health include the use of herbal medicines, mind/body approaches such as meditation, physical therapies including massage, acupuncture, exercise programs, and approaches that address both physical and spiritual well-being. These methods incur limited costs, are available locally, and, according to WHO, are utilized as the primary source of health care by 80 percent of the world's population.

An essential feature of traditional systems of health is that they are based in cosmologies or paradigms that take into account mental, spiritual, physical, and ecological dimensions in the conceptualization and evaluation of health and well being. Assumptions of causality frequently differ from those of Western medicine, and treatments are designed to reflect those underlying theories of causality. Indeed, classification of diseases, medicinal plants, and ecosystems in traditional knowledge systems may vary substantially from those of Western taxonomies.

A fundamental concept found in many systems is that of balance: the balance between mind and body; between different dimensions of individual bodily functioning and need; between individual and community; individual, community, and environment; and individual and the universe. Disease is understood to arise from a breakdown in the state of balance in one or more of these areas. Treatments are designed not only to address the locus of the disease, but to restore a state of systemic balance to the individual and his or her inner and outer environment.

Historically, the paradigms of traditional knowledge systems have been considered "primitive" by modern or Western science. However, recent advances in environmental sciences, immunology, medical botany, and pharmacognosy have led to a new appreciation for the precise descriptive nature and efficacy of many traditional taxonomies, as well as for the efficacy of the treatments employed. There

is an emerging awareness that any meaningful appraisal of a traditional system of health and its contribution to health care must take into account the paradigm or cosmology that underlies diagnosis and treatment.

Organizational Relationships Between Modern and Traditional Medicine

Under colonial influence, traditional medical systems were frequently outlawed by authorities. In the postcolonial era, the attitudes of Western medical practitioners and health officials have maintained the marginal status of traditional health care providers, despite the role that these practitioners play in providing basic health care to the rural of majority, developing countries and within indigenous communities.

Traditional medicine and modern medicine have interfaced with each other in four broad ways (Stepan 1983).

1. Monopolistic: Modern medical doctors have the sole right to practice medicine.
2. Tolerant: Traditional medical practitioners are not officially recognized, but are free to practice on the condition that they do not claim to be registered medical doctors.
3. Parallel: Practitioners of both modern and traditional systems are officially recognized. They serve their patients through separate but equal systems, such as India.
4. Integrated: Modern and traditional medicine merged in medical education and jointly practiced within a unique health service, such as in China and Viet Nam.

Factors Influencing Policy Development

Despite the historic suppression of traditional medicine by modern medical interests, an increasing number of developing countries are displaying policy interest in traditional approaches to health care that has led to a resurgence of interest in research, investment, and program development in this field. Several factors underlie this new interest.

Economic Factors

The majority of the rural populations of developing countries cannot afford Western medical health care. In Vietnamese peasant communities, there is a common saying that traditional medicine costs one chicken, modern medicine costs one cow, and modern hospital treatment costs many cows. Rural people may have to travel for a day or more to reach a modern medical clinic or pharmacy. This results in lost wages, which is compounded by the cost of transport and the relatively high cost of medicines themselves.

Typically, more than 80 percent of health budgets in developing countries are directed to services that reach approximately 20 percent of the population. Of this, 30 percent of the total health budget is spent on the national pharmaceutical bill (Bannerman 1983).

In Asia, traditional systems of health have been incorporated as formal components of national health care for approximately 20 years. The Indian Medicine Central Council Act of 1970 gave an official place in national health programs to the Ayurvedic and Unani medical systems of India. India now has over 200,000 registered traditional medical practitioners, the majority of whom have received their training in government colleges of Ayurvedic or Unani medicine. China has had a policy of integrating traditional medicine into national health care for more than three decades, and has an extensive national program in which modern and traditional medicine are combined as formal components of health care provision. In both India and China, the traditional health sector provides the majority of health care to the poor and rural communities.

In recent years, other countries have begun to provide increased support for their long-standing traditional medical systems, recognizing that they cannot afford Western medicine. In Thailand, for example, the Ministry of Health promotes the use of 66 traditional medicinal plants in primary health care, based on scientific evidence of the efficacy of these plants, as well as on traditional patterns of utilization. The Fourth Public Health Development Plan of Thailand (1977–1981) stated the country's general policy to promote the use of traditional medicinal plants in primary health care. The Seventh Plan (1992 to 1996) promotes the integration of traditional Thai medicine into community health care and prioritizes research on medicinal plants. The Thai Ministry of Public Health also promotes the use of medicinal plants in state-run hospitals and health service centers (Koysooko 1993). A study by the Royal Tropical Institute of the Netherlands found that traditional herbal medicines were used most effectively in primary health care in Thailand when self-administered. Since most rural people treat themselves before seeking help from either modern or traditional medical practitioners, herbal medicines offer a low-cost intervention in the early treatment of disease, and provide a safe alternative to the growing problem of self-medication with inappropriate doses and harmful combinations of over-the-counter drugs (Le Grand 1990).

In Korea, between 15 percent and 20 percent of the national health budget is directed to traditional medical services, and government reports indicate that traditional medicine is favored equally by all levels of society. Health insurance coverage is available for Oriental medical treatments. In Japan, where physicians have been authorized to prescribe and dispense medications, over two thirds of all physicians reportedly prescribe herbal medications (Norbeck 1987).

Cultural Factors

Cultural factors play a significant role in the continued reliance on traditional medicine. Often villagers seek symptomatic relief with modern medicine, and turn to traditional medicine for treatment of what may be perceived as the "true cause of the condition" (Kleinman 1980). Traditional medical knowledge typically is coded into household cooking practices, home remedies, and health prevention and health maintenance beliefs and routines. The advice of family members or other significant members of a community has a strong influence on health behavior, including the type of treatment that is sought (Nichter 1978).

Decolonization and increased self-determination for indigenous groups has led some countries to reevaluate and promote their traditional medical systems. At a 1993 Pan American Health Organization conference on indigenous peoples and health, representatives from South America reported increasing activity and interest in traditional medicine in their countries (Zolla 1993). Several Latin American countries have departments or divisions of traditional medicine within their health ministries.

Mexico has undertaken an extensive program of revitalizing its indigenous medical traditions: over 1000 traditional medicines have been identified as a result of a program of ethnomedical and pharmacognostic research; training centers have been established by the government to pass traditional medical knowledge on to new generations of health care workers; and hospitals of traditional medicine have been established in a number of rural areas. The Mexican Constitution is currently being revised to include traditional medicine in the provision to national health care (Argueta 1993). Nongovernment organizations (NGOs) have played a strong role in revitalizing traditional health in Mexico, organizing national and international meetings on traditional approaches to health care. More than 50 different traditional medicine associations were represented at a 1992 meeting of the Instituto Nacional Indigenista.

Native North American communities have been incorporating traditional forms of treatment into health programs for some years. In the United States, Indian Health Service (IHS) alcohol rehabilitation programs include traditional approaches to the treatment of alcoholism. An analysis of 190 IHS contract programs revealed that 50 percent of these programs offered a traditional sweat lodge at their site or encouraged the use of sweat lodges (Hall 1986). Treatment outcomes improved when a sweat lodge was available. Often these sweat lodges include the presence of medicine men or healers, and the presence of a traditional healer greatly improved the outcome when used in combination with the sweat lodge. In northern Canada, The Inuit Women's Association developed a program to revitalize traditional birth practices (Flaherty 1993). Women who were midwives in their own communities for many years were interviewed and recorded on videotape, and these tapes are being used to train young midwives in the use of traditional methods.

National Crises

In addition to economic and cultural factors, national crises have spurred governments to evaluate their indigenous medical traditions as a means of providing affordable and available health care to their citizens. War and national epidemics are two common crises faced by these nations.

War

During the recent war in Nicaragua, there was an acute shortage of pharmaceutical supplies. In 1985, out of necessity, the country turned to its herbal traditions as a means of fulfilling the country's medical needs. A department was established within the health ministry to develop "popular and traditional medicine as a strategy in the search for a self-determined response to a difficult economic, military and political situation" (Castellon 1992).

The new department of traditional medicine initiated a program of ethnobotanical research, in the midst of war. More than 20,000 people nationwide were interviewed regarding their use of traditional and popular remedies, the methods of preparing these remedies, and the sources of plant ingredients. Previously, nurses and health workers in rural areas frequently manned outposts without medical supplies. They often were surrounded by medicinal herbs of which they knew nothing.

A national toxicology program was begun, based on the extensive survey. Over a period of six to seven years, pharmacognostic studies attempted to determine the chemistry and medicinal properties of commonly used plants. As a result of this effort, inexpensive medicines were produced locally and sustainably in rural areas to treat a wide range of conditions including respiratory ailments, skin problems, nervous disorders, diarrhea, and diabetes.

Following Vietnam's war of independence from France, an official policy was articulated by President Ho Chi Minh in 1954, asserting the importance of preserving and developing traditional medicine as a basic component of health care throughout the country, because a significant proportion of the population could not afford modern medicine.

A national heritage program in traditional medicine was established to ensure that the medical knowledge of experienced practitioners was gathered, recorded, and passed on to future generations through formal training programs. Simultaneously, a policy was developed to promote the modernization of traditional medicine and to incorporate it into health service provision integrated with modern medicine. This policy was expanded and strengthened during the 1960s and 1970s, during the war between the North and the South. Emergency medical strategies were generated, including the development of a traditional medical program for the treatment of burns.

After several decades of pharmacognostic and toxicological research, the National Institute of Materia Medica in Hanoi has developed a list of 1869 plants of known safety and efficacy in the treatment of common medical conditions. Traditional medicine now accounts for one third of all medical treatments provided (Institute of Materia Medica, Hanoi 1990).

Epidemics

In Africa, governments face huge drug bills for the growing AIDS crisis, and are looking to their indigenous medical traditions and medicinal plants for inexpensive and effective methods of at least alleviating the suffering of AIDS victims. The Health Ministry of Uganda has been active in generating research into the role of traditional medical practitioners in treating people with AIDS. The Uganda AIDS Commission and the Joint Clinical Research Centre in Kampala have worked with traditional healers' associations to evaluate several traditional treatments for opportunistic infections associated with HIV/AIDS. An official of the Uganda AIDS Commission commented on research findings, saying that traditional medicine is better suited to the treatment of some AIDS symptoms such as herpes zoster, chronic diarrhea, shingles, and weight loss (Kogozi 1994).

International support also has been provided for a project in Ethiopia, which has resulted in the development of a cultivated and produced molusciscide that has proven to be effective against the endemic water-borne disease schistosomiasis. Support for this project has included investments from IDRC of Canada, the Rockefeller Foundation, and the World Bank. Linking traditional medicine to biodiversity conservation and economic factors such as affordable health care appears to have attracted a new form of international investment in traditional medicine.

The outbreak of chloroquine-resistant malaria also has inspired a number of countries to re-examine traditional methods of treating malaria. Artemisinin programs, based on an extract of the traditional Chinese anti-malarial plant *artemisia annua*, are being used in Africa, China, and Vietnam.

With approximately 30 percent of the health budgets of developing countries being directed to the cost of drugs produced in industrialized countries (Bannerman 1983), the prospect of dealing with epidemics such as AIDS, malaria, and tuberculosis, is forcing many governments to look to their indigenous systems of medicine and medicinal flora for low-cost solutions.

International Pressure to Conserve Biodiversity

Traditional health systems intersect with areas of the national economy other than health care: they interface with environmental concerns as well.

Environmental factors, such as land degradation through erosion or development, have contributed to the loss of natural habitats. Loss of natural habitats can affect the availability of medicinal plants, hence, local health standards. In countries where this has occurred, herb gatherers must walk increasingly longer distances to find herbs that previously grew nearby. This contributes to increasing the cost, availability, and sustainability of naturally occurring sources of medicines that traditionally provided basic health care to rural communities.

National economic development may be linked to the cultivation and use of traditional medicines. Wild harvesting of medicinal plants can provide an additional source of family income and also saves expenditure on other forms of medicine. However, overharvesting constitutes a serious threat to biodiversity. Overharvesting of medicinal plants occurs in China, where approximately 80 percent of the raw materials (animal and plant) for traditional medicines come from wild sources, raising the need for new policies to integrate health, environmental, and economic perspectives. Investments are needed to develop appropriate cultivation and harvesting strategies that will meet the demand for inexpensive and accessible medicines, while ensuring the conservation of diverse biologic resources.

Most developing countries lack the information and resources to apply the contemporary methods of studying the inventory of flora and fauna. It has not been possible to track resource depletion systematically in medicinal plants or in animal species that are used in traditional formulae. International collaboration in developing taxonomic capabilities of environmental and forestry departments is one means by which donor agencies can protect diverse medicinal plant species, thus influencing the long-term health of local populations in developing countries.

Although local health needs have constituted the primary beneficiary of the world's medicinal plant resources, there has been a recent growth of interest in traditional medicine from the international pharmaceutical industry, as well as from the natural product industry in Europe and America. Traditional medicine has come to be viewed by the pharmaceutical industry as a source of "qualified leads" in the identification of bioactive agents for use in the production of synthetic, modern drugs. The National Institutes of Health (NIH) in the United States initiated two drug discovery projects along these lines.

The 1992 NIH "Biodiversity Project" was developed by a consortium of United States Government agencies, including the National Cancer Institute, the National Science Foundation, and the United States Agency for International Development. The project was designed to develop partnerships among the agencies, pharmaceutical companies, and the governments of developing countries. It has three main goals: drug discovery; economic development in developing countries through the establishment of economic programs related to the pharmaceutical production process; and conservation of diverse biologic resources in developing countries.

These projects promote the conservation of biodiversity through a model of drug discovery. This model has several important components. First, the local plant knowledge of traditional medical practitioners is made accessible through the use of ethnobotanists. Second, samples of plant materials are tested in laboratories for bioactive properties. If a plant contains molecules that are found to have initial effects, further laboratory research is undertaken, including the modeling of apparently active molecules for synthetic reproduction. Once a molecule is reproduced, it can be patented and commercial production is protected.

The other source of interest in traditional medicine is the natural products industry in Europe and the United States. In Europe, where there is a large industry in phytomedicines, extracts of medicinal plants are sold in purified form to treat and prevent a wide variety of conditions.

These trends have led to a situation where traditional medicine is viewed as a source for the production of other medicines, rather than in terms of its intrinsic value. These concerns have been expressed by the traditional medicine community. A prevailing view is that this trend does not contribute to the development of traditional medicine as a health care system for poor or rural communities, the main constituency of traditional medical care. Rather, the international drug development initiative is seen to take medicinal knowledge from these communities to serve the demand for new drugs in industrial countries. The drugs that are being developed are for the treatment of cancer and heart disease, which are the major killers in industrialized societies, rather than for the treatment of malaria and other endemic diseases that decimate the populations of the developing countries from which the knowledge derives.

There has been no attempt, to date, to develop a scientific understanding of the efficacy of medicinal plants in addressing the primary health care needs of the populations in the areas from which the plants derive. Some projects, however, have recognized this imbalance, the New York Botanical Garden's ethnobotany program in Belize, for example, and are addressing the situation through community-based projects to produce natural medicines for local consumption. They also are working to include knowledge of medicinal plants in school curricula as a means of conserving endangered traditional medical knowledge, as well as to conserve medicinal plants and rain forest areas. In a recent international initiative, the NIH has funded research and policy evaluation on the role of traditional medicine in the provision of cost-effective primary health care in developing countries.

Myths Contributing to the Marginalization of Traditional Health Care

Myth 1. Traditional medicines are of value only when their active ingredient is known and they are purified for mass production.

The reductionism of Western science leads to the search for a single element which can be identified as the sole or the primary cause of an effect. In pharmacology, this has led to an emphasis on identifying one chemical or compound as the cause of a plant's medicinal properties. This "active ingredient" approach to medicinal plants and traditional medicines reflects a particular paradigm, rather than a particular truth about the way in which natural medicines work. This approach also reflects commercial considerations. For commercial purposes, a single ingredient can be replicated in a laboratory easily, synthesized, patented, and mass-produced. In the United States, however, a drug company cannot obtain a patent on a natural product; without patent protection, drug companies have no commercial incentive for producing medicines.

Practitioners of traditional medicine view the active ingredient approach as reductionistic and oversimplified. In the Ayurvedic tradition of natural health care of India, there is an expression that this approach takes the knowledge from the plant and throws away the wisdom. The multiple ingredients in a traditional prescription might include some plant materials that have been selected to address the particular site of pathology, others to stimulate a general immune response, and still others to offset side effects or to increase cellular uptake. This complex approach to pharmacology is based on the concept of "synergistic activity."

Traditional pharmacologies emphasize a principle of synergistic activity among the components of plant ingredients of herbal mixtures. This assumes that, just as the body is designed to extract multiple components from food, it is also designed to do so from medicinal plant materials. Traditional medicines typically use complex mixtures of plants, which are prepared through a process that might include drying, crushing, heating, boiling, and even burning. Consequently, the chemical structure of the plant materials is transformed, producing a set of compounds that may differ from that of each plant in the prescription.

The principle that enduring effectiveness can be found in a complex mixture of chemicals rather than in a single molecule is best demonstrated in the case of malaria. In recent years, new strains of the parasite have developed that are resistant to the antimalarial

drugs, chloroquine and mefloquine. However, these are still not resistant to the antimalarial activity of the original cinchona bark—the natural source of quinine, on which the synthetic antimalarials were modeled (Wyler 1992).

In conclusion, it is interesting to note that the principle of synergistic activity also serves as the basis for Western pharmacology's use of multiple drug treatments in cancer chemotherapy. Here, there is a principle that a single compound is not sufficient to produce an overall systemic change, and that a complex of chemical inputs are required to fight the disease. Although the types of chemicals used clearly differ from those traditional medicines, there is a common principle that multiple ingredients produce a greater effect than the sum of the effects of individual components.

> **Myth 2. Based on findings from the plant screening programs of the pharmaceutical industry and national drug development programs, the therapeutic benefit of traditional medicines is limited.**

This view sometimes is espoused by those familiar with plant screening programs, such as those run by the National Cancer Institute in America, where tens of thousands of medicinal plants have been screened for anticancer effects, and only a handful have been identified as having therapeutic potential. It is important to note, however, that the screens used test only for cytotoxicity, the ability of a chemical to kill cancer cells. Any plant or plant-based compound that does not show a cytotoxic effect—that does not kill cancer cells—is considered to have no anticancer properties.

The mechanisms by which natural medicines work might be more sophisticated than a simple mechanism of killing wayward cells. This has been illustrated by a series of experimental studies on Ayurvedic herbal preparations Maharishi Amrit Kalash 4 and 5, which have looked at the effect of these preparations on a range of cancers. The studies (which include research conducted by a different division of the National Cancer Institute) have found that Maharishi Amrit Kalash 4 and 5 have marked anticancer effects. Cancer prevention effects have been shown with experimental breast cancer (Sharma 1990), lung cancer (Patel 1992), and liver cancer. There has been no evidence of cytotoxicity in these effects. A study on the effects of these herbal preparations on neurological cancer cells found that there was a transformation, or morphological differentiation, of the neurological cancer cells (neuroblastoma) into normal healthy nerve cells (Prasad 1994). These herbal preparations did not kill cancer; rather, they produced a process of transformation in cancer cells that some researchers have proposed may be activated at the molecular level.

These examples illustrate that the methodologies utilized in modern medical science completely overlook the effects by which natural medicines produce their effect, due to a fixed and limited view of what constitutes therapeutic action. To address this neglect, the new, Congressionally-mandated NIH Office of Alternative Medicine is working to develop a series of methodologies appropriate for the evaluation of nonWestern or complementary medical therapeutic approaches.

> Myth 3. Traditional health systems may have some use in the provision of care for chronic, low-level conditions, but they are of no value in providing acute or emergency care.

The conventional view is that traditional health care is best used for chronic, low-level conditions, rather than for the treatment of acute conditions. However, in some countries, traditional medicine is used in the treatment of trauma and major diseases.

In Vietnam, the National Institute of Burns conducts an active program of research to evaluate traditional medicinal formulae in the treatment of burns (Institute of Burns 1993). Traditional medicines now are utilized in combination with modern medicine, widely and effectively, in the treatment of burns. This direction was developed as a matter of necessity during the war with South Vietnam and the United States, when burn treatments needed to be available immediately in remote jungle locations. Traditional medicinal plants were utilized, and resulted in a national program of research and the development of over 60 medicines for use in different aspects of burn therapy. These medications are effective in generat-

ing membrane formation, inhibiting bacterial growth, and stimulating the formation of scar tissue on burn lesions. The treatment time with traditional medicine is markedly shorter than that of conventional burn medication (The Trungh 1993).

The Vietnamese Institute of Acupuncture in Hanoi uses acupuncture analgesia in place of general anesthesia for major surgery. The Institute for Burns also uses this approach. Both institutes report that with perioperative acupuncture, patients experience minimal or no pain, have fewer postoperative complications, and their wounds heal more quickly than when general anesthesia is used (Tai Thu 1993).

In April 1991, the National Council of Ministers in Hanoi renamed the Institute of Burns after an early Vietnamese physician, Le Huu Trac. According to Vietnamese health officials, this is the first time that a national institute has been named after a prominent figure in traditional medicine—a development that reflects a commitment to integrating traditional medicine into national health care, including emergency treatment.

> Myth 4. Little scientific knowledge is available on the safety and efficacy of traditional medicine, and all international efforts regarding traditional medicine should be directed to toxicity and efficacy research.

It is not correct to state that there has been little or no research done on traditional approaches to health care; studies have been done in many countries. However, the level of research sophistication, the language in which studies are published, the focus of this research, and the bias of the scientific establishment as to what constitutes a published study—all have contributed to these studies being overlooked or, on occasion, rejected by the wider scientific community.

In some countries—India, China, Korea, Vietnam, Mexico, to name a few—a substantial body of toxicity data has been gathered on medicinal plants and traditional medicines. In addition, international botanical research has identified the chemistry, including the toxicity, of many plants used in traditional medicines. Entire journals are dedicated to pared with traditional approaches. Ann NY Acad Sci 472:168–178

Institute of Burns. 1993. Establishment of a new scientific center of Vietnam—The National Institute of Burns, named LE HUU TRAC—that needs much support. Institute of Burns, Hanoi

Institute of Materia Medica, Hanoi. 1990. Medicinal Plants in Viet Nam, WHO Regional Publications. Western Pacific Series No. 3, Manila

Kleinman A. 1980. Patients and Healers in the Context of Cultures. University of California Press, Berkeley

Kogozi J. 1994. Herbalists open hospital. The NEW VISION, Kampala, February 4, 14

Koysooko R, Chuthaputti A. 1993. Promising practices in the use of medicinal plants in Thailand. Presented at The WHO Symposium on the Utilization of Medicinal Plants, Philadelphia, April 19–21

Le Grand A, Wondergem P. 1990. Herbal Medicine and Health Promotion. KIT Press Royal Tropical Institute, Amsterdam

Nichter M. 1978. Patterns of curative resort and their significance for health planning in south Asia. Med Anthropol 2:29–58, 1978

Norbeck E, Lock M. 1987. Health, Illness and Medical Care in Japan. Honolulu, University of Hawaii Press

Patel V, Wang J, Shen RN, et al. 1992. Reduction of mouse Lewis lung carcinoma (LLC) by M-4 rasayana. Nutr Res 12:667–676

Prasad KN, Edwards-Prasad J, Kentrotti S. 1992. Ayurvedic (Science of Life) herbal agents induced differentiation in murine neuroblastoma cells in culture, Neuropharmacol 31:6;9–607

Reid W, et al. 1993. Biodiversity Prospecting. World Resources Institute, Washington DC

Sharma H, et al. 1990. Effect of MAK (M4 & M5) on DMBA-induced mammary tumors. Eur J Pharmacol 183:2;193

Sok CW. 1995. Country report, In Proceedings of WHO Symposium on the Utilization of Medicinal Plants, Philadelphia, April 19–21, 1993. University of Pennsylvania Press, Philadelphia

Stepan J. 1983. Patterns of legislation concerning traditional medicine. In: Bannerman R (ed.) Traditional Medicine. WHO Publication, Geneva

Tai Thu, N. 1993. Personal communication with the director of the Vietnamese Institute of Acupuncture. July

The Trungh L, et al. 1993. Personal communication with the director of the Le Huu Trac Institute for Burns. July

Vidal J. 1993. Whose new lease on life? The Guardian, May 21

World Bank. 1993. World development report on health: World Bank, Washington DC, July

WHO Traditional Medicine. WHO Publications, Geneva

Wyler DJ. 1992. Editorial: bark, weeds and iron chelators—drugs for malaria. N Engl J Med, Nov. 19

Zoll AC. 1993. Proceedings of Conference on Indigenous Peoples and Health, Winnipeg, Canada, April 13–18

research on the chemistry of medicinal plants, and studies are referenced in databases such as NAPRAL-ERT, a natural products research database located at the University of Illinois. Other databases contain collections of studies in the area of "complementary" medicine, a term that includes many traditional systems of medicine as they are utilized in industrial countries. These include the British Library's Complementary Medicine Index and the research database of the British Research Council for Complementary Medicine. On review, this collective body of data may well satisfy questions regarding the safety of commonly used herbal treatments.

More data may ultimately be needed on a country by country basis, in order for lending or donor agencies to be able to determine the extent of utilization and treatment, the preventive efficacy, and the suitability and form of investment in this sector. However, existing data needs to be evaluated for safety and efficacy.

Regarding the question of efficacy: as noted above, many countries have a body of scientific research on the medical properties of many plants utilized in traditional medicine. It is important to give credit to the countries and the scientists involved in this undertaking, which is partly necessitated by the lack of available Western medicines. Research has been conducted under circumstances such as lack of equipment and chemical supplies—these are far from conducive to the production of Western-style research. However, it would be unscientific to dismiss these studies in making a determination of the availability of effectiveness data of traditional herbal medicines. Although much of this research is not available in English, scientists familiar with Chinese, Hindi, Korean, Vietnamese, Spanish, or Portuguese languages could be called on to evaluate this body of research as a means of supporting international investment. In addition, abstracts could be translated into English for a first level of review.

Finally, to place the Western concern about potential toxicity of herbal medicines in perspective: in the United States, where one in three people report using some form of "alternative" medicine (Eisenberg 1993), plant poisonings in 1989 were due almost exclusively to consumption of toxic ornamental plants, not herbs. Such poisonings resulted in only one fatality. In the same year, fatal, nonsuicidal poisonings by antidepressants, analgesics, sedatives, and heart drugs totaled 414 (Fugh-Berman 1993).

> Myth 5. The global value of traditional medical knowledge is twofold: it serves as a source of leads for the development of new Western drugs, and the potential medicinal value of tropical rain forest species provides a basis for generating international support to preserve the world's rain forest areas and to conserve regional biodiversity.

Early colonial views construed developing countries in terms of the commodities that would benefit colonial interests, such as minerals, timber, spices, rubber, copra, farm lands, and people. Prospecting for treasure—including silver and gold in the Americas, gems in the Far East, and gold and diamonds in Africa—contributed to the widespread exploitation of local peoples and the loss of their resources.

The term *biodiversity prospecting* has appeared recently in the lexicon of conservation and drug development. It refers to the search for commercially useful medicinal plants in the world's rain forest areas. Using the analogy of gold prospecting, this model looks at methods of harnessing the biological treasures of forest areas for the medicinal needs of the world (Reid 1993).

The engine behind the growth of the biotechnology industry and the race to patent life forms with new chemicals and new genetic structures. The increase of activity in this field is illustrated by the fact that, although very few international companies and "no U.S. company was working on higher plants" in 1980 (Farnsworth 1985) in 1990, 223 companies worldwide were investigating medicinal plants as the source of new pharmaceutical leads (Fellows 1991).

A widely-publicized ethnobotanical program in Costa Rica involves a partnership between Merck Pharmaceutical and a local nongovernment organization, INBio, to develop drugs from traditional sources. In this agreement, $1.135 million was provided to Costa Rica by Merck for rain forest conservation activities, and a certain percentage of profits from drugs developed through this program will be returned to the country.

There were large public demonstrations on the streets of Costa Rica in protest of the government forming this kind of relationship with Merck. While this project, and others using this model, may recognize the intellectual property rights of traditional custodians of medical knowledge, concern has been expressed by indigenous organizations about the priorities involved in strategies of this kind. Some critics view this as a form of neocolonialism in which the wealthy countries are still looking at the poorer countries as a source of raw materials to be used to develop products for industrialized societies. These critics argue that, as in other colonial initiatives, the real profits will go elsewhere, rather than to the countries from where the initial material and knowledge originated. Representatives of the biotechnology industry argue that life forms, including medicinal plants, are part of a global commons and are thus available for exploitation.

The traditional perspective is that biotechnology skews public understanding of the importance of preserving tropical rain forest areas. The emphasis on preserving forests for their potential in producing new pharmaceuticals induces governments to focus on pharmaceutical development rather than on developing sustainable, affordable, and locally available medicines from their own indigenous medical traditions. This is a loss both for the present and the future.

Domestic garden and community-based cultivation programs have been developed in several countries; these offer a viable solution to the need for locally accessible and affordable medicines. Research mentioned earlier by the Royal Tropical Institute of the Netherlands concluded that countries focus too much on the role of health care providers, including traditional practitioners, whereas studies show that the majority of health activities involve self-medication. People treat themselves and their family members with medicines that they grow, produce, or buy locally, before they seek help from a health care practitioner. In this light, the domestic garden programs of countries such as Vietnam and Nepal, and the community garden programs of Belize, offer an important model for conservation and sustainable medicinal plant use. In these programs, the use of wild sources of plants is reduced, self-suffi-

ciency in health care is strengthened, and each family or communal garden can serve as a miniature conservatory of medicinal plants that otherwise might be endangered. Thus, biodiversity issues can be addressed through community development initiatives that encourage sustainable and effective health care.

To reiterate, then, the "biodiversity prospecting" argument overlooks the role of traditional medical knowledge in addressing the health needs of the communities from where the medicinal plants and the knowledge about their appropriate use and harvesting derive. As has been noted in recent press reports, "the rush of interest in prospecting for new chemicals is taking place in a policy vacuum" (Vidal 1993). With no clear national or international policies or regulations, the marketplace becomes the final arbiter of procedure. Inevitably, the most powerful players prevail.

A broader economic perspective would recognize that the health status of developing countries is central to the economic health of those countries, and thus to the world economy. Traditional medicine and medicinal plants, play an important role in meeting the basic health needs of the majority of the world's population. This is an equally, if not more potent argument than the biotechnological case for preservation of the world's medicinal plant species.

Summary

Currently, there is wide variability in the consideration given by health planners to traditional health systems. In some countries, traditional medicine is incorporated routinely into health planning. However, this occurs in only a minority of cases, primarily in Asia. In most cases, the revival has come from nongovernment organizations, particularly in Latin America. Most health ministries continue to overlook the fact that basic health care is provided to the majority of the population by traditional practitioners and budgets and that national health plans lack any reference to traditional medicine.

National and international funding currently is directed to the provision of Western-style health services in developing countries and indigenous com-

munities. Research consistently links reductions in morbidity and morality rates to economic conditions, educational levels, particularly to years of female education and large scale public health measures such as sanitation and water supply (World Bank 1993). While these factors—rather than the availability of Western medicines—have been found to lead to improved levels of health, health planners continue to operate under the view that Western medicine provides the primary means of improving health in these communities. This belief is not based in a scientific appraisal of the world's natural systems of health. Some traditional treatments are still more effective than modern treatments, as is the case with South American indigenous preparations of cinchona bark against new strains of malaria, the use of traditional burn medications in Vietnam, and the powerful cancer-prevention effects of Ayurvedic herbal preparations.

While old and limited views of traditional systems of health continue to exist, there is an emerging intellectual and policy climate that is giving expression to a fresh perspective. Whereas the old view favors the marginalization of traditional systems of health, the new view looks to them to provide complementary therapy, and in some cases, new solutions to major health crises.

The scientific paradigm for evaluating traditional systems of health has been called into question and a search has begun, including an important endeavor by the United States National Institutes of Health, to identify and develop methodologies that, according to the mission statement of NIH's Office of Alternative Medicine, "respect the paradigms" of traditional systems. The paradigm of health and medicine that has prevailed in this century, namely that of a molecular approach to human biology and the treatment of disease, also is being called into question by new findings from mind/body medicine and environmental health that promote a more integrated and holistic view of human health. This new view is consonant with the ancient or traditional concepts of health and human potential that underlie many of the world's traditional systems of health. The list below presents an outline of how this shift affects perspectives of traditional health care systems.

Old and New Perspectives on Traditional Systems of Health Care

Old	New
Primitive	Holistic
Ineffective	Cost-effective
Marginalized	Locally available
Becoming extinct	Undergoing renewal
Need to be regulated	Need to be promoted
Source of leads for pharmaceutical industry	Valid in their own right, with local economic value
Active ingredient model	Synergistic activity concepts

References

Argueta A. 1993. Presentation to World Bank Conference on Indigenous Knowledge and Sustainable Development. Washington DC. September 28

Balick M. 1995. Conservation in today's world. Proceedings of WHO Symposium on the Utilization of Medicinal Plants, Philadelphia, April 19–21. 1993. University of Pennsylvania Press, Philadelphia

Castellon U. 1992. Report of the fundacion centro nacional de medicina popular tradicional. Dr. Alejandro Davila Bolanos. Nicaragua

Eisenberg D et al. 1993. Unconventional medicine in the United States: prevalence, costs, and patterns of use. N Engl J Med, 328:4

Farnsworth N, Soejarto D. 1985. Potential consequences of plant extinction in the United States on the current and future availability of prescription drugs. Econom Botany 39:231–240

Fellows LE. 1991. Pharmaceuticals from traditional medicine plants and others: future prospects. A paper presented at the New Drugs from Natural Sources Symposium. London, June 13–14

Flaherty M. 1993. Proceedings of Conference on Indigenous Peoples and Health. Winnipeg, Canada. 13–18, p. 1–72

Fugh-Berman. 1993. The case for natural medicine. Nation, September 6 and 13.

Hall RL. 1986. Alcohol treatment in American communities: an indigenous treatment modality

Index

Page numbers followed by f *indicate figures; those followed by* t *indicate tables*